NURSING HISTORY REVIEW

OFFICIAL JOURNAL OF THE
AMERICAN ASSOCIATION FOR THE HISTORY OF NURSING

1062-8061 2009 – Volume 17

CONTENTS

SPRINGER PUBLISHING COMPANY

NEW YORK

BOOK REVIEWS

Cover Photo: The Ottawa General Hospital Training School graduation class of 1912. This photograph is part of the collection of the AMS Nursing History Research Unit at the University of Ottawa School of Nursing and reprinted with permission.

Nursing History Review is published annually for the American Association for the History of Nursing, Inc., by Springer Publishing Company, LLC, New York.

Business Office: All business correspondence, including subscriptions, renewals, advertising, and address changes, should be sent to Springer Publishing Company, LLC, 11 West 42nd Street, New York, NY 10036.

Editorial Office: Submissions and editorial correspondence should be directed to Patricia D'Antonio, Editor, *Nursing History Review,* University of Pennsylvania, 420 Guardian Drive, Room 307, Philadelphia, PA 19104-6096. See Guidelines for Contributors on page 8 for further details.

Members of the American Association for the History of Nursing, Inc. (AAHN) receive *Nursing History Review* on payment of annual membership dues. Applications and other correspondence relating to AAHN membership should be directed to: Janet L. Fickeissen, Executive Secretary, American Association for the History of Nursing, Inc., P. O. Box 175, Lonoka Harbor, NJ 08734-0175.

Subscription Rates (per Year): Volume 17, 2009. For institutions: Print, $150; Online, $105; Print & Online, $225. For individuals: Print, $85; Online, $65; Print & Online, $130. Outside the United States—for institutions: Print, $160; Online; $115; Print & Online, $240. For individuals: Print, $105; Online, $85; Print & Online, $160. Payment must be made in advance by check (in U. S. dollars drawn on a U.S. bank) or international money order, payable to Springer Publishing Company, LLC, or by MasterCard, Visa, American Express, or Discover.

Indexes/abstracts of articles appear in: CINAHL® print index & database, Current Contents/Social & Behavioral Science, Social Sciences Citation Index, Research Alert, RNdex, Index Medicus/MEDLINE, Historical Abstracts, America: History and Life.

Postmaster: Send address changes to Springer Publishing Company, LLC, 11 West 42nd Street, New York, NY 10036.

ISSN 1062-8061

GUIDELINES FOR CONTRIBUTORS

Nursing History Review, the official publication of the American Association for the History of Nursing, is peer-reviewed and published annually for subscribers and members of the Association. Original research manuscripts are welcomed in broad areas related to the history of nursing, health care, health policy, and society. The *Review* prefers manuscripts of approximately 40 pages, inclusive of endnotes.

Submitted manuscripts must be prepared using the guidelines specified in the *Chicago Manual of Style,* 15th edition. Manuscripts must have a title page that contains the full title of the manuscript, the author(s) name(s) as they are meant to appear in print, institutional affiliations and preferred mailing addresses *for all authors,* and relevant contact information for the corresponding author. The title page must be followed with an abstract of approximately 150–200 words.

Manuscripts must be double-spaced and of letter-quality print. They must also use a type size of at least 12 characters per inch or 10 points. Please leave generous margins of at least 1 inch. All pages, including text, notes, and reference pages, must be numbered consecutively. All notes must be double-spaced and placed at the end of the manuscript as endnotes rather than footnotes.

Authors are responsible for securing permissions for all materials submitted. If more than 500 words of text are quoted from a book, or more than 250 words from an article, or if a table or figure has been previously published, the manuscript must be accompanied by written permission from the copyright owner.

Initial submissions of manuscripts may be sent by e-mail to nhr@nursing.upenn.edu. All submissions will be acknowledged when received. *Final versions of manuscripts accepted for publication* should be prepared in MS Word. The final packet must be submitted via e-mail to nhr@nursing.upenn.edu. Photographs or other figures accompanying the final manuscript must be attached as TIF files with resolutions of at least 600 dpi.

Copyright Agreement

The following dated agreement signed by all authors must accompany each manuscript submitted for publication:

> The undersigned author(s) transfers all copyright ownership of the article entitled [title of article] to the Springer Publishing Company, LLC, in the event that the article is published in **Nursing History Review.** This transfer of copyright includes, but is not limited to, the worldwide rights to any and all forms of publication now known or hereafter developed, including all forms of print and electronic media. The undersigned author(s) warrants and represents that the article is original, is not under consideration by another journal, has not been published previously, and contains no matter that is libelous, unlawful, or that infringes upon an other copyright.

All correspondence regarding manuscripts should be sent to: Patricia D'Antonio, RN, PhD, FAAN, Editor, *Nursing History Review,* University of Pennsylvania School of Nursing, 420 Guardian Drive, Room 307, Philadelphia, PA 19104–6096. Phone: 215/898–4502. Fax: 215/573–2168. E-mail: dantonio@nursing.upenn.edu or nhr@nursing.upenn.edu.

AMERICAN ASSOCIATION FOR THE HISTORY OF NURSING, INC.

EDITOR'S NOTE

As I write, the 25th Annual Research Conference of the American Association for the History of Nursing looms large in my future. As you read, I hope you have returned safely home, impressed with the scholarship and with the work of a new generation of scholars. Books, articles, impact factors (more on that later) are important metrics of success. But the nurturing of what I count as a third generation of historians is, to my mind, the most important one. We—those of us from the first and second generations—have written nurses into the historical record and, admittedly in some areas more than others, we have changed the historical record. There is still much work to be done, but we came of age armed with tools forged in the "rights" revolution and with frameworks—most notably that of social history—upon which we constructed "stories from the bottom up."

To my newest colleagues: our tools and frameworks may not be yours. If we believe, as does historian Nancy Hewitt, "that all history is written in a dialogue with current issues, concerns, and perspectives," then use your histories to talk to yours.[1] Think big and move beyond, for example, the obvious nursing shortages and rise in chronic illnesses. Think about what shortages and such illnesses *mean* and *represent.* Ellen DuBois, for example, has suggested that if women's history was once the child of social history then today it may well be the mother of a new political history—one interested in interrogating not only what actors did but also in the values that distinguished how they thought about their world and how they negotiated among themselves and that world.[2] To turn this toward the history of nursing: our past tools and frameworks may be the mother of an epistemological stance that explores the ways in which nurses thought, acted, and interacted among themselves and their constituents.

Recently, Arlene Keeling, Meryn Stuart, Cynthia Connolly, Barbra Mann Wall, Julie Fairman, and I tried to give some form to this idea when we were asked to present a panel on "Nursing and Activism" to the Sigerist Circle, an affiliated organization of the American Association of the History of Medicine. But rather than present the usual *activist* nurses, we tried to unpack the trope of *activism* by wondering about the ways in which the more ordinary nurses we studied theorized (or thought about) the social and political implications

Nursing History Review 17 (2009): 11–13. A Publication of the American Association for the History of Nursing.
DOI: 10.1891/1062–8061.17.11

of their own actions. And there are many more such tropes waiting to be unpacked. *Care* is one such trope.

Globalization is another. We have a rich, still growing, and still needed body of knowledge about nursing is this country or that country; and we have a smaller but as important body of knowledge comparing a particular practice in country A with that in country B. We are becoming more comfortable with the theoretical implications and the idioms of *colonial* and *postcolonial* discourses and histories. We do know we need to know more about the conversations nurses had that crossed national boundaries. But we have not yet moved to where we need to be: *globalization* will remain too narrowly defined until we realize its potential for framing new kinds of questions. What kinds of historical questions will allow us to transcend traditional nation-state boundaries in our work? What kinds of questions will allow us to bring a transnational framework into the homes and the communities within which our historical nurses live and work? And what kinds of questions will allow us to bring it into our historical workplaces—sites of men and women maintaining social identities and real communication with more than one real or imagined nation?

There are other challenges awaiting you as well. We know that such concepts as gender, race, and class are not additive but intersectional. And we know that there are significant differences among actors we might assign to specific gendered, raced, and classed categories. But how do we write about such complexity? How do we write histories, as S. Jay Kleinberg, Eileen Boris, and Vicki L. Ruiz challenge us, "in which identity covers multiple dimensions so that one is not merely gendered, or raced, or classed, or abled, but all of these factors combine and refract upon each other in a *mezcla* (or mixture) of self and society"?[3]

This is, I believe, an exciting time to be rethinking, once again, nursing's history. The project is in good hands.

Patricia D'Antonio

From the Editor: Nursing History Review's *Impact Factor*

An impact factor, calculated yearly by the Institute for Scientific Information (ISI) for a carefully selected group of health care journals, currently stands as a statistical proxy for a research journal's prominence. While the precise meaning, reliability, and validity of an impact factor (which measures the number of times articles from a journal are cited) remains very controversial, the *Nursing History Review* was one of the original nursing journals (and is now one of only 40 international nursing journals) for which ISI calculates an impact factor.

In 2008, Thomson Scientific (who creates the impact factor) has moved the *Nursing History Review* out of the nursing category and into that of the "History of the Social Sciences." This, I think, is a testament to the multidisciplinary nature of the *Review*; according to my calculations: we are the only truly multidisciplinary journal in nursing and 33% of our authors in the last five years (volumes 12–16) are historians and social scientists.

Our 2006 (this is the latest) impact factor is 0.222. That is below the median for the category, but we are a small and specialized journal. I might add that the *Review's* actual (or raw) impact factor is relatively meaningless: many of our articles are cited in books and humanities and nursing journals that are not indexed by ISI. However, our listing is among a very select number of journals: this suggests the prominence (a more reliable relative measure) of the *Review* relative to peer journals such as *Nursing Research, Research in Nursing and Health,* or the *Journal of Advanced Nursing.*

From the Editor: In Appreciation to Our External Reviewers

On behalf of the Editorial Review Board, I thank the following colleagues who gave generously of their time and expertise in the review of manuscripts: Geertje Boschma, Jacqueline Brooks, Karen Buhler-Wilkerson, Winifred Connerton, Katy Dawley, Mary Gibson, Madeline Healy, Arlene Keeling, Stephanie Kirby, Brigid Lusk, Susanne Malchau, Ann McMahon, Ann Marie Ryan, Christoph Schweikardt, Cynthia Toman, and Jean Whelan.

Notes

1. Nancy Hewitt, quoted in Nancy F. Cott et al., "Considering the State of U.S. Women's History," *Journal of Women's History* 15, no. 1 (2003): 155.
2. Ellen DuBois, quoted in Nancy F. Cott et al., "Considering the State of U.S. Women's History," *Journal of Women's History* 15, no. 1 (2003): 157.
3. S. Jay Kleinberg, Eileen Boris, and Vicki L. Ruiz, "Introduction: Narratives, Intersections, and Dialogues," in *The Practice of U.S. Women's History: Narratives, Intersections, and Dialogues,* ed. S. Jay Kleinberg, Eileen Boris, and Vicki L. Ruiz (New Brunswick, N.J.: Rutgers University Press, 2007), 4.

Nursing History: An Irrelevance for Nursing Practice?

Anne Borsay
Professor in the School of Health Science

It was a great privilege for me as a non-nurse to be invited to deliver the Monica Baly Lecture for 2006. Though I did not have the pleasure of meeting Monica, we shared a love of Georgian Bath and in the early 1990s corresponded over a short article of mine on corruption at the famous Mineral Water Hospital in the city, which was duly published in the *History of Nursing Society Journal*.[1] Even in that brief exchange of letters, Monica's commitment to and enthusiasm for historical research were immediately striking. I cannot do full justice to her memory. I want to attempt, however, to spell out the relevance for nursing practice of the approach to nursing history that she pioneered. To do this, I shall be exploring three principal themes: the development of nursing history since 1900; the origins of the medical model that continues to inform the British health care system; and the ways historical scholarship can offset the worst effects of this model by facilitating critical reflection on professional identity, patient perspectives, and evidence-based decision making.

The Development of Nursing History

Like women's history, nursing history had its origins in Victorian biography, which celebrated "women worthies" whose good example was seen as an exemplar for female readers.[2] With this agenda, it is not surprising that the "iconic figure of Florence Nightingale" reigned supreme.[3] Sarah Tooley's *Life,*

Nursing History Review 17 (2009): 14–27. A Publication of the American Association for the History of Nursing.
DOI: 10.1891/1062–8061.17.14

for instance, was a romantic tale, written in 1904 to coincide with the 50th anniversary of Florence's departure to the Crimea. A simple chronology, short on insight into her personality and motivation, it emphasized the self-sacrifice to which all women were expected to aspire, along with their duty to supply physical and spiritual sustenance.[4] During the course of the 20th century, the genre of *critical* biography emerged from this hagiographic approach.[5] Even Sir Edward Cook's official biography of 1913, though eulogistic, flagged less favorable qualities: Florence's domineering personality; the long and bitter struggle with her family; her cavalier treatment of friends; her calculated decision not to marry. Cook even discreetly suggested that the relentless pursuit of public activity was a product of frustrated sexuality![6] Almost 40 years were to elapse before Cecil Woodham-Smith produced her much-acclaimed biography. Woodham-Smith insisted in her "Note of Acknowledgement" that she was offering "a complete picture of Miss Nightingale"—a recreation of her personality that not only brought out Florence's inner conflict with herself and outer conflict with her family, but also showed how she was able to operate effectively in a world controlled by men.[7]

Biography has many virtues as a historical tool. First, individuals come alive. Second, criticisms are voiced, despite fears that negative comment may be suppressed. Thus in *Eminent Victorians,* published in 1918, Lytton Strachey penned a scathing essay on Florence, indulging in wit and mocking sarcasm: "At times Mrs Nightingale almost wept. 'We are ducks,' she said with tears in her eyes, 'who have hatched a wild swan.' But the poor lady was wrong; it was not a swan that they had hatched, it was an eagle."[8] Third, biography is able to challenge biography. Witness how Jane Robinson's recent study has rehabilitated Mary Seacole[9]—quickly forgotten after her death though greeted with "rapturous enthusiasm" at the public banquet held in London to honor Crimean soldiers. Now she has been featured on a postage stamp, issued in July 2006 to commemorate the 150th anniversary of the National Portrait Gallery.[10] Nevertheless, biography does have limitations. In particular, it overlooks "the more ordinary lives" of nurses and patients, and prevents a comprehensive analysis of the economic, social, political, and cultural environments in which they lived.[11] Therefore, a contextual approach is essential to counterbalance these shortcomings.

The first attempt at contextualization came in 1960 with Brian Abel-Smith's *History of the Nursing Profession,* which looked at the politics of *general* nursing and assessed the role of structure, recruitment, terms and conditions, professional associations, and trade unions. But, as Abel-Smith himself admitted, nursing as "an activity or skill"—and "what it was like ... to nurse ... or to receive nursing care"—were largely absent from his story.[12] It was Monica

Baly who started the process of filling these gaps in the first, 1973 edition of *Nursing and Social Change.* For her,

> the development of nursing ... [was] like weaving a cloth with social change as the warp and, running to and fro with the weft ... [was] the shuttle of care ... only by tracing the threads to their historical origin ... [could] we begin to understand the confusion and profusion of health services in the twentieth century.[13]

Implicit in this narrative was a progressive, humanitarian ethos that reached its high point during the postwar consensus: the market economy was subjected to government intervention in the public interest; social relationships were heavily influenced by social class; liberal democracy granted nominal political equality through universal suffrage; and the welfare state was lauded as the means to guarantee all citizens a minimum level of income, education, housing, and health.[14]

By the late 1970s, however, this consensus was falling apart as the economy went from crisis to crisis, class relations led to industrial conflict, political institutions and procedures lost public credibility, and the welfare state—including the National Health Service (NHS)—failed to deliver effective services.[15] Celia Davies captured this loss of confidence for nursing history in 1980, when she attacked the assumption that "progressive and humanitarian ideas ... [would] eventually win out against the opposition of vested interests." Quite the opposite: reforms were "double-edged, always in part at least reflecting the views of the most powerful."[16] This assault on the inevitability of progress was derived from "the application of concepts and methods from the social sciences to original [historical] sources."[17] Since emerging in the late 19th century, the social sciences had concerned themselves with the structure of modern societies: with themes like the nation-state, industrialization, social class, family and community, science and religion. But with the changes that were undermining the postwar consensus, these "grand narratives" became less plausible. National autonomy was being eroded by economic globalization, for example. Personal identities were being designed from the consumption of material goods. Political identities were being constructed around lifestyles, regions, and particular issues. Above all, confidence in the rational society, planned and managed by experts, was faltering.[18]

Neither history nor the social sciences nor the health care professions were immune to these *postmodern* trends. Full-blown postmodernism rejected the possibility of any objective truth, stressing moral relativity and reducing knowledge to power. "We should admit ... that power produces knowledge," insisted Michel Foucault, "that knowledge and power directly imply one another."[19] Accordingly, the past could not be understood in a rational way because every interpretation was merely the outcome of its perpetrator's political values. But postmodern history has never been more than a marginal force in Britain. What it has done is leave mainstream history with three important legacies. First, there is a commitment to global or international perspectives. Second, the dead weight of deterministic social structures has been lightened by a new recognition of individual identity and agency; in other words, space is being made for personal contingency within the old grand narratives. Third, with determinism in retreat, a constitutive role for cultural artefacts—previously regarded as only reflective or derivative—is possible. Consequently, history has escaped from the fetish of the document to embrace a rich variety of primary sources: visual, oral, literary, and material.[20]

Today the best nursing history displays all these characteristics, as we see in volumes like *New Directions in the History of Nursing*, edited by Barbara Mortimer and Susan McGann in 2005.[21] The "myths and legends" accumulated over "a century of anecdotal writing have been chipped away to reveal the complex story of an occupation shaped and reshaped by social and technological change."[22] As the editors of *Nursing History and the Politics of Welfare* concluded, there has been a transformation from "an internalist and triumphalist form of professional apologetics to a robust and reflective area of scholarship."[23]

The Relevance of the Past

Research of this caliber makes an important contribution to the academic community, its impact extending beyond women's history to the discipline as a whole. But is it germane to nursing practice? For Sioban Nelson, this question is redundant. "History," she declares, "is always relevant."[24] Yet nursing and history do sit on opposite sides of the science/arts divide, what in the 1950s C. P. Snow called "the two cultures of Western civilization."[25] Nurses are pictured at the forefront of scientific knowledge, applying their expertise to urgent patient needs. Historians are pictured stuck in the past, digging around in dusty archives to produce books and articles that nobody ever reads. Given this polarity, the point of nursing history for nursing practice has to be demonstrated rather than assumed. Learning from the past in a simplistic way is not an option because, contrary to the popular adage, history never repeats itself. As John Tosh has argued, "nothing in human society … ever happens twice under exactly the same conditions or in exactly the same way."

Nonetheless, though we cannot "trawl" the past for "solutions to current problems," we can use it to enhance our understanding of the present.[26]

There are occasions when historical data and historical methods are of direct relevance to nursing practice. Health care records from the past can be used to study the trajectories of genetically transmitted diseases or the impact of new drug regimes. Historical methods—notably oral testimony—may also be of value in professional practice, building the self-esteem of patients damaged by illness or harmful service provision.[27] But at least as important as the direct application of records and methods is the indirect way in which history facilitates critical reflection.

The Medical Model of Health Care

At the core of this facility for critical reflection is history's capacity to counterbalance the medical model, which has dominated the delivery of health care in Britain. The medical model endorses "anatomical, physiological and biochemical malfunction as the causes of ill-health [and] encourages a *disease-orientated* approach to care that stresses the structure and function of the body ... rather than the uniqueness or integrity of the individual."[28] There has been a tendency to attribute this reductionism to the growth in molecular medicine that has occurred during the last 15 years, and the resulting shift in focus "from the whole patient and whole organs to diseases of molecules and cells."[29] The real roots lie far deeper. They go back to the Renaissance, when the static, God-centered world-picture of the medieval era was displaced by a dynamic, secular one in which the world was construed as a working machine of divine design that was subject to a degree of human control.[30] This mechanistic mentality had two implications that were particularly consequential for health care: the mind/body split of René Descartes (1596–1650) and the experimental methodology of Francis Bacon (1561–1626).

Descartes endorsed the machine model with enthusiasm, advocating a rigid division between body and mind. As the late Roy Porter explained, Descartes

> postulated two radically different entities, extension (material) and mind (immaterial). Only the human soul or mind possessed consciousness. Literally everything else in Nature, including the human body ... , formed part of the realm of what Descartes called "extension" (obeying the laws of mechanics). "Extension," which included all other living creatures, was a legitimate terrain for scientific investigation.

> By Descartes' deft manoeuvre, mind had, so to speak, been mystified, whilst the body was laid bare.[31]

The tools with which the material body was to be scientifically investigated were derived from the observational and experimental methodologies promoted by Francis Bacon. Bacon was committed to inductive logic; he "believed that only a pre-theoretical gathering of bare facts could guarantee that the explanation of a natural phenomenon would not be pre-judged, or prejudiced." In other words, he was an empiricist for whom the deductive reasoning of the medieval world was no longer acceptable.[32]

The legacies of the Renaissance for health care were far-reaching. Of course, change did not happen immediately. Over time, however, doctors secured a monopoly over the mechanical functioning of the body that excluded theologians and moralists as well as other practitioners: nurses and midwives, cunning men and wise women, bonesetters and truss-makers, vendors of ubiquitous unorthodox cures. Furthermore, the conception of the body and its treatment also evolved. Before Descartes and Bacon, the holistic humoral theory of Hippocrates and Galen prevailed: good health was enjoyed when the four natural humors—blood, phlegm, yellow bile, and black bile—were in equilibrium with each other and with a set of "non-natural" external factors—air, diet, exercise, climate, and weather. Ill health struck when this happy balance was disturbed.[33]

By 1800, however, a new, localized pathology was well established in which the body was isolated from its environment and tissue became the unit of analysis. "The more one will observe diseases and open cadavers," declared one French surgeon of this school, "the more one will be convinced of the necessity of considering local diseases not from the aspect of the complex organs but from that of the individual tissues."[34] Whereas Harvey had earlier understood the heart as a single mechanical entity, localized pathology reduced every body part to a collection of different membranes.

There were serious ramifications for clinical relationships. From the 1750s, doctor and patient began to inhabit different conceptual worlds of illness. Increasingly, the doctor came to rely on "signs and symptoms" that were conducive to a "disease-orientated diagnosis." Alien labels were thus attached to patients' conditions as their narratives disappeared first from hospital and later from community consultations.[35] Statistical analysis was associated with this new mindset. Doctors quantified from the early 18th century onward, and the voluntary hospitals founded from the same period kept data on patients that were used for studies of clinical efficacy. The body's functioning was thus measured and tabulated, mortality statistics were collected, and the success of medical innovations was tested.[36] Therefore, by the beginning of the 19th century, the foundations of the modern medical model and its attendant problems had already been laid.

Professional Identity

There are at least three areas in which history may help to offset the worst excesses of this medical model for nursing practice: professional identity, patient perspectives, and evidence-based decision making. The emergence of the nursing profession after 1850 was a chance to challenge the supremacy of medical knowledge and practice. After all, Florence Nightingale was skeptical of medicine's claim to be "a curative process." It was, she insisted in *Notes on Nursing,* "no such thing." "Surgery removes the bullet out of the limb, which is the obstruction to cure, but nature heals the wound." The distinctive responsibility of the nurse was to put "the patient in the best condition for nature to act upon him." Yet despite advocating a separate role, nurse education under Nightingale's influence inculcated obedience to the doctor, drawing on the military and religious roots of the profession to foster "hierarchy" and "duty," "service," and "sisterhood."[37]

This missed opportunity was captured in Mick Carpenter's characterization of how nursing became professionalized in Britain. Carpenter identified "three main attempted transformations." Nightingale's name was attached to the first era or phase, which "lasted from the mid-nineteenth century to around the time of the First World War" and tried to establish an autonomous "nursing structure," despite "subordination" to "the managerial needs of the local hospital" as well as to medicine. The second phase—"the professionalization of care"—was "initiated in the late nineteenth century by Mrs. Bedford Fenwick" and tried to achieve the "social closure" of nursing "as an exclusively middle-class occupation." As Carpenter elaborated, "This sought professional autonomy for the nursing structure from the state and local managements, an extension of the domination of general nursing over the nursing universe, and a complementary but still subordinated position of nursing to an ascendant medicine." The third phase—"the new professionalism"—crossed the Atlantic to Britain in the early 1970s and was predicated on a "renewed" effort "to achieve the longstanding goals of professionalization," which were eventually manifest in Project 2000. But "whereas previous movements . . . sought to professionalize the whole occupation," the new professionalism concentrated on clinical nurses, seeking to provide them with a knowledge base—independent of medicine—that challenged biomedicine in the name of the patient by developing nursing plans that were "rational, rigorous and individualized."[38]

In her 2005 Monica Baly Lecture, Celia Davies recommended that we "ditch the concept of professionalization" and think instead in terms of "professional identity," which is better able to comprehend the complexities of "nursing knowledge, practice, regulation and caring."[39] The fragmentation implicit in Carpenter's third phase—where "an elite corps" of clinical nurses merely supervise the basic care delivered by "assistants" with limited training—endorses the validity of this conclusion. Despite the aspirations of the second phase, nursing never became a monolithic profession of white middle-class women, and by 1939 the majority of recruits were still being drawn from "the lower middle and respectable working classes," just as they had been at the end of the 19th century. From the mid-1940s, chronic staff shortages encouraged hospitals to rely on a "steady flow" of Black nurses from the former British colonies, who—congregated in poorly paid but often physically and emotionally demanding jobs—faced institutional racism both at work and in the community. Moreover, the stereotypical image of the profession was further undermined from the late 1960s when men—never entirely absent but largely employed in the psychiatric sector—were deliberately targeted in recruitment campaigns for general nursing.[40]

In recent years, multidisciplinary working and the destabilizing effects of new technology and rapid social change have compounded the complexities of class, race, and gender. Therefore, like members of other professions, nurses are no longer ascribed a single identity by virtue of their membership in this particular occupational group. Rather, they are forced to construct their own identities on an ongoing basis by thrashing out the multiple meanings of their changing roles. History can contribute to this critical reflection, enabling the compilation of a professional narrative by exploring contemporary experiences with reference to the past.

Patient Perspectives

The individual nursing plans—a key feature of Carpenter's third, "new professionalism" phase—were also an attempt to escape from the reductionism of the medical model by ensuring that patient perspectives were at the center of the caring process.[41] In Britain, Roper, Logan, and Tierney redefined nursing to underline its role in—first—"preventing, alleviating or coping with problems of activities of living"; and—second—promoting "a greater awareness of the cultural, environmental, political and economic factors affecting health." In the United States, where theorizing attained a higher level of abstraction, the nonphysical needs of patients achieved a higher profile. Neuman's model, for instance, envisaged people as "*open systems* in interaction with their environments" with four "*variable areas*" over and above "the physiological": "the psychological, the socio-cultural, the developmental and the spiritual."[42] But being far removed from "real" patients, nursing theory is now less widely regarded as an effective defense of their perspectives. History, on the other hand, offers flesh and blood examples to keep the recipients of health care in the frame as a consideration of the patient-practitioner relationship shows.

On June 7, 1749, Richard Kay—a local doctor from Bury in Lancashire (UK)—was visited by Mrs. Driver, whose cancerous breast he had removed in December of the previous year. This is how he described the encounter in his diary:

> Mrs Driver came here for us she being determined to undergo a second amputation, [.] upon dissecting the knot I soon found I had more work to do than was expected as there appeared other kernels closely joined together which lay down to the abdomen and the compass of six or seven inches square, [.] in some parts I took off the skin, in others dissected them from under the skin, so that below where her breast formerly was down her ribs to her belly I dissected from her at a moderate computation five hundred different distinct knots or young cancers; she was sick and very poorly after the operation.

Richard Kay was a dedicated doctor who worked long hours traveling to his patients on horseback. He was also a deeply religious man whose professional commitment was underscored by a strong Nonconformist faith. And when Mrs. Driver died, he took the trouble to attend her funeral.[43] Yet from this account we get no sense that the surgery was conducted without effective anesthetic.

Historical narratives of the nurse-patient relationship are more difficult to come by. In 1809, however, a minor actor called Joseph Wilde was admitted to the Devon and Exeter Hospital with an injured knee. In a long poem describing his experiences, Wilde told of the camaraderie among patients, the ambulant of whom helped to clean the wards and look after their bedridden fellows. In contrast, relations with the staff were cold and impersonal. Allocated to an upper floor despite his physical impairment, he thus saw "Signs of impatience ... but none of pity" in the "stormy eye" of the nurse who accompanied him as he climbed the stairs "with painful steps and slow"—"presage," he thought, of "trouble to ensue."[44]

The purpose of these examples is not to denounce health care practitioners as callously indifferent to the pain of their patients. What they flag is the psychological distance that may open up in all professional relationships, be they past or present. Confronting this issue historically will not necessarily foster "empathy and tolerance" as a result of "identifying with other persons, times and beliefs."[45] And neither attitudes nor behavior will necessarily change because the effect of any individual engagement with a historical episode is unpredictable.[46] But by creating opportunities for professional reflection, less threatening due to their location in the past, history offers a device for imagining the delivery of care from the patient's perspective.

Evidence-Based Decision Making

The evidence-based practice that "rose to prominence in the late 1990s" was not an inevitable threat to patient orientation. Indeed, Judith Parker has suggested that nurses "acquired a language for placing aspects of their practice into a more public domain," allowing "formerly taken-for-granted and routine practices to be opened up for inspection, discussion and possible change. Evidence-based nursing thus empowers nurses to speak coherently and authoritatively and to defend practices or argue for change using tools increasingly acceptable to policy-makers and fund-holders."[47] Additionally, the evidence-based approach itself embodies a commitment to personalize the patient. As the architect of the methodology, David Sackett, and his colleagues have said: "Good doctors use both individual clinical expertise and the best available external evidence. Without clinical expertise, practice risks becoming tyrannised by evidence, for even excellent external evidence may be inapplicable to or inappropriate for an individual patient."[48]

But evidence-based health care does not have an entirely clean bill of health. Critics have questioned "the primacy accorded … [both] to the randomized control trial for assessing the efficacy of interventions, and to epidemiological data for predicting the course of illness."[49] Even Judith Parker has admitted that it is a mechanism for exerting "fiscal constraint upon health expenditure." And, most important, the exhortation to protect the individual patient from generalized decision making is easily subverted in a busy health care system where the reductionist medical model holds sway.[50] History provides a template for decision making in this uncertain environment.

Although clinical decisions are assumed to rest on firm foundations, surveying the past reveals present practice to be a temporary phenomenon in an evolving chronology—not an unsurpassable pinnacle of achievement. Just as state-of-the-art treatments from 50 years ago are today discredited, so our own innovations will in their turn become outmoded.

Amid these shifting sands, "evidence-based practice requires a blending of the research-based and experiential knowledge of professionals with the individualised personal knowledge of patients and their carers."[51] The strategies that historians adopt to cope with similarly complex scenarios may be helpful in achieving this synthesis. Historical decision making draws on two types of raw material: primary sources—documents, plus the oral testimony, visual images, literary texts, and artefacts that postmodernism has advanced—and secondary sources—the books, articles, and dissertations in which previous historians have distilled their thinking. Following T. E. Christy, John Sweeney sets out a procedure to "determine a historical fact": "two independent primary sources must concur or one independent primary source and one independent secondary source must concur without disagreement or conflicting evidence."[52] In reality, the decision-making process is more intuitive—albeit "anchored in empirically available phenomena," as nursing philosophers have argued.[53]

Historians seep themselves in the debates that surround their subject. They familiarize themselves with its economic and political, social, and cultural context. They consider how far their primary sources support or conflict with established positions. They try to explain the discrepancies. And after carefully weighing up the pros and cons, they construct an argument that aspires to internal consistency—in other words, does not contradict itself—and resonates with their understanding of the world. There is no one right answer. But in struggling to accommodate a wide variety of sources, historians employ a methodology consistent with the messy nature of the human condition and with the uncertainty that is also inherent in clinical decision making.

In this article, I have examined three main themes: the evolution of nursing history from hagiographic biography to the contextualized analysis of the past that Monica Baly instigated; the influence of the medical model in the professionalization of nursing; and the part that history can play in challenging its reductionism: in relation to professional identity, to patient perspectives, and to evidence-based decision making. *Nursing* history, now a mature area of specialization within historical scholarship, has the research to resource critical reflection on these issues. Therefore, it is not an irrelevance for nursing practice.

ANNE BORSAY, B.Sc. Econ (Wales); M.Litt (Oxon.), Ph.D (Wales)
Professor of Health Care and Medical Humanities
School of Health Science
Swansea University
Singleton Park
Swansea SA2 8PP
United Kingdom
a.borsary@swan.ac.uk

Acknowledgments

This paper is a revised version of the Monica Baly Lecture given at the Third Annual Conference of the Royal College of Nursing (RCN) History of Nursing Society, held at the Royal College of Nursing in London on November 14, 2006.

Notes

1. Anne Borsay, "'Persons of Honour and Reputation': The Voluntary Hospital in an Age of Corruption," *Medical History* 35, no. 3 (1991): 281–94. An abbreviated version was reprinted in *History of Nursing Society Journal* 3, no. 6 (1991): 1–15.

2. June Purvis, "From 'Women Worthies' to Poststructuralism? Debate and Controversy in Women's History in Britain," in *Women's History: Britain, 1850–1945,* ed. June Purvis (London: UCL Press, 1995), 1–2.

3. Barbara Mortimer, "Introduction—The History of Nursing: Yesterday, Today and Tomorrow," in *New Directions in the History of Nursing: International Perspectives,* ed. Barbara Mortimer and Susan McGann (London: Routledge, 2005), 1. For an excellent overview of the biographical literature on Florence Nightingale, see Lilli Sentz, "Focus on Nursing," *Watermark, Newsletter of the Association of Librarians in the History of the Health Sciences* 13, no. 2 (Winter 1989): 9–14.

4. Sarah Tooley, *A Life of Florence Nightingale* (London: S. H. Bousfield, 1904).

5. See, for example, Stephen Davies, *Empiricism and History* (Basingstoke, UK: Palgrave, 2003), 43–55.

6. Edward Cook, *The Life of Florence Nightingale,* 2 vols. (New York: Macmillan, 1913).

7. Cecil Woodham-Smith, *Florence Nightingale, 1820–1910* (London: Constable, 1950).

8. Lytton Strachey, *Eminent Victorians* (1918; repr., London: Penguin, 1986), 111–61, 115.

9. Jane Robinson, *Mary Seacole: The Charismatic Black Nurse Who Became a Heroine of the Crimea* (London: Constable, 2005).

10. "Mary Seacole, 1805–1881," *Medi Theme* 25, no. 3 (August 2006): 98. Albert Charles Challen painted the portrait in 1866.

11. Mark Jackson, "Biography as History," *Journal of Medical Biography* 12, no. 2 (2004): 63–65.

12. Brian Abel-Smith, *A History of the Nursing Profession* (London: Heinemann, 1960), xi.

13. Monica Baly, *Nursing and Social Change,* 3rd ed. (London: Routledge, 1995), xiii.

14. See, for example, Dennis Kavanagh and Peter Morris, *Consensus Politics From Attlee to Thatcher* (Oxford: Blackwell, 1989).

15. For an overview of this political situation, see Peter Clarke, *Hope and Glory: Britain, 1900–1990* (London: Penguin, 1996), 283–357.

16. Celia Davies, "Introduction: The Contemporary Challenge in Nursing History," in *Rewriting Nursing History,* ed. Celia Davies (London: Croom Helm, 1980), 12.

17. Robert Dingwall, Anne Marie Rafferty, and Charles Webster, *An Introduction to the Social History of Nursing* (London: Routledge, 1988), back cover.

18. For accessible accounts of this *postmodern* condition, see David Lyon, *Postmodernity* (Buckingham, UK: Open University Press, 1994); Martin O'Brien and Sue Penna, *Theorizing Welfare: Enlightenment and Modern Society* (London: Sage, 1998), 184–207; Steven Pinch, *Worlds of Welfare: Understanding the Changing Geographies of Social Welfare Provision* (London: Routledge, 1997), 112–27.

19. Michel Foucault, *Discipline and Punish: The Birth of the Prison,* trans. Alan Sheridan (Harmondsworth, UK: Penguin, 1977), 27.

20. Richard J. Evans, *In Defence of History* (London: Granta, 1997), 243–44; Arthur Marwick, *The Nature of History* (London: Macmillan, 1970), 136–37.

21. Mortimer and McGann, *New Directions in the History of Nursing.*

22. Dingwall et al., *Introduction to the Social History of Nursing,* back cover.

23. "Introduction," in *Nursing History and the Politics of Welfare,* ed. Anne Marie Rafferty, Jane Robinson, and Ruth Elkan (London: Routledge, 1997), 1.

24. Sioban Nelson, "The Fork in the Road: Nursing History Versus the History of Nursing," *Nursing History Review* 10 (2002): 175.

25. C. P. Snow, *The Two Cultures,* intro. Stefan Collini (1964; repr., Cambridge: Cambridge University Press, 1993).

26. John Tosh, *The Pursuit of History: Aims, Methods and New Directions in the Study of Modern History,* 2nd ed. (London: Longman, 1991), 9–20.

27. See, for example, Herman P. Meininger, "Narrating, Writing, Reading: Life Story Work as an Aid to (Self) Advocacy," *British Journal of Learning Disabilities* 34, no. 3 (September 2006): 181–88.

28. Peter Aggleton and Helen Chalmers, *Nursing Models and Nursing Practice,* 2nd ed. (Basingstoke, UK: Palgrave, 2000), 28.

29. J. Wyn Owen, "Art, Health and Well-Being: Why Now? The Policy Advisor's View," in *Medical Humanities: A Practical Introduction,* ed. Deborah Kirklin and Ruth Richardson (London: Royal College of Physicians, 2001), 81.

30. Mary Midgley, *Science and Poetry* (London: Routledge, 2001), 24–25.

31. Roy Porter, "What Is Disease?" in *The Cambridge Illustrated History of Medicine,* ed. Roy Porter (Cambridge: Cambridge University Press, 1996), 93–95.

32. John Henry, *The Scientific Revolution and the Origins of Modern Science* (Basingstoke, UK: Macmillan, 1997), 53.

33. N. D. Jewson, "Medical Knowledge and the Patronage System in Eighteenth-Century England," *Sociology* 8, no. 3 (1974): 369–85; Roy Porter and Dorothy Porter, *In Sickness and in Health: The British Experience, 1650–1850* (London: Fourth Estate, 1988), 30–31; J. C. Riley, *The Eighteenth-Century Campaign to Avoid Disease* (London: Macmillan, 1987), 89–90, 145.

34. Roy Porter, *The Greatest Benefit to Mankind: A Medical History of Humanity From Antiquity to the Present* (London: HarperCollins, 1997), 265.

35. Mary E. Fissell, "The Disappearance of the Patient's Narrative and the Invention of Hospital Medicine," in *British Medicine in an Age of Reform,* ed. Roger French and Andrew Wear (London: Routledge, 1991), 92–109.

36. Anne Borsay, "An Example of Political Arithmetic: The Evaluation of Spa Therapy at the Georgian Bath Infirmary, 1742–1830," *Medical History* 45, no. 2 (April 2000): 149–72.

37. Hugh McKenna, *Nursing Theories and Models* (London: Routledge, 1997), 85–87.

38. Mick Carpenter, "The Subordination of Nurses in Health Care: Towards a Social Divisions Approach," in *Gender, Work and Medicine: Women and the Medical Division of Labour,* ed. Elianne Riska and Katarina Wegar (London: Sage, 1993), 115–25.

39. Helen Sweet, "And Our Own Conference . . . ," *History Info, Newsletter of the Royal College of Nursing History of Nursing Society* (Winter 2005/6): 8.

40. Julia Hallam, *Nursing the Image: Media, Culture and Professional Identity* (London: Routledge, 2000), 84–129.

41. McKenna, *Nursing Theories,* 85–91.

42. Aggleton and Chalmers, *Nursing Models,* 45, 149, 151.

43. *The Diary of Richard Kay, 1716–51, of Baldingstone, Near Bury: A Lancashire Doctor,* ed. William Brockbank and Fred Kenworthy (Manchester, UK: Chetham Society, 1968), 134, 135, 136, 141–42, 146, 147, 151.

44. W. B. Howie, "Consumer Reaction: A Patient's View of Hospital Life in 1809," *British Medical Journal* 3 (September 8, 1973): 534–36.

45. John Sweeney, "Historical Research: Examining Documentary Sources," *Nurse Researcher* 12, no. 3 (2005): 64.

46. For a similar point in relation to reading poetry, see Neil Pickering, "The Use of Poetry in Health Care Ethics Education," *Medical Humanities* 26, no. 1 (June 2000): 35.

47. Judith M. Parker, "Evidence-Based Nursing: A Defence," *Nursing Inquiry* 9, no. 3 (2002): 139.

48. David L. Sackett, William M. C. Rosenberg, J. A. Muir Gray, R. Brian Haynes, and W. Scott Richardson, "Evidence Based Medicine: What It Is and What It Isn't," *British Medical Journal* 312 (January 13, 1996): 72.

49. Trisha Greenhalgh, "Intuition and Evidence—Uneasy Bedfellows?" *British Journal of General Practice* 52 (May 2002): 396.

50. Parker, "Evidence-Based Nursing," 139; see also Greenhalgh, "Intuition," 396.

51. Kate Gerrish, "Evidence-Based Practice," in *The Research Process in Nursing,* 5th ed., ed. Kate Gerrish and Anne Lacey (Oxford: Blackwell, 2006), 496.

52. Sweeney, "Historical Research," 71, citing T. E. Christy, "The Methodology of Historical Research," *Nursing Research* 24, no. 3 (May–June 1975): 182–92.

53. See, for example, Steven Edwards, *Philosophy of Nursing: An Introduction* (Basingstoke, UK: Palgrave, 2001), 52–53, 58–60.

"Do Trained Nurses . . . Work for Love, or Do They Work for Money?" Nursing and Altruism in the Twenty-First Century

Ellen D. Baer
Professor Emerita of Nursing, University of Pennsylvania
Visiting Professor of Nursing, Florida Atlantic University

A dear friend of mine was hospitalized in the summer of 2007 with renal artery narrowing, for which she received a stent. She is 81 years old, and had several postdischarge setbacks that required a second hospitalization in one of New York's most prestigious hospitals. (Please note: as has been shown in multiple nursing research studies regarding transitional care, had she had proper nursing care and appropriate discharge planning during the first event, the second hospitalization would not have been needed at all.[1]) I visited her several times and was overwhelmed by the absence of any sign of nursing care. Endless streams of individuals entered her room, each doing some tiny little job—filling a water pitcher, taking a temp, delivering a tray, mopping a floor, emptying a wastebasket, and so on. None of these individuals could answer any question from her; none would agree to do anything for her other than their assigned task. They barely looked at my friend. Had she been in extremis they would not have noticed.

My esteemed colleagues, this is 21st-century sick care without nursing. And why has our nation systematically eliminated nursing care from our hospitals? Because of money. Nursing care is the largest budget item in hospital care. So the health care profiteers systematically strip nursing budgets, insisting

Nursing History Review 17 (2009): 28–46. A Publication of the American Association for the History of Nursing.
DOI: 10.1891/1062–8061.17.28

that hordes of less costly, untrained individuals can perform all the nursing tasks.[2] This short-sighted behavior on the part of unschooled business people would not be possible if society fought it.

For my whole nursing career I have been consumed (obsessed?) by society's inability to understand what nursing is; to recognize the expertise that good nursing entails and its critical importance to health care outcomes.[3] Why do people insist on seeing nurses as nice people mopping fevered brows instead of highly skilled experts giving life-saving, highly technical care? I think the answer lies in society's and nursing's history.

The story of nursing is, of course, a story of gender. But I also think it is a story of ideological debate. Is it science or art, a profession or vocation, independent or dependent, possessed of its own expertise or handmaid to medicine, or, is it in fact degrees of each of these? Those questions lead to others: how to prepare to do nursing, where to do it, who is in charge of it, how much to pay for it, what are proper nurse/patient ratios, and how important it is to patient morbidity and mortality. These are the debates that reflect what I call ideological conflict.

I and others have researched many of these issues.[4] I have examined the concepts themselves—science, autonomy, professionalism—to see whether nursing can be defined by those concepts.[5] All this research was helpful, but it actually increased my frustration, because we have shown that nursing *does* make a difference and *can* be defined by those concepts. The fact that it can be highlights the question as to why it is not, except with reservations. That discovery led me to social history, which examines issues in the context of society's customs and mores in various time frames. I chose to focus on the 1890s, the close of nursing's first generation in the modern era. That research proved more fruitful, although it provided no simple answers. The most general conclusion that emerged from my research is that from the outset of modern nursing there was no consensus among the nurses themselves, or their sponsors, as to their ideological convictions.[6] Nursing was, and is, a house divided, with strong leaders and convincing arguments existing on all sides of each issue.

Because of the competing definitions, philosopher of science Thomas Kuhn might say that nursing lacks a paradigm or unifying principle. But I disagree. Among nurses there is a basic consensus that patients are at the center of nursing's work and that patients' needs drive its practice, education, and research. It is that consensus that holds nursing together and provides the central paradigm. The divisions exist a step removed from that center, the work, and have more to do with the status of the work and whether it is professional work or missionary work. I have concluded that society has difficulty assigning expert status to a role that is practiced primarily by women and that says its primary purpose is caring for people.

Origins

Nursing is said to have developed in response to the need of the sick for care. As a general statement that is probably correct, but there have always been sick people in need of care. The significance of the emergence of modern nursing in the mid-19th century in the Crimea with Florence Nightingale was that it represented a substantive change in the manner in which the sick were cared for: the introduction of a system of caring for the sick, and the recognition and acceptance of the need to prepare (or "train") the people who would deliver the care.

Prior to the advent of the "trained nurse," the sick at home were cared for by what Linda Richards, America's first trained nurse, described as "the so-called *born nurse*" (emphasis in the original). In Richards's words, these women, who

> by their kindness of heart and cheerful service gained for themselves this title were by no means wholly untrained. Experience, which is a most excellent teacher, together with the instruction of older women and of the family doctor, provided a practical and efficient training. A love for the work and a strong desire to alleviate suffering had made most of them excellent nurses. These women, one or more of whom could be found in every village or community, . . . were always subject to call.[7]

The role was identified as a woman's role containing certain personal qualities and quasireligious ideals: kindness of heart, cheerfulness, a love of the work, a willingness to be "on call," and a desire to alleviate suffering—all without consideration of remuneration.

One hundred and fifty years later, nursing is still grappling with those origins. The origins established nursing as work done out of love, of caring for friends and family, work done without consideration of pay. But, over the intervening century and a half, nursing has become highly skilled work, expertise gained in years of study and further years of experience. Now we see it as work in which philanthropic and altruistic ideals conflict with professional self-determination. As I have argued elsewhere, "philanthropic and altruistic agents do not usually seek economic gain or even parity for their efforts. But, professionals who have spent years developing a particular expertise do expect to be paid for their work and recognized in other ways as well."[8]

The public nature of this debate about nursing and money is longstanding. In 1890 a nursing journal named *The Trained Nurse* responded to an article in the *Buffalo Courier,* an upstate New York newspaper. "Do trained nurses," the editorial wondered, echoing back the question raised in the article, "work for love or do they work for money?"[9] But the journal turned this question on its head:

> And why should [this question] be asked of nurses more than of any other class of wage earners? ... Is untiring devotion and consecration incompatible with commensurate pecuniary returns for the same? ... No one hears that physicians should grandly ignore money; on the contrary, the practice of medicine is one of the best paying of the professions. Why should nurses lower their prices that the doctors can extract more from their patients' pockets?

And this debate has not gone away. In 1998 the *Wall Street Journal* asked, "How did the Daughters of Charity—an order whose nuns live on $40 a month, wear modest blue habits and pray and light candles daily in their provincial house—come to be known as the Daughters of Currency?"[10] The *Journal*'s complaint was that the Sisters' health care institutions actually made money, money that the nuns used to subsidize their charity work among the poor. The two articles demonstrate the century-long inability of nursing to satisfy economic complaints. Criticized equally for making money or costing money, nurses occupy the unenviable position of being wrong no matter what their economic state is.

And so to the purpose of this article: What is it that nurses do their work for? Is it for love or money? And does the answer to that question have an impact on the quality of the nursing care?

Catastrophe, Charisma, and Reform

Self-interest is fundamental to human nature. An ideology exists when people are persuaded to go beyond that individual self-interest and coalesce, even if only for the moment, around a larger interest. The agent of persuasion may be a catastrophic event, a charismatic leader, a noble cause. Dr. Albert Worcester pointed out in 1914,

> In times of war and pestilence, and of other national disasters, helpers in abundance volunteer. But in eras of peace and prosperity the common forms of helplessness do not so surely stir the hearts of those able to give the help that is needed.[11]

The ideology of modern nursing was born through catastrophes of war, at the Crimea for the English, on the battlefields of the Civil War for America. It was nourished in its infancy by the charisma of reformer Florence Nightingale. But, as these forces faded at the 19th century's close, the fledgling, awkward, youthful nursing group sought a new frame around which to collect. The noble cause, embodied by missionary Linda Richards, was persuasive for some nurses and suited the 19th-century emphasis on the authority of religion and the role of the Victorian woman. In the early 20th century the professional ideology of Isabel Hampton gained strength. Hampton, a Canadian former teacher, was superintendent of nurses at the Johns Hopkins Hospital, certainly the most prestigious hospital and arguably the most influential nurses' training school in the early 20th century. Her ideology was persuasive to other nurses and suited the rising authority of science and expanding opportunities for women.

The particular perspective one adopted dictated other, related choices: the kind of person who would do the work, the type of reward that would be satisfactory, the preparation required, even the organization of the work and who would direct it. Few nurses defined their ideological choices as explicitly as had the early leaders, Nightingale, Richards, and Hampton. As time went by, the more common practice was to debate the secondary choices regarding levels of independence, education, and pay.

The particular research I am presenting now emerged from an investigation that analyzed the nursing speeches and discussions at the 1893 Chicago World's Fair. The Fair, timed to celebrate the 400th anniversary of Columbus's discovery of America, provided modern nursing, at the very tender age of 21, with its first formal meeting, chaired by Hampton. Hampton set the agenda and chose the speakers, ensuring the predominance of nurses of a professional mindset and deliberately setting aside Nightingale's emphasis on calling and Richards's actions as missionary. My article seeks to capture a moment in time, as nursing came of age and tried to grapple in public with its identity, educational priorities, and organizational construct.

The article focuses on the debate at the Fair surrounding two ideological themes pertinent to this study. I will talk first about the place of religion and the moral guardian role in nursing, and then about the social class issues surrounding nursing as work and related economic considerations. Please note that such a separation is clearly artificial, for the issues really swirled into and about each other. The product was usually a blend, but often there was conflict among the several issues. By dealing with them separately, the conflictive product among the competing ideals, and within each, can be more easily seen and understood.

The Place of Religion and Religious Ideals

The affiliation between religion and the care of the sick is as old as recorded history. From early beliefs in witchcraft and magic came an association between the functions of the priest and those of the physician.[12] As Adelaide Nutting and Lavinia Dock, our first historians, noted, at times in some groups "the advice of women was honoured because it was believed that something prophetic and divine dwelt in them."[13] In Europe, the care of the sick by religious orders became commonplace. In the United States, an 1869 American Medical Association report of the Committee on the Training of Nurses recommended, "That, while it is not at all essential to combine religious exercises with nursing, it is believed that such a union would be eminently conducive to the welfare of the sick in all public institutions."[14]

It seems, then, not surprising that nursing would reflect such a history, described at the Fair by Mrs. Baker, Medical Matron of the Surgical Department at Seventh Day Adventists' Battle Creek Sanitarium:

> if we work "as unto Him," seeking to leave, as results of our effort, healthier bodies, purer homes, sweeter lives and nobler aspirations as we go from home to home we can safely leave the results with the Great Physician under whom we serve.[15]

By the late 1880s the place of religion in nursing had assumed certain distinctive characteristics. It was always a Christian, mostly Protestant, form. The predominant form of Protestantism was evangelism, whose foundations lay in strict adherence to the Bible and whose procedures included proselytizing, conversion, and revivalism. While it afforded its women members opportunities to be assertive in the interests of advancing Christianity, evangelism was, as historian Joan Brumberg argued, "at the same time ... an impediment to the development of any widespread acceptance of political feminism."[16] Biblical patriarchy, with women subject to their husbands, was too critical to the evangelical belief system to allow for women's autonomy on a general basis.

Other religions created their own hospitals and training schools, with similar constraints. The Training School for Nurses of St. Joseph's (Catholic) Hospital in Philadelphia noted in its bulletin that "Recommendation of a clergy-man ... or other well-known citizen, is always expected."[17] In addition, St. Joseph's stated as its purpose: "It is the plan of the school to furnish every essential equipment and privilege accorded by the best of modern training schools, and, in addition, to furnish the guarded moral environment of a religious order."

Association with religion prior to entering nursing was considered serious testimony to one's good character. Continued association with religion during nursing life was considered to provide the guarded moral environment in which one was less likely to do wrongful acts. The various training school entrance requirements and daily routines dramatized these uses of religion. Even ostensibly secular, scientific hospitals sought religious references for candidates. Every applicant to the Johns Hopkins Training School for Nurses, for example, was required to submit a letter of support from her pastor or minister.[18] Only Quaker applicants were not so obliged, as they had no ministers. Friends of their Societies wrote instead.

America's first hospital, the Pennsylvania Hospital in Philadelphia, founded by Benjamin Franklin, had on its seal, which formed the motif for the nurses' pin, the Good Samaritan parable: "Take Care of Him and I Will Repay Thee."[19] The aura of religion was woven into the students' lives as nurses in other ways as well. The hospital brochure stated that the school "starts the day with chapel." At capping ceremonies students recited the Florence Nightingale Pledge:

> I solemnly pledge myself before God and in the presence of this assembly: to pass my life in purity and to practice my profession faithfully. I will abstain from whatever is deleterious and mischievous, and will not take or knowingly administer any harmful drug. I will do all in my power to maintain and elevate the standards of my profession, and will hold in confidence all personal matters committed to my keeping and all family matters coming to my knowledge in the practice of my profession.
>
> With loyalty I will endeavor to aid the physician in his work, and devote myself to the welfare of those committed to my care.[20]

One student's letter reminded her classmates: "There was a holy example set us 1900 years ago in Galilee which I know you are trying to follow and which I was trying to follow too."[21]

In her influential book *Nursing Ethics,* the first of its kind to instruct nursing students on proper behavior above and beyond clinical skill, Isabel Hampton Robb described

> the nurse's work as a ministry; it should be consecrated service, performed in the spirit of Christ who made himself of no account but went about being good. . . .
>
> The nearer to her heart she keeps the teachings and the life of Christ in her everyday work, the greater will be her strength to overcome difficulties and to forget herself in helping others.[22]

Cardinal Gibbons of Baltimore provided a summary of the many 1893 Fair reports that spoke to this ideal in nursing:

> When the desire of relieving the sufferings of humanity is prompted and ennobled by the love of God, it keeps alive that spirit of self-sacrifice and devotedness which we so admire in those who consecrate their lives to the care of the sick.[23]

There were several very practical reasons for infusing spiritual precepts into nursing work. First, the almshouse hospitals into which the pupil-nurses were sent in 1873 to perform their nursing work have been described by historian Charles Rosenberg as essentially "low dens of vice."[24] Prostitution, drunkenness, thievery, and every sort of immoral activity were known to be rampant among the inmates as well as their untrained attendants, called "nurses." The only previous nurses who had escaped the harshness of this fate were religious protected by the armor of their habits. As a substitute, the new "trained" nurses were given by their sponsors an armor of moral rectitude with which to shield themselves.

Second, as nursing work gained acceptance and success, the sponsors and nursing leaders hoped to attract better-educated, more genteel candidates to nursing. There was little in the work itself to warrant such ambitions. Attaching nobility and "higher rewards" to the menial work had the very practical result of gaining the interest of some women of this desired sort.

The third very practical consideration was economic. If one can be convinced that the reward for one's service comes from other than monetary sources, one will likely not press for monetary compensation quite as fiercely. Furthermore, there was the notion of control through obedience to authority. Religion offers a kind of control available to no other authorities. It is invisible, does not require logical proofs or reasons, and carries hidden, uncertain punitive measures to those in violation. Finally, the women nurses were fulfilling the task assigned women by society of protecting and promoting the moral values.

On a larger scale, the training school, functioning in those years as the actual and only nursing department, was described by Lavinia Dock as "a moral force within the hospital," which exerted a "purifying influence" in city and municipal hospitals where "the misery of the neglected sick was one thing, the depravity and moral degradation another."[25] As Dock said,

> Of all the attributes of the school its moral strength is the most easily demonstrable, and its reformatory work is the part of its whole work in which it can most securely stand on its own merits.

This moral purpose had existed from the reform beginnings of formal nursing in America. The Constitution and By Laws of the Visiting Committee for Bellevue Hospital listed as its primary purpose to visit "with a view to mental, moral and physical improvement of the patients, and to bring about such reforms as may be practicable."[26]

This purpose reflected, in essence, the sexual romanticism characteristic of feminists of the 1880s and 1890s, whereby women used their moral guardian societal role as the legitimating principle of their reform work. Moving out of traditional roles in their homes, they entered the work world under the auspices of charity work with reform goals. This was a helpful interpretation for nurses because it gained them entry into almshouses and hospitals. It was less successful in later years when professionalizing issues emerged. Having gained entry on a basis that reinforced certain elements of women's dependent societal role, it was difficult to reject those pieces when nurses later sought greater independence and self-determination.

Economics and Social Class

Now to my second theme: the economic aspects of social class. Here I would argue that the predominant social view of nursing in the last half of the 19th century was determined through its linkage to money paid, or not, for the services rendered. Dr. Charles Krafft, director of La Source Normal Evangelical School for Independent Nurses for the Sick in Lausanne, Switzerland, explained in a speech at the Fair. If a woman chose "to employ some part of [her] time in the gratuitous care of the sick," the work was ennobled and admired.[27] If she did so for remuneration, she was in danger of being considered to "think more of her own comfort than of the beauty of self-sacrifice, and of the amount received for her services rather than of her resolution to give the best that she has cheerfully and ungrudgingly to her work."[28] Hampton Robb later described in *Nursing Ethics* the source she believed gave rise to this feeling:

> The care—or perhaps we might say the criminal negligence—accorded to poor patients in hospitals in days gone by had made the name "hospital" a by-word and a term of reproach which is not yet wholly eradicated. . . .
>
> [the terrible nature of nursing in that era] . . . accustomed people to regard paid nurses as self-seeking menials engaged in something far lower than domestic work, and whose only object was to benefit by others' misfortune at the least expenditure of care and trouble on their own part.[29]

As the nation underwent the Industrial Revolution, it began to experience new arrangements between those who owned or organized commercial capital enterprises and those who worked in those enterprises for wages. Upper-class people owned the enterprises; working-class people worked in the enterprises for wages; and a new group, the middle class, emerged to organize and manage the enterprises.

In the Fair speeches, presenters consistently identified class distinctions as of primary interest in the selection of nurses. Hampton advised watchfulness against admitting "the commercial woman, who enters the school ... only seeking ... future dollars and cents, never working for the love of her work."[30] Such regular references to the income derived from nursing as a job have class-consciousness as their implicit shadow, for such admonitions would apply only to women who needed money, who were not of the leisure class.

The schools had the same difficulty: "that of obtaining pupil nurses of the right stamp—young women of good education, refinement and strong physique."[31] They all agreed on this point. The prominent American schools requested evidence of these characteristics through personal letters by the candidates, documenting their backgrounds and education. Schools sought supportive letters from clergy, influential citizens, and physicians to substantiate the rest. But the difficulty of attracting such women was great, and for good reason, for as Dr. Horatio Storer, one of Boston's strongest medical supporters of formal nurses' training, described it,

> A nurse's toil is great, her duties often disgusting, her pecuniary remuneration small in comparison with her requirements and her labors; so that there is nothing to invite the cooperation of the better class of women, save the highest motives which can influence the true Christian.[32]

The problem became circular in nature, for if "the services of gentlewomen" could be obtained, "to be a nurse [would] impl[y] a certain social status" and others would follow.[33] The converse was equally potent.

Schools, sponsors, and physicians such as William Richardson fervently hoped that as "the supply comes more nearly to equal the demand, the public and the profession will be able to exercise more choice in the matter; and then the best nurses will come to the front."[34] Abraham Jacobi hoped that those "from better stock ... [will] raise themselves to higher ambitions, ... spend money and two years of their lives for the purpose of learning" the care of the sick.[35]

The Fair presentations and discussions traced this problem through many nations. Mrs. Dacre Craven, a prominent spokesperson for district nursing in England, described a history in which "the first paid secular nurses for the poor in England . . . were taken from the lower grade of women." After a study of the services, a recommendation was made "to recruit the [district] nurses entirely from the class known as gentlewomen" for these reasons: the district nurse practiced alone frequently, so had greater responsibility; she therefore needed greater education; such requirements would attract "ladies"; such ladies would have a greater influence over their patients, and would raise the opinion of nursing held by the public. Further, it would be possible to give more advanced lectures to such ladies "than were available in hospitals where lectures had to be adapted to women of a lower grade and education."[36]

Luise Fahrmann, superintendent of Victoria House in Berlin, explained that nursing the sick poor in Germany was designed "to open to young women [& widows] of the educated ranks of life (but in poor circumstances and without occupation) an honorable, gratifying and blessed vocation."[37]

Dr. Krafft outlined the French system that institutionalized the division between paid and unpaid nurses. Paid *internes* were selected on the basis of their need for self-support; *externes* were leisure-class participants. But the French made a particular effort not to value one more or less than the other:

> Our school holds it honorable for women and for men alike to earn their daily bread . . . we render homage to those who, placed in a position of great wealth, consecrate it to the gratuitous care of the poor. But, if we see in this a privilege, we do not see in it a superiority. In our eyes, each nurse should remain free, either to accept remuneration or to refuse it.[38]

The United States, consistent with its political ideology of thought (if not always of fact), attempted to define nursing socially as a unitary and standardized entity to which any woman could aspire should she meet the requirements. Hampton presented the highlights:

> She must be strong mentally, morally, and physically, and to do thorough work she must have infinite tact, which is another name for common sense. . . . [with] no general rule governing the special attainments or degree of education required from the women who present themselves as candidates.[39]

Applicants for admission to the Hopkins Training School represented many strata of American social life: one was "a lady of fine social position and family"; another was described as an "Educated, ladylike, sympathetic and active" member of a farming family; a third applicant's "parents were industrious and well to do farmers, of good reputation"; a fourth "belongs to a very respectable old family in Philadelphia. She is a young lady of refinement and integrity and the best standing in a large family connection." Several were described as having been reared in well-to-do circumstances and left without funds unexpectedly.[40]

But we also know these were not the only kinds of nursing students. Anna Turner, a Bellevue pupil, described her farming origins, her grandfather a "hard worker," the orchard and animals with which they lived, the neighbors who were

> nearly all of pioneer stock, kind and helpful to each other. There were only a few who had good finished houses but they were never thought of as being socially above the poorest. The morale was higher than in any place I have ever been since. Character was the thing that ranked highest. . . .
>
> My parents were too poor to have a home so we never lived long in one place. There was also a new baby about every two and a half years—no two being born in the same house. I was the oldest and often much in the way so I would be sent to my already much outnumbered grandparents.[41]

When Turner was almost 10, a fifth baby arrived and she went permanently to live with her grandparents, eventually doing "most of the work in the house."

These class considerations and differences contained very difficult conflicts. On the one hand, all the schools, doctors, sponsors, and nursing leaders were seeking a "higher type" of woman to do nursing work. They considered more educated women more able to teach hospital patients the values of health and cleanliness and impose the desired moral order. Yet nursing was paid work, in which the higher classes were not likely to engage. In addition, hospital patients were cared for by pupil-nurses who carried no authority. As graduates, nurses entered private nursing, where the social relationship was reversed. In private nursing, the patient was usually the higher-class participant. How could a nurse of a "higher type" work comfortably after graduation in situations where she was specifically instructed not to expect equality to the family with which she worked?

The emergence of the middle-class worker was the only possible solution. A nurse who could be "higher" in the hospital and "lower" in private nursing was what was really wanted. In the language of the new economic order of capitalism, this nurse would be the middle manager: not the owner of the enterprise; not the lowly laborer of the enterprise; but the organizer of the enterprise, the manager and arranger of the work of lower laborers, for the benefit of owners, shareholders, and sponsors of various sorts. These characterizations were not addressed directly, but were implicit in the Fair debates.

Shifting Ideological Patterns

As I have argued before,

> It has taken almost 150 years for nursing to evolve from an assumed part of the private role of women in their homes to a paid work of educated professional [men and women] in public institutions. This evolution has occurred haltingly, awkwardly, and with difficulty and dismay on the parts of many who preferred to view the role romantically as the loving acts of caring people unattached to fees.[42]

What I hope to add here is a more nuanced understanding of that halting, awkward, and often difficult evolution. That evolution did not occur in a social vacuum; it took place within a tapestry of conflicting social mores and it remains imbedded in these mores as it struggles with its current identity.

As a 19th-century phenomenon, nursing was caught between the shifting ideological patterns of that era and was fraught with conflict. Different nurses, sponsors, physicians, and groups of each, espoused different ideologies. A competition emerged in the late 19th century as to which ideological pattern nursing would embrace. There was no resolution. Without a generic consensus regarding these issues, nursing could assert only partial authority in the health care field, assume only partial control of its own work, and propose only partial remuneration for its own expertise and services. Specifically regarding money, whichever direction nursing took, the opposing force levied its critique. When nurses sought more remuneration for their critical knowledge and skill, they were, and are, accused of trying to capitalize on the misfortunes of others. When nurses remained steadfast to their patients, resisting strikes and other labor mechanisms to attain parity, they were, and are, left behind in salary, benefits, and other attributes of professional recognition.

By 1893 approximately 150 hospital nurse training schools had been established in a mere 20 years, and nursing had become an acceptable occupational alternative for women.[43] The first generation of nurses and their sponsors were satisfied to have accomplished their reform goal: establish the nursing work and make hospitals places that "did the sick no harm."[44]

The second generation of nurses had a new agenda. They sought more systematic training for pupil-nurses, full control over their nursing (nonmedical) work, job protection for the graduate nurses who still competed with untrained nurses for private nursing, recognition, and reward for their nursing work. This agenda provided the framework for the nursing programs and discussions at the 1893 World's Fair in Chicago. The problem, though, was that the agenda was neither unanimously nor even consistently supported by all the nurses. Nursing had achieved significant diversity of membership. Variations in every datum of demography were the norm and fluctuation in ideals within the group was the consequence. The conflicts so spawned within nursing itself were a chief obstacle in achieving the goals of the second generation of nurses and the attainment for nursing of legitimacy as an authoritative professional group. The result of this chain of circumstance was the prevention of nursing from achieving a clear identity within the advancing scientific authority.

Thus, even now, in the 21st century, although nursing is expected to work within science, and participate in enacting the results of science, it is not expected to know science or be science. It therefore remains on the threshold between the religious legitimacy from which it emerged and the scientific legitimacy into which it has never achieved full entry, even with its increasingly impressive research productivity. The result is a peculiar sort of autonomy whereby nurses act independently most of the time, but dwell within a pretense of dependence. The label *semiprofession* or *paraprofession* or some other quasiterm is attached to this strange arrangement with all the ramifications such a predicament implies.

To conclude regarding the research question: Do nurses work for love or money? The answer seems to be both. One goal without the other to balance it seems to create a predominance of one value and structure, to the detriment of the patient, the work, and the nurse.

On one hand, surely few people choose a nursing career for financial gain. But every nurse needs to earn a fair and equitable wage. Through their educational programs nurses have to become and remain aware of the economics of health care without being corrupted by that awareness. Because most nurses do not bill directly for their services, they are free to express their expertise in ways that are unfettered by concerns about costs and benefits. Yet, they cannot be completely impervious to the economic constraints that are close to crippling the industry. They have to find a way to practice nursing within fiscally sound parameters while still making patient needs their central focus.[45]

On the other hand, nurses currently occupy a distance from money that seems to contribute to nursing's "most trusted" status in national polls. According to nurse historian Marcie Rutherford (who also has an MBA):

> [Most] Nurses ... neither gain from the profits nor suffer from company losses. [Because most nurses are] ... employees, paid an hourly or salaried rate, the public

> does not see nurses directly linked to money. There is no conflict of interest. Nurses' pay remains stable no matter how many patients they treat or the [number] ... of supplies they dispense. The services nurses provide are directed by the patient's plan of care and/or in response to the patient's health care needs. [Therefore] Patients trust nurses' motives and see their services as genuine and not affected by any connection to personal gain.[46]

This is a powerful finding that all health care providers would do well to listen to. Because, now that hospitals are methodically doing away with the very nursing care that people like my dear friend enter hospitals to obtain, people will stop using them. The absence of trusted experts at their bedsides will scare patients away, just as hospitals are already scaring nurses away—nurses who fear they cannot do their jobs responsibly in the current hospital environment and so take their nursing skills to other health care settings, such as homes.

With that in mind, I'd like to end with two prophecies from Florence Nightingale that touch on these issues. The first, from *On Trained Nursing for the Sick Poor* (1881), stated:

> Hospitals are but an intermediary stage of civilization. At present hospitals are the only place where the sick poor can be nursed, or, indeed, often the sick rich. But the ultimate object is to nurse all sick at home.[47]

The second, in a conversation with Henry Bonham Carter (1867), Nightingale said:

> My view you know is that the ultimate destination of nursing is the nursing of the sick in their own homes.... I look to the abolition of all hospitals and workhouse infirmaries. But no use to talk about the year 2000.[48]

Ellen D. Baer, RN, PhD, FAAN
Professor Emerita of Nursing, University of Pennsylvania
Visiting Professor of Nursing, Florida Atlantic University
732 Village Road, North Palm Beach, FL 33408
561–622–2151
ellendbaer@aol.com

Acknowledgments

This paper was first presented at the Zula Mae Baber Bice Memorial Lecture at the University of Virginia School of Nursing and Medical Center Hour, November 7, 2007.

Notes

1. Nurse researchers like Dorothy Brooten and Mary Naylor have repeatedly demonstrated that significantly improved patient outcomes and cost savings occur using specific nursing interventions with various patient populations during transitions.

2. Ellen D. Baer and Suzanne Gordon, "Money Managers Are Unraveling the Tapestry of Nursing," *American Journal of Nursing* 94, no. 10 (1994): 38–40. See also Ellen D. Baer, Claire M. Fagin, and Suzanne Gordon, eds., *Abandonment of the Patient: The Impact of Profit-Driven Health Care on the Public* (New York: Springer, 1996).

3. Ellen D. Baer, "Women and the Politics of Career Development: The Case of Nursing," in *Nursing History and the Politics of Welfare,* ed. Anna M. Rafferty, Jane Robinson, and Ruth Elkan (London: Routledge, 1997), 242–58.

4. Linda Aiken and others have demonstrated significantly reduced patient mortality in care units that have increased nurse staffing. See Linda H. Aiken, Sean P. Clarke, D. M. Sloane, Julie Sochalski, and J. H. Silber, "Hospital Nurse Staffing and Patient Mortality, Nurse Burnout, and Job Dissatisfaction," *Journal of the American Medical Association* 288, no. 16 (2002): 1987–93. See also Sean P. Clarke and Linda H. Aiken, "Failure to Rescue: Needless Deaths Are Prime Examples of the Need for More Nurses at the Bedside," *New England Journal of Medicine* 346, no. 22 (2003): 42–47.

5. Ellen D. Baer, "Philosophical and Historical Bases of Advanced Practice Nursing Roles," in *Nurse Practitioners: Evolution of Advanced Practice,* ed. Mathy D. Mezey, Diane O. McGivern, and Eileen M. Sullivan-Marx (New York: Springer, 2003), 37–53.

6. Ellen D. Baer, "Nursing's Divided House—An Historical View," *Nursing Research* 34, no. 1 (1985): 32–38; Baer, "'A Cooperative Venture' in Pursuit of Professional Status: A Research Journal for Nursing," *Nursing Research* 36, no. 1 (1987): 18–25; Baer, "Nursing's Divided Loyalties: An Historical Case Study," *Nursing Research* 38, no. 3 (1989): 166–71; Baer, "American Nursing: 100 Years of Conflicting Ideas and Ideals," *Journal of the New York State Nurses' Association* 23, no. 3 (1992): 16–21; Baer, "Aspirations Unattained: The Story of the Illinois Training School's Search for University Status," *Nursing Research* 41, 1 (1992): 43–48. Baer, "Nurses," in *Women, Health, and Medicine in America: A Historical Handbook,* ed. Rima D. Apple (New York: Garland, 1990), 459–75.

7. Linda Richards, *Reminiscences of Linda Richards, America's First Trained Nurse* (Boston: Whitcomb & Barrows, 1911), 3–4.

8. Ellen D. Baer, "Introduction: Nursing's Ambivalent Relationship with Money," in *Nurses' Work: Issues Across Time and Place,* ed. Patricia D'Antonio, Ellen D. Baer, S. D. Rinker, and Joan E. Lynaugh (New York: Springer, 2007), 82.

9. Editorial, *The Trained Nurse* 5 (July–December 1890): 96. Annette M. Summer, ed., "A Monthly Magazine, consecrated to those who minister to the sick and suffering, in Hospital and Home. The Recognized Organ of the Nursing Profession" (Buffalo, N.Y.: Lakeside Publishing).

10. Monica Langley, "Money Order: Nuns' Zeal for Profits Shapes Hospital Chain, Wins Wall Street Fans," *Wall Street Journal,* January 7, 1998, cited in Marcella Rutherford, "More Than Good, Kind Angels: The Daughters of Charity's Relationship to Valuation, Mission, and Money, 1916–1994" (PhD diss., Florida Atlantic University, 2007), 158.

11. Alfred Worcester, AM, MD, *Nurses for Our Neighbors* (Boston: Houghton Mifflin, 1914), 2.

12. J. D. Gatewood, MD, "Notes on Naval Hospitals, Medical Schools and Training Schools for Nurses, with a Sketch of Hospital History," in *Hospitals, Dispensaries, and Nursing,* ed. John S. Billings, MD, and Henry M. Hurd, MD, Papers and Discussions in the International Congress of Charities, Correction and Philanthropy, Section III, Chicago, June 12–17, 1893, under the Auspices of the World's Congress Auxiliary of the World's Columbian Exposition (Baltimore: Johns Hopkins Press, 1894; repr., New York: Garland, 1984), 213–17.

13. M. Adelaide Nutting and Lavinia L. Dock, eds., *A History of Nursing,* 2 vols. (New York: G. P. Putnam's Sons, 1907), 1: 96.

14. Nutting and Dock, *A History of Nursing,* 2:368, quoting from *Proceedings of the American Medical Association* (May 1869); repr., *Medical News* (Philadelphia) 20 (1869): 339, 351.

15. Mrs. S. M. Baker (Medical Matron of the Surgical Department of the Battle Creek Sanitarium), "Nursing in Homes, Private Hospitals and Sanitariums," in Isabel Hampton et al., *Nursing of the Sick 1893,* Papers and Discussions from the International Congress of Charities, Correction and Philanthropy, Chicago, 1893, published under the Sponsorship of the National League for Nursing Education (New York: McGraw-Hill, 1949), 201.

16. Joan J. Brumberg, *Mission for Life: The Story of the Family of Adoniram Judson, the Dramatic Events of the First American Foreign Mission, and the Course of Evangelical Religion in the Nineteenth Century* (New York: Free Press, 1980), 104.

17. Training School for Nurses of St. Joseph's Hospital, *Announcements for 1895–6,* 6, Memorabilia maintained by Southeastern National League for Nursing, History of Nursing Museum, Pennsylvania Hospital, Philadelphia.

18. Personal Letters of Applicants, Record Group 3, ser. a, Box 1, School of Nursing Papers, Alan Mason Chesney Medical Archives in Turner Auditorium, Johns Hopkins Medical Institution, Baltimore.

19. Nursing School Papers, Pennsylvania Hospital Historic Library, Philadelphia.

20. Mary Cora McNinch, Capping Ceremony, Pennsylvania Hospital Historic Library. The Pledge seems to have originated at Bellevue in 1893 and was used at most capping ceremonies by the early 1900s. See Box 2, Folder 38, Hunter-Bellevue Archives, 440 E. 26th St., New York (administered by Hunter College Library, 695 Park Ave., New York).

21. Letter dated August 17, 1900, MHW Folder, Pennsylvania Hospital Historic Library.

22. Isabel Hampton Robb, *Nursing Ethics: For Hospital and Private Use* (Cleveland: E. C. Koeckert, 1916) (Copyright 1900 Mrs. Robb), 38.

23. Cardinal Gibbons (of Baltimore), "Work Done by Religious Communities Devoted to the Relief of the Sick," in Billings and Hurd, *Hospitals, Dispensaries, and Nursing,* 473.

24. Charles E. Rosenberg, "From Almshouse to Hospital: The Shaping of Philadelphia General Hospital," *Milbank Quarterly* 60 (1982): 108–54.

25. Lavinia L. Dock (Asst. Superintendent of Nurses, Johns Hopkins Hospital), "The Relationship of Training Schools to Hospitals," in *Nursing of the Sick 1893,* 13–14, 21.

26. Bellevue Hospital—Notes of Eliza Perkins, Superintendent 1876–1888, Constitution and By Laws of the Local Visiting Committee for Bellevue Hospital, New York City, organized January 26, 1872, Article II, p. 2, Hunter-Bellevue Archives.

27. Dr. Charles Krafft (Director), "La Source Normal Evangelical School for Independent Nurses for the Sick at Lausanne, Switzerland," in Billings and Hurd, *Hospitals, Dispensaries, and Nursing,* 505.

28. Irene Sutliffe (Directress, New York Hospital Training School), "The History of American Training Schools," in Billings and Hurd, *Hospitals, Dispensaries, and Nursing,* 512.

29. Robb, *Nursing Ethics,* 28.

30. Isabel A. Hampton (Superintendent of Nurses and Principal of the Training School, Johns Hopkins Hospital), "Educational Standards for Nurses," in *Nursing of the Sick 1893,* 2, 9.

31. *The Nightingale* 1, no. 4 (June 1886): 24, "A Paper in the Interests of Methodical Nursing of the Sick" (New York: Sara E. Post, MD, Publisher).

32. H. R. Storer, *On Nurses and Nursing With Especial Reference to the Management of Sick Women* (Boston: Lee and Shepard, 1868), 11.

33. *The Nightingale* 2, no. 4 (June 1887): 2.

34. William R. Richardson, MD (Visiting Professor at Massachusetts General Hospital), "The Duties and Conduct of Nurses in Private Duty," Address delivered at the Boston Training School for Nurses, June 18, 1886 (London: Field and Tuer, 1887), 8.

35. Abraham Jacobi, MD, "The Historical Development of Modern Nursing," Address delivered at the First Commencement of the Mt. Sinai Training School for Nurses, May 12, 1883 (pamphlet reprinted from *Popular Science Monthly,* October 1883).

36. Mrs. Dacre Craven (née Florence S. Lees), "On District Nursing," in Billings and Hurd, *Hospitals, Dispensaries, and Nursing,* 547–49.

37. Luise Fahrmann (Superintendent of Victoria House, Berlin), "The Victoria House for the Care of the Sick at Berlin," in Billings and Hurd, *Hospitals, Dispensaries, and Nursing,* 481–82.

38. Krafft, "La Source Normal Evangelical School," 505, 501.

39. Hampton, *Nursing of the Sick 1893,* 3, 4–5.

40. Johns Hopkins School of Nursing Papers, Personal Letters of Applicants, Record Group 3, Folders 3, 5, 4, 3, 1, 14.

41. Diary of Anna Turner, Bellevue Hospital Training School for Nurses, Hunter-Bellevue Archives, 5, 6, 10.

42. Baer, "Ambivalent Relationship . . . , Introduction," 85.

43. Arlowayne Swort, "The ANA: The Formative Years, 1875–1922" (EdD diss., Teachers College, Columbia University, 1973), 16, reports that 12 schools existed in 1880, 45 in 1885, 132 in 1890, and 358 by 1896. Lavinia L. Dock, ed., *A History of Nursing* (New York: G. P. Putnam's Sons, 1912), 3: 141, reports 15 schools in 1880, 35 in 1890, 432 in 1900, and 1,023 in 1907. Elizabeth Hobson, *Recollections of a Happy Life* (New York:

G. P. Putnam's Sons, 1916), 112, reports 3 schools in 1873, 30 in 1898, and 1,100 in 1911. Although the figures vary, the evidence of overwhelmingly rapid growth is substantial.

44. Florence Nightingale, *Notes on Hospitals,* 3rd ed. (London: Longman, Green, Longman, Roberts, and Green, 1863), Preface.

45. Rutherford, "More Than Good, Kind Angels," 197–200.

46. Rutherford, "More Than Good, Kind Angels," 197.

47. Florence Nightingale, *On Trained Nursing for the Sick Poor* (London: Spottiswoode & Co., 1881), 10.

48. Monica Baly, *As Miss Nightingale Said—Florence Nightingale Through Her Sayings: A Victorian Perspective* (London: Scutari Press, 1991), 68–69. Special thanks to the University of Virginia Center for Nursing Historical Inquiry for alerting me to this wonderful quote.

ARTICLES

"The Reflection of England's Light": The Instructive District Nursing Association of Boston, 1884–1914

CARRIE HOWSE
External Member, University of Gloucestershire

Abstract. This article examines the extent to which the Instructive District Nursing Association (IDNA) of Boston was influenced by the English system of district nursing. The schemes had the same aims and motivation, but the differences in their organizational structures, in particular the lack of specialist training and professional supervision of the Boston nurses, affected the IDNA's work with its poor, mainly immigrant patients. It is clear that much was achieved, but it is also apparent that problems increased as the work expanded. Attempts to solve these difficulties can be traced through the introduction of a nurse supervisor, establishment of a training school, and eventual radical reorganization. The IDNA also had a leading role in the expansion of the visiting nurse movement throughout the United States. I discuss attempts to establish national standards, particularly through the formation of the National Organization for Public Health Nursing (NOPHN). With the disparate arrangements in the U.S. health care system, the NOPHN was unable to reach a workable consensus and failed to produce a comprehensive and cohesive national system similar to that which had been established in England.

At a conference of nurses held in Chicago in June 1893, Calina Somerville, who worked for the Instructive District Nursing Association (IDNA) of Boston from 1886 to 1890, described district nursing in America as "the reflection of England's light," and expressed a hope that "the new century will find us in the full blaze of sunlight, and that the darkness, disease, and foul air

Nursing History Review 17 (2009): 47–79. A Publication of the American Association for the History of Nursing.
DOI: 10.1891/1062–8061.17.47

of our tenements will have been dispelled and purified through the systematic efforts of organized trained nursing."[1] While her words were somewhat florid, the sentiments she expressed were well received by her audience at a time when philanthropists and leading nurses on both sides of the Atlantic saw nursing the sick poor in their own homes as a means of providing social improvement as well as professional care.

This article examines the extent to which the IDNA of Boston was influenced by the English system of district nursing. District, or visiting, nursing in the United States has received attention from American historians, and some of these studies acknowledge the influence of the English system,[2] but they describe and discuss the American system separately. Analyzing reports, minutes books, rules and regulations, correspondence, and contemporary journals makes it possible to discuss the similarities and differences between the two systems. I consider the degree to which this contrast affected the progress and problems of the IDNA, from 1884, when Abbie Howes paid her first fact-finding visit to England, to 1914, by which time Mary Beard's radical reorganization of the IDNA had taken effect. This period coincided with the formation of the National Organization for Public Health Nursing (NOPHN), when leading nurses, including Beard, attempted to consolidate their past experience and influence the future role of public health nursing through the establishment of national standards. With the expansion of visiting nursing throughout the United States, the need had arisen to balance charitable intentions with sound financial practice, cases of acute illness with chronic conditions, and nursing care with public health education. However, with the disparate arrangements in the U.S. health care system, NOPHN was unable to reach a workable consensus.

In England, by contrast, standardization had been achieved with the formation of Queen Victoria's Jubilee Institute for Nurses (QVJI) in 1889. Based on Florence Nightingale's definition of the dual aims of district nursing as curative care and preventative education, which she had first formulated in the 1860s, QVJI unified existing philanthropic schemes through its system of standardized training, local supervision, and national inspection. Its rules for affiliation recognized diverse local circumstances and arrangements of District Nursing Associations (DNAs), which served communities from inner-city slums to isolated rural villages. Its organizational structure acknowledged the importance of the social elite as local administrators, while also providing professional monitoring of the nurses' work. Thus, each DNA functioned within a supportive framework, but with individual responsibility for its day-to-day operational issues.

The criteria QVJI produced for its so-called ideal DNA make it possible to gauge the progress of the IDNA of Boston in terms of its aims and organization. Comparing a single U.S. agency with an English national standard does not provide a commensurably detailed analysis of care at a local level, but it does enable the similarities and differences between the fundamental elements of the two schemes to be explored. The philanthropic founders of the IDNA sought the advice of their English counterparts and shared their ideals, but their approach to the work in Boston lacked both the administrative efficiency and the professional uniformity of QVJI. Identifying these differences and analyzing their effects on the IDNA's work adds a new dimension to the understanding of the relationship between these two distinct yet interrelated schemes of district nursing.

The English System

District nursing in England began in Liverpool, a prosperous commercial port in the northwest of the country, when William Rathbone (1819–1902), a philanthropic merchant, resolved to set up, at his own expense, a scheme to provide home nursing for the sick poor. In 1861, he wrote to Florence Nightingale asking for her advice and support. Nightingale suggested that the only way to ensure an adequate supply of suitable nurses was to set up a special training school at the Liverpool Royal Infirmary, where Rathbone was a member of the management committee. In 1862, the Liverpool Training School & Home for Nurses was duly opened, under a superintendent who had trained at the Nightingale School at St. Thomas's Hospital in London. Thus the precedent was set that district nurses should be hospital trained, preferably under the Nightingale reformed system, before being specially trained in district work. By 1867, the city of Liverpool had been divided into 18 districts, each with its own nurse and each organized by a philanthropic lady volunteer and lay committee.

The success of the Liverpool system proved a stimulus to other large towns and cities. Manchester and Birmingham founded similar schemes, but in London sparse care was provided by religious and philanthropic organizations whose nurses were only partially trained or had no training at all. When Rathbone became a Liberal Member of Parliament (MP), and consequently spent part of each year in the capital, he and Nightingale worked together "to try to get for London a scheme for organising the disjointed efforts in the metropolis into our plan."[3] To this end, Nightingale wrote a pamphlet, *Suggestions for Improving the Nursing Service for the Sick Poor,* and selected Florence Lees (later Mrs. Dacre Craven) to carry out a detailed survey of the existing district nursing provision and needs in London. Lees, an experienced nurse who had trained at the Nightingale School, produced a meticulous report, as a result of which the Metropolitan Nursing Association (MNA) was formed in 1875. Lees was appointed superintendent general, responsible for recruiting and supervising the trainees, who, after completing the standard one year's training as Lady Probationers at the Nightingale School, paid to be trained specifically as district nurses at the MNA Central Home. By 1886, seven branches had been formed in various parts of London, and the following year the opportunity arose to extend the MNA's work throughout the country.

In 1887, as part of the celebrations for Queen Victoria's Golden Jubilee, the women of England were invited to make donations to a Jubilee Fund, and the Queen was asked to decide how the money should be spent. From various plans submitted to her, she chose a national scheme produced by Rathbone and Nightingale to provide professionally trained and supervised district nurses for the sick poor in their own homes, based on the rules and standards of the MNA. In 1889, a Royal Charter was issued, formally establishing Queen Victoria's Jubilee Institute for Nurses (QVJI), with Rathbone as vice-president and Florence Craven as a member of the Queen's Council. Existing urban district nursing associations, that conformed to the general principles of the Institute, were invited to apply for affiliation; rural areas were brought into the scheme by the affiliation in 1892 and eventual amalgamation in 1897 of the Rural Nursing Association, a national charity that had been founded in Gloucestershire in 1890.

Whereas the central administration of QVJI was endowed by the Jubilee Fund, each district nursing association (DNA) was responsible for raising its own funds. The QVJI rules of affiliation stated that "the services of the nurse shall be for cases of the sick poor and working classes in their own homes." However, it added that patients "may be attended who, though unable to incur the expense of a private nurse, are able to make some contribution to the funds of the Association." Most DNAs therefore adopted a sliding scale of annual subscriptions, dependent on income, with the poorest patients receiving free care.[4] At the local level, each DNA was run by a volunteer lady manager and committee; each county had a County Nursing Association (CNA), made up of representatives of the DNAs; and overall, QVJI was controlled by the Queen's Council (personally appointed by Queen Victoria), to which all DNAs and CNAs were required to submit annual reports. Each DNA was responsible for employing its own nurse, while each CNA employed a county superintendent whose appointment required approval of the Queen's Council. Finally, the Council employed inspectors who toured the country and, like the superintendents, were trained and experienced Queen's Nurses.[5] In this way, the English system of district nursing was consolidated and regulated, with a central governing body and national standards.

The Boston System

By the last quarter of the 19th century, northeastern U.S. cities, particularly those on the coast, were experiencing problems similar to those that had existed in England since the beginning of the Industrial Revolution 100 years before. The rapid expansion of industrial towns and prosperous cities attracted an influx of the poor in search of work in England, migrants from the countryside; in the United States, immigrants from overseas. In both cases, this led to a clear separation of classes, with the poor living in overcrowded, dirty, disease-ridden conditions. As William Rathbone had been inspired by the plight of the poor in Liverpool, so Abbie Crowell Howes was motivated to help the poor of Boston.

Howes was a member of a prominent Boston family and a supporter of the Women's Education Association (WEA), an offshoot of the New England Women's Club founded in 1868. The WEA promoted and funded women's involvement at every level of education, and in 1873 it helped found the Nurses' Training School at Massachusetts General Hospital. In 1884, with this dual interest in education and nursing in mind, Howes visited England to observe the work of the district nurses in Liverpool. This, of course, was before the formation of QVJI, but more than 20 years after the opening of the Liverpool Training School and 9 years after the founding of the MNA; district nursing under the Nightingale/Rathbone system was, therefore, well established in parts of England, if not the whole country, at this time. In 1885, Howes wrote to Emily Mansel, who had succeeded Craven as Superintendent of the MNA Central Home. In reply, Mansel sent a report of the MNA's work, some pamphlets, and a letter in which she suggested that

> the best way for starting District Nursing in Boston would be, if you could hear of some lady who has received a year's Hospital training and whom you could send *here* to this Home, for three months training in District work. She would then understand all the working of it and be able to start it in America. . . . I think you would find it would lead to the work being more successful in the long run.[6]

Howes also communicated with Dr. W. H. H. Hastings, superintendent of the Boston Dispensary, who approved of the plan to establish a system of district nursing in the city, and offered a small room in the Dispensary building as a temporary office.[7] As the district doctors, with whom the nurses were to work, visited only patients who were unable to afford private medical care, so the nursing would also be available only to the poor.

On January 19, 1886, representatives of the WEA met to form the new Instructive District Nursing Association committee and to appoint the first nurse. Amelia Hodgkiss had already worked with the poor patients of the Dispensary of the New England Hospital for Women & Children, where she had trained. She began work in Boston on the morning of Monday, February 8, 1886, and visited the sick in 2 of the 10 districts covered by the Boston Dispensary. In her first 10 days on duty, Hodgkiss made 31 visits, but by March she was obliged to take a rest for a fortnight, as it was "found she has been undertaking to do too much among the sick in two districts." She was dismissed on November 1, and her place was taken by Calina E. M. Somerville, a graduate of Boston City Hospital Training School. Another Boston graduate, Elizabeth Rinker, began work on June 15, 1886. During that first year, these pioneer district nurses among them made 7,182 visits to 707 patients.[8]

The following year, on May 1, 1887, Emma Gordon, another graduate of the Boston City Hospital, joined the IDNA staff and was sent to London to train with the MNA. That same year, the Board of Managers voted to separate from the WEA and become an independent charity. A total of four nurses were employed that year, with a fifth for six months, who among them made 17,056 visits to 1,836 patients. With this change of status and rapid increase in work, it became necessary in 1888 to rent a room at 2 Park Square as an office and appoint an agent who received applications for visits and kept the records of the association. In addition to five district nurses, a "nurse-at-large" was provided to work under doctors not employed by the Boston Dispensary, with the intention of extending the availability of the service. However, the calls on this nurse proved insufficient to justify the expense of her employment, and the experiment was given up the following year; temporary agency nurses from the city's Directory for Nurses or the Nurses' Club were hired for additional cases and emergency work as required. By the end of 1889, six district nurses were employed; 26,056 visits were made that year to 2,131 patients.[9] Thus, in the first four years of the IDNA's work, the numbers of nurses and patients both tripled and the number of visits increased 360%.

Boston was not the first or only American city to found a system of district nursing in the 1880s. The Women's Board of the New York City Mission had employed a hospital-trained missionary nurse as early as 1877, the same year the city's Charity Organization Society was formed. Based on the English society of the same name, formed in 1869, it coordinated the philanthropic activities of overlapping, individual charitable groups. The first Visiting Nurse Association (VNA) was founded in Buffalo, New York, in 1885.[10] The Visiting Nurse Society of Philadelphia followed in February 1886, and the VNA of Chicago in 1889. These associations developed and operated separately, though a loose network made possible the exchange of ideas: Helen Jenks, founder and president of the Philadelphia organization, visited Boston in March 1887 and "gave the committee some interesting details of the work carried on there."[11] Jenks herself had been inspired by a houseguest from England who had described the district nursing system in her hometown of Manchester. It is clear, then, that the philanthropic ladies of Boston and other American cities were inspired in their charitable work by their English counterparts. By the time QVJI was founded in England in 1889, the culmination of 30 years of experience, district or visiting nursing in Boston was still in only its earliest stage, yet fundamental differences as well as similarities already existed between the two systems.

Aims and Motivation

At the first meeting of the IDNA Board of Managers in 1886, it was recorded that "This Committee consider the name *Instructive* should be given to the District Nurse, as in her visits to the sick she should endeavor as far as possible to instruct members of the family visited to care for their sick."[12] This statement reflected Nightingale's dual aims of district nursing, whereby the nurse should "nurse the room as well as the patient" and teach the whole family by example.[13] To achieve these aims, Emily Mansel explained in her reply to the initial request for information from Abbie Howes, the MNA "consider it much more desirable to have *ladies* to nurse among the poor than people of a lower class."[14] She expanded on this point in an article in the *Nursing Record,* stressing that district nurses "should be of a refining and elevating character" if they were to "leave their patients in a more wholesome atmosphere, morally as well as physically, than they found them. The seeds of cleanliness and self-respect have been sown, and a wish for better things inculcated." While "sound health of body and mind" were considered "absolutely essential" for the nurse, her attitude toward her work and patients were equally important:

> She must have enthusiasm, energy and the spirit that will not shrink when difficulties arise. Many come to the work with grand and high-flown ideas. For a time they seem to enter into it, but when they find that the work is of an exceedingly

> practical character, the novelty wears away and interest fails. These do not make good District Nurses. What we want are good women, with earnestness and steadfastness of purpose. Women prepared to throw their whole heart into the work.[15]

These views were formally embodied in *A Guide to District Nurses and Home Nursing,* a manual Florence Craven was asked to write for the use of QVJI nurses in 1889, and which Nightingale proofread. Craven emphasized that a district nurse must be motivated by "a real love for the poor, and a real desire to lessen the misery she may see among them. . . . Her aim must be not only to aid in curing disease and alleviating pain, but also through the illness of one member of a family to gain an influence for good so as to raise the whole family." Craven saw district nursing as "too high and holy" a calling to warrant any aim other than the highest possible standards, and she expected QVJI nurses to share her views: "No nurse should take up district work unless she feels that 'to serve the poor' is her vocation."[16]

The objectives of the IDNA nurses echo those of their English counterparts: "by precept and example to give such instruction to the families which they are called upon to visit as shall enable them thenceforwards to take better care of themselves and their neighbours, by observing the rules of wholesome living and by practising the simplest arts of domestic nursing."[17] The nurses of Boston were also expected to be motivated by a sense of missionary zeal:

> A work like this demands for its perfect fulfillment women with a real vocation for visiting the poor. A nurse may have proved herself most excellent in the hospital, she may have been thoroughly successful in private nursing, and yet utterly fail in District Nursing simply because she has not that spirit of self-sacrifice which is not content with a merely perfunctory performance of her duties. A woman with a high sense of her vocation will go into the poor tenement and by her quick eye and ready tact will discern not only how the present emergency of illness can be met, but also how the whole status of the family can be permanently improved.[18]

Under the rules of both QVJI and the IDNA, nurses were forbidden to give monetary aid to their poor patients—needy cases were to be referred to other, relevant agencies. The nurses were not permitted to interfere with the religious opinions of the patients, nor could they accept presents of any kind from patients, families, or friends. In these ways, the English and Boston systems had the same aims and motivation. The most important differences between the two schemes were the lack of special training for the nurses in Boston and the absence of a nurse supervisor in a central home.

Training and Supervision

In England, Nightingale and Craven both emphasized the importance of specialist training for district nurses. In 1876, Nightingale wrote that "a district nurse . . . must be of a yet higher class and of a yet fuller training than a hospital nurse."[19] In Craven's manual, the opening sentence reiterated and stressed this belief: "For district nurses a higher education and higher grade of woman are required than for the hospital nurse or even hospital superintendent."[20] The standard qualifications for a Queen's nurse (QN) were a minimum of one year's training in a general hospital, followed by six months' training in district nursing under trained district superintendents. To work in a rural district, a QN also had to complete three months' training in midwifery. QVJI's syllabus, which Craven helped to adapt from the MNA training scheme, included sanitary reform, teaching health matters, ventilation, drainage, water supply, diets for the healthy and sick, feeding of infants, infectious diseases, and nursing of mothers and their infants after childbirth. These subjects, complemented by practical work, were tested by a three-hour written examination.

Once qualified, a QN would be sent for one year to a post arranged by QVJI, after which she was free to apply for a vacancy of her choice. In urban areas, the nurses lived together in a central home with a head nurse. This arrangement was considered essential for their health, morale, and reputation, as Nightingale strongly believed that "district nurses . . . deteriorate if they have no *esprit de corps,* no common home under wise and loving supervision."[21] Throughout her career, a QN's work was closely monitored by local superintendents and national inspectors, whose reports were held at QVJI's head office in London. Thus, any problems were identified and dealt with to ensure that standards were maintained.

In Boston, the IDNA emphasized that all its nurses must be graduates of a hospital training school, and preference was given to those who had trained in Boston. Testimonials were required and a personal interview was considered essential, but once appointed, each nurse was allowed a degree of "elasticity within limits." While "a certain prescribed routine" was necessary "to avoid confusion and waste of time," it was felt that "any set of hard-and-fast rules would be a hindrance to effective service in work where the demands differ so widely as they do in the Dispensary districts."[22] Two lady managers were in charge of each Boston district, and a five-member Executive Committee had the authority to make decisions between the Board of Managers' monthly meetings. Each nurse gave a detailed weekly report to her managers, who presented a summary to the Board, and each nurse also produced a detailed written report each month for the president, with whom all the staff met at the association office for a general monthly consultation and discussion. In 1890, President Phoebe Adam asked each nurse in turn to prepare a paper on some aspect of the work, to be read at these monthly meetings. In this way, it was hoped that "the varying experience of each nurse has been of assistance to all the others through suggestions and discussions."[23]

A course of lectures was given by local doctors during the winter of 1893 and each subsequent year, on subjects including "Duties of Nurses," "Surgery & Bacteriology," and "Diseases of the Throat & Nose."[24] This arrangement caused some concern, and one manager queried the possible "effect of these lectures on the nurses; whether it made them feel too much as if they were doctors." The president thought not, and "said that the lectures waked the nurses up."[25] Similar fears were expressed when a library was planned for the nurses; it was agreed that it should contain "everything possible on nursing," but no medical books, as "the constant danger with trained nurses is that they shall usurp the doctors' position and prescribe for the patients."[26]

With no specialist training for their nurses and no agreed standards, the IDNA managers determined association policy. As we have seen, volunteer lady managers and lay committees were an important part of QVJI's organizational structure, particularly in isolated rural areas, where the local "Lady Bountiful" remained an influential figure. Their organizational, administrative, and fund-raising skills were vital, and the national system of district nursing could not have been so successfully established in England without them.[27] However, Nightingale stressed that a district nurse "must always have the supervision of a trained superior."[28] Therefore, QVJI's local superintendents and national inspectors had to be experienced QNs, not philanthropic ladies who knew little or nothing of nursing.

This hierarchical arrangement was seen as essential to the efficient running of the scheme, and leading figures in the English system assumed it would be adopted in other countries. A nurse from Germany trained with the MNA before being appointed as the first superintendent in Berlin, and there was clearly some confusion when Emma Gordon was sent from Boston to London in 1887. Emily Mansel wrote to Abbie Howes, "We always thought and Miss Gordon herself seemed to think that the object of her coming here was to qualify her for the post of Superintendent on her return to America ... but somehow we seem to have got hold of a wrong idea." When Gordon returned to Boston, she was appointed nurse for the South End district of the city, but she resigned in May 1888 after she was put on probation for leaving her post without permission to nurse a sick friend.[29] The IDNA managers had the opportunity to establish a supervisory post with an English-trained nurse within two years of the association's foundation, but they chose to reject this vital element of the English system.

Relationship With Doctors

Whereas the IDNA nurses lacked a nurse supervisor, they did work more closely with the doctors than did the QNs. QVJI recommended that, when starting a DNA, the local committee should hold "one or more small meetings to discuss the matter with those interested, especially the medical men of the district," and doctors, particularly the County Medical Officer of Health, should be invited to become members of the CNA General Committee. Furthermore, QVJI rules specifically stated that, "The general sick nursing of the patients shall be carried out under the direction of the medical practitioners."[30] In their day-to-day duties, however, the doctors and district nurses worked separately. This was the very reason that Nightingale stressed the importance of specialist training for a district nurse: "because she has not the doctor always at hand; … and because she has to take notes of the case for the doctor who has no one but her to report to him."[31] Craven added, "the district nurse rarely sees the doctor, and in many cases not at all. His orders are given in writing."[32]

Under the QVJI rules, the initial application for the services of the nurse could be made directly to her or to the DNA Committee, but after that first visit, "she must not continue to visit without informing a medical man and receiving his instructions, if any." The nurse could only dispense drugs that had been prescribed by the doctor; "when the nurse has anything to communicate to the doctor she shall do so in writing, and it is hoped that the doctor will do the same to avoid leaving messages with patients or their friends."[33] In England, the officially recommended working relationship between doctors and district nurses was, therefore, one of cooperation and communication.

In Boston, the nurses worked in conjunction with the Dispensary doctors, though the IDNA rules made it clear that the nurses were employed by the association and worked under the control of their managers: "Nurses shall be under the authority of the Board of Managers of the Association. . . . The authority of the physicians over the nurses is limited to the carrying out of orders by the nurses in the care of the patients entrusted to them."[34] A nurse could not accept a direct request for a visit, from herself or a doctor; all such applications had to be referred to the offices of the IDNA or the Dispensary. Each day, the nurse and doctor would meet in their district, often at the local druggist's shop. The nurse would report on the previous day's work and receive her new orders. The doctor and nurse would then visit new and very sick patients together, after which the nurse would continue on her rounds alone, returning to the most seriously ill patients for a second visit in the afternoon. In the five years from 1889 to 1893, the nurses made an average of 28.2% of their visits with doctors.

However, while in theory the IDNA nurses worked more closely with the doctors than did their QVJI counterparts, they did not always work in harmony. The Annual Reports regularly included letters and comments from the Dispensary doctors, praising the nurses and their work: "The nurse is indispensable"; "She is of the greatest service"; "I could not do without her"; "The nurse knows every street and house in the District, and everybody knows her and relies upon her"; "The nurse does a great amount of work; has tact and good judgment. She is invaluable."[35] But other records, such as the minutes of board and committee meetings, reveal problems behind the scenes. The Dispensary doctors varied in their skills and attitudes; not all the nurses proved suitable for the work; some found the work too physically strenuous or emotionally demanding; there were clashes of personality, and problems caused by misunderstandings and lack of communication.

Kate Rogers, who began work in March 1888, disappeared eight months later with her nurse's bag; it was noted that "her work has not been satisfactory."[36] Elizabeth Rinker, one of the earliest recruits to the IDNA staff, resigned "in despair" in October 1889 when a physician, Dr. Sargent, newly appointed to the North End district, gave her "nothing to do." Five months later the replacement nurse was removed from the district, as Dr. Sargent made things so difficult that "she found it impossible to work satisfactorily" with him. The Board of Managers voted that the doctor "should be fully informed of all the charges against him and told that if a nurse were again employed there, it would be conditional upon his behavior."[37] When, in 1891, the doctor in the Central district asked the nurse to report for duty at 7:30 instead of 8:00 A.M. each morning and to undertake all his work on Sundays, the president sent him a copy of the association rules, duly marked.[38] Some doctors strongly opposed the rule that the doctor and nurse should make the first visit to each patient together; in 1892, a new doctor appointed to the South Cove district did not "care for the services of a nurse" at all, and she was transferred to another district.[39] The same year, the doctor in the South Boston district was reported as making "an impression of great incompetency and sometimes does not meet the nurse for several days, but leaves notes for her instead."[40] Conversely, in 1897, it was reported that one nurse had not been meeting the doctor of her district regularly. Although "Miss Welch did not think that she had been remiss," she was informed in writing by the president "that she had no right to work independently."[41]

Such varied reactions by the doctors to the district nurses were certainly not unique to Boston. In England, the introduction of a Queen's nurse into a district was often met with hostility by the local doctors. Many of these nurses, trained and educated under the Nightingale system, were from an equivalent social background to the doctors and were seen as potential rivals in a society and profession where men still expected to dominate. Doctors felt defensive of both their knowledge and their position. In 1896, one doctor wrote to the *British Medical Journal* condemning "that craze which is at present affecting a certain section of fashionable society for putting women in positions of authority . . . which practically place them on a level with . . . the medical staff. . . . It is a most unfortunate movement . . . [and] it is our duty to make a distinct stand against this sort of thing."[42] Another doctor dismissively referred to "the Jubilee midwifery nurses (I am not sure of the name they bear)," and condemned their work as "an outrage on the medical practitioner." When he was asked to cooperate in the work of his local DNA, he "declined emphatically" to the secretary, a lady of social standing in the area and the wife of an eminent barrister. As a result, he was boycotted both socially and professionally.[43] Thus, in both countries, the working relationship between the doctors and nurses was influenced by the social position and connections of the lady managers.

Relationship With Managers

Like their English counterparts, most IDNA managers were clearly well intentioned, but initially there were some complications caused by different managers working "on different lines."[44] They were expected "to give all the aid and interest the district may need, at times visiting the homes of the patients to judge more wisely of their condition," but one doctor complained that the managers of his district expected to accompany him on his rounds.[45] It was, therefore, "thought best to restrict any visiting by the Managers, by rules and regulations." These were to be printed and given to each manager, and included the pointed direction: "Do not give help without an intelligent understanding of the case." Each manager was also expected to make the nurse "feel your interest in her and her work."[46] Some managers suggested that this aspect of their role included a moral and pastoral duty to the nurses outside their working hours, while others maintained a more distant relationship: one doctor complained that, until he saw a copy of the Annual Report, he did not even know that his district had two managers for the nurse.[47]

The majority of these wealthy, philanthropic women were genuinely concerned for the nurses' health and welfare, as well as caring about their work among the poor. They recognized the nurses as professionals and believed that the authority this enabled them to exert over their patients, together with their "refinement and higher social standing," was essential in teaching to "the poor those rudimentary principles of the laws of physical well-being that are household precepts with the well-to-do."[48] However, the managers were, in turn, socially superior to the nurses, and without the advice and superintendence of a nurse supervisor and the unifying, communal atmosphere of a central home, they expected the nurses to defer to their judgment and accept their decisions without prior consultation.

This approach proved problematic. When the first president, Phoebe Adams, retired in 1898 due to failing health, a three-woman Committee on Nurses and Physicians, later renamed the Committee on Nurses, was appointed, responsible for appointing and discharging the nurses and receiving their monthly reports. Their first act was to inform the nurses that they would all be moved to different districts. The nurses and doctors were clearly not impressed: "With but one exception the nurses expressed themselves as believing the change fatal to their work," and several of the doctors either visited or wrote to the Committee Chairman "expressing their feelings as to the inadvisability of the change." So great was their concern that at the next full Board of Managers meeting the new president, Elizabeth Cordner, moved that the plan should be reconsidered. The "power of the Committee on Nurses" was discussed, and it was voted that, "owing to the many expressions of regret received from the Doctors and Nurses relative to the proposed changes, the Managers decide to . . . allow things to remain as they are at present." In a clear fit of pique, the chairman of the Committee on Nurses promptly resigned.[49] While, on this occasion, the nurses had joined forces with the doctors to express their concerns, the managers still made the final decision and controlled the future development of the work.

The Patients

Despite such problems, the work of the IDNA progressed steadily throughout the 1890s. By 1891, 7 of the 10 Dispensary districts were served by the nurses. The following year, a nurse was employed to follow up cases discharged from the Children's Hospital and to treat those designated as pediatric outpatients, though this work was given up in 1895 and transferred to the nurses of the hospital's own Training School. In 1893, Roxbury and Cambridge were added as additional districts, but it did not prove possible to provide them both with nurses immediately. By the end of 1895, all 10 of the original Dispensary districts and Cambridge were covered. A sudden increase of 800 patients and more than 5,000 visits in 1896 was caused by "a large number of very ill children, bronchitis and pneumonia being the prevailing diseases."[50] Even after the outbreak was over, a heavy workload remained, and at the end of 1898 one physician suggested that attendants should be employed "to do such work of a kind such as the fully trained district nurses have not the time to do."[51] After much discussion and with the approval of the Dispensary physicians, it was agreed that some "chronic cases, and other cases that the nurse was unable to attend" should be handed over to the Massachusetts Emergency & Hygiene Association.[52] All applications for an attendant were to be made by the doctor directly to the association's supervisor, Miss Strong, and the attendant would work entirely under the order and direction of the district physician.[53]

Even with this new arrangement, by 1899, the first year in which nurses were employed in all 12 districts, the total number of visits exceeded 50,000. In addition, the number of visits the nurses made with doctors had fallen to 17%. With the IDNA organizational structure, this increase in visits made by the nurses alone does not indicate a greater degree of autonomy, but it does suggest increased individual responsibility. In the words of one doctor, each nurse stood "as a fortunate medium between the doctor and those large numbers of the poor who regard the Dispensary as a *right:* believing that it and the physicians are generously supported by the City government so that all citizens may demand and get whatever they choose to exact from it."[54]

Another physician, Dr. George Craigen, was even more critical of the patients, condemning them as ignorant ("they know nothing of sanitary or hygienic laws"), indifferent ("life is often held at a low estimate"), and stupid ("so dense as to be almost incredible").[55] However, the nurses themselves expressed more sympathy for the poor. Calina Somerville reported: "There seem to be three classes to deal with in our work—a few who are too old to change their ways, a few who are indifferent through intemperate habits, and a large number who are grateful for the help and instructions given."[56]

Somerville's views corresponded with the findings of distinguished QN Margaret Loane, whose handbook superseded Craven's manual at the turn of the century. Loane identified seven categories among the English poor, from fatalists "convinced that to attempt to alter the course of a serious illness is not only useless but impious," via those "who have a physical disgust for all forms of illness, and who allow that disgust to overpower the feelings of common humanity," to the class "more numerous by far than all the others put together, . . . who are ignorant, but willing and able to learn."[57] The educative aspect of the nurses' work in England was further complicated by local traditions and regional traits, and Loane stressed the importance of effective communication with the patients' family and neighbors. Similarly, Amy Hughes, Superintendent General of QVJI from 1905 to 1917, earlier wrote in the first issue of the *Queen's Nurses' Magazine* (*QNM*): "The Queen's Nurse is face to face with the ignorances and prejudices of generations, whether she is working in town or country." In particular, Hughes warned of "the tyranny of custom exercised by the *grandmother* of the family," and she urged the nurse to "speak to the *mother* in simple language" and thus gradually "to produce an effect on the community at large."[58]

In Boston, these class differences were exacerbated by race and language: in one year alone, patients were recorded of more than 20 nationalities.[59] In Dr. Craigen's North End district, the patients were

> largely of foreign stock—Portuguese, Italians, Russian and Polish Jews, with a considerable number of Irish, and a scattering of almost every other nationality. Many can neither speak nor understand English. . . . They are strongly prejudiced by tradition, sometimes of family, sometimes of race; and their traditions frequently run directly counter to our efforts.[60]

In some cases, the attitude of the poor proved impossible to overcome. When one Dispensary physician, accompanied by the district nurse, arranged for a child with diphtheria to be admitted to the City Hospital, the entire family fled overnight, "and no trace of them could be found. Their ignorant dread of a hospital induced them to flee with their sick child rather than allow it to be taken where they felt sure it would die."[61] One case was abandoned when the nurse was assaulted by the patient's drunken husband, and another was given up because the patient was "most trying and difficult to get along with, and finds fault with every thing that is done for her."[62]

On a positive note, several nurses commented in their reports on the willingness of Italians to care, not only for their own people, but also for neighbors of other nationalities, while other nurses found that children and young girls were "our most apt and willing pupils. It may be that they learn faster and remember better than their elders because they have fewer prejudices to overcome."[63] Describing a typical working day during her time as an IDNA nurse, Somerville recalled that almost every day she had found family and neighbors caring for a patient by "carrying out many of the simple directions that have been given during some former sickness."[64]

The Need for Change

By the time the Conference of Nurses was held in June 1893 (as part of the International Congress of Charities, Corrections & Philanthropy at the Chicago World's Fair), Boston, Philadelphia, and Chicago operated the largest district or visiting nurse associations in America. Smaller societies existed in New York, Brooklyn, Buffalo, Baltimore, Kansas City, and Newport, Rhode Island. After the conference, the president of the IDNA received "letters from Western and Southern cities, and also from Canada, asking for advice and information as to the best methods of starting similar organizations,"[65] and a Lucy B. Fisher asked permission to visit with some of the IDNA nurses, as she was hoping to establish district nursing in California.[66] Direct contact was maintained with leading figures of the district nursing movement in England, thus emphasizing not only the established authority of the English system, but also its continuing influence on American nursing.[67] Abbie Howes, founder of the IDNA, died in London in April 1895 during a trip to study methods in English cities, "hoping to apply the results of her investigations here at home."[68] Clearly, the Boston IDNA was at the forefront of the development and expansion of district nursing in America throughout the 1890s, and in the spring of 1900 the Board of Managers made a significant decision that marked a major change in the organizational structure of the IDNA—to appoint a nurse superintendent.

As the number of nurses employed by the IDNA increased, the Board of Managers had also grown. By 1900, it consisted of 27 ladies and the president, too large a body to work efficiently and effectively, but made up of individuals confident of their own ability and reluctant to relinquish any of their authority. Therefore, when the Executive Committee first recommended that a nurse superintendent should be appointed, the Board objected that "it would be an unnecessary change as the managers ought to be able to look after their districts." The Executive Committee replied that, "The Managers are none of them expert nurses and without that it is impossible to see that the *very best* work is done." After much discussion, the Board would only agree that an Assistant Agent should be engaged to oversee the nurses during the summer months when many of the managers were away on vacation. President Elizabeth Cordner was empowered to offer the post to Miss Strong, supervisor of the Massachusetts Emergency & Hygiene Association, and it was only when Strong refused the position that Cordner was able to convince the Board that the post of Assistant Agent would not attract a nurse of suitable caliber. She gave "many strong reasons to show the necessity of having a Superintendent," and stressed that the work of the managers would be "in no way supplanted." It was only then that the managers accepted the Executive Committee's recommendation and approved Cordner's choice, Annie Ethel Beer, a "singlewoman of Boston."[69] It would appear that the nurses themselves were not consulted, and while it was recorded that they "had accepted the need of the Superintendent being placed over them quietly," it was also noted that two nurses had resigned in protest: Miss McBride, the longest-serving member of staff, who had joined the IDNA in May 1888, and Miss White, who had written to the president to complain that "the nurses' honor had been questioned."[70]

Beer began work on May 16, 1900, on a one-year contract, under the charge of the Committee on Nurses and the president. She was responsible for ensuring "that each nurse does her duty promptly and efficiently" and had the power to suspend a nurse and recommend her dismissal. She appointed temporary substitute and emergency nurses, or if necessary, undertook such work herself. Significantly, it was specified that "she shall give probationers six months or more training" and recommend those she considered suitable for permanent appointment to the staff.[71] This was the first reference in the IDNA records to provision of specific training in district nursing, but no syllabus was devised or standards agreed on. The inclusion of teaching probationers as a specific clause in Beer's contract marked an important stage in the development of the IDNA, but it did not compare with the systematic training and demanding examinations undertaken by QVJI nurses in England.

Beer's initial impression of the IDNA nurses and their work was not encouraging. She visited each nurse in her district, inspected their books and supply closets, and heard their verbal reports. She found "a lack of uniformity in the work, each nurse doing much as she pleased … [with] a lack of attention to the details of district nursing, and in some cases to the personal appearance of the nurse." Aprons were not always worn as part of the uniform, and some nurses were careless about disinfecting their hands and thermometers. Beer considered the cotton bags the nurses carried unsuitable and unhygienic, and suggested leather replacements. The nurses' books were not kept neatly, and the closets were dusty and untidy. In particular, she believed that the arrangement of the nurses visiting with the doctors resulted in a waste of "a great deal of unnecessary time." Overall, she found the nurses "taken as a class" were generally good nurses, but some were "Sallies too old to do justice to the work."[72]

In addition, Beer expressed concern regarding the arrangement of employing temporary agency nurses. She described to the president how, on one occasion, it took three days to find a substitute after one district nurse resigned. The agency nurse "remained only four days and then left to take a case, saying the work was too hard." Beer experienced great difficulty finding another substitute, and eventually "succeeded in getting a nurse only to spend a day showing her how to do the work and then have her tell me the walking was too much."[73] Unfortunately, Beer's views and recommendations were not well received by the managers, and it was pointedly noted that: "It was decided that the work of the Association shall go on as it has in the past until Miss Beer shall thoroughly understand its methods."[74]

Beer did succeed in introducing improved, more detailed record-keeping. She "did not think the nurses spent as much time with their patients as they might," and "thought there should be some method of telling how much time a nurse spent in her district and a record of such made each day."[75] She therefore suggested that each nurse should be issued a casebook, to be submitted to her managers weekly when giving her report. At the end of each month, Beer collected and inspected the books before they were forwarded to the Committee on Nurses.[76]

Beer approached her duties with enthusiasm and gradually began to win the respect and support of the nurses. Under the terms of her contract, she was available at the association's office from 2:30 to 3:00 P.M. each day "to advise the nurses";[77] after six months in her post she was able to report that "The half hour which I spend at the Office has not until the last few months been taken much advantage of but the spirit of opposition is fast becoming a thing of the past."[78] However, most of her recommendations were ignored by the managers, and their view of her position was made clear by an amendment to the Rules for Nurses, which read that, while "the nurses shall be subject to the authority of the superintendent, they shall also be subject to the superior authority of the Board of Managers."[79] Clearly, Beer was expected to conform to the wishes of the Board rather than the ladies cooperating with the new superintendent.

Beer resigned at the end of her contract in May 1901, and her place was taken by Martha H. Stark, who was already a staff member. Stark was a graduate of Massachusetts General Hospital and the Boston Lying-in Hospital. She had been head nurse at MGH for a year and a half, and joined the IDNA in 1898 as nurse for the East Boston district. She was described by Beer as "an excellent district nurse, ... very neat and also particular about details."[80] In addition, as an experienced staff member, Stark was already familiar with the routine and methods of the IDNA, and during 10 and a half years in her post she neither changed the former nor challenged the latter.

Progress and Problems

The most significant development during the first decade of the 20th century was the opening of a Training School of District Nursing in October 1906.

It was accommodated in the house at 561 Massachusetts Avenue where the association's office had moved the previous year. Initially, the house was rented, but it was bought in 1911. It was large enough to accommodate 14 nurses—5 staff nurses, 8 pupils, and a House Superintendent—with domestic staff consisting of a cook, a maid, and a chore boy, with a laundress giving three days' service a week. Charlotte Macleod was appointed House Superintendent, responsible for the pupils, while Stark continued as District Superintendent, overseeing the work of the trained nurses. Macleod was a graduate of Waltham Hospital, Massachusetts, with 13 years of nursing experience in the United States and Canada. Importantly, she had also trained at a QVJI school in England.

The IDNA training course, the first of its kind in the United States, lasted four months and offered "thorough instruction in district nursing." The objective was not only to increase the number of nurses available to the poor, but in particular to provide for "the lodging house population, and others who can and are really able to pay small fees." In the first four months after the school opened, the pupils paid 2,525 visits to 212 patients throughout the city, making many of the calls of the "work at large," which formerly had to be given to agency nurses.[81]

In 1906 the Executive Committee also voted "that the nurses shall discontinue the custom of meeting the physicians and making the visits with them and that it shall be left to the Superintendent to make the proper arrangements in regard to communicating with the physicians."[82] This, of course, had been one of Beer's recommendations six years earlier, but it was only with the continuing expansion of the work that it was finally adopted by the Executive Committee. However, the decision was made without consulting the Boston Dispensary or the nurses. On being informed of the change, Dr. Williams, secretary of the Dispensary, wrote to the IDNA president "to protest most earnestly . . . that your Board should have passed a decisive vote upon a matter of such importance . . . without conferring with us." In a four-page letter, he set out 16 objections to the change and requested a joint conference of the Boards.[83] This was held in September, but the Dispensary's concerns were overruled and the new system was put into effect in October.

From that date, Stark arrived at the District House at 8:30 A.M. each day, heard the reports of the five nurses in residence, communicated by telephone with each of the other nurses, and arranged their day's work. This method was intended to save time, but it was clearly not met with universal approval—within a year, seven nurses, who had worked for the association for one to six years, had resigned, along with the vice-president, the treasurer, and two of the managers.

It is possible that Stark's personality and approach to her duties may have added to feelings of discontent. Her monthly reports to the president certainly convey her energy, but they also suggest a lack of sympathy toward the nurses and the pressure under which they worked, despite her own experience in a Boston district. She described one nurse as oversensitive—"sometimes, when simply talking with her, her eyes fill with tears quickly"; another (whom Beer had described as "a splendid nurse"[84]) was said by Stark to have "the air of a martyr." During the winter of 1902, she unequivocally informed the president that "I hold the nurses responsible if they do not notify me any week when they find their districts too heavy, it being quite impossible for me to visit every district each week."[85]

By 1910, the work of the IDNA had expanded to cover ante- and postnatal cases; tuberculosis care; inspecting children attending kindergartens and day nurseries; visiting settlement houses; running three milk stations; inspecting factory employees in their workplace; nursing policyholders of the Metropolitan Life Insurance Co; and attending cases of contagious diseases, particularly scarlet fever and diphtheria, throughout the city. In England, a comprehensive national program of government-funded Public Health Work was introduced in 1908, which included health visiting, maternity and infant welfare clinics, inspection of schoolchildren, and tuberculosis care. As QVJI was recognized as one of the country's main agencies of care and health education, these duties were added to the district nurses' work. This clearly caused some resentment as a contributor to *QNM* noted that "each development on the social side has met with a certain amount of opposition at its first introduction, but each succeeding year has shown how indispensable the new departure has proved to the health of the community." She acknowledged that a district nurse "will not get the same kudos" for preventative work as she would "for one patient snatched from the Gates of Death," but she urged each nurse to realize "that the 'health' work she may be called upon to do ... [is] as important as that which is generally regarded as 'more interesting'."[86]

Thus, in England, health work was seen as an integral part of a district nurse's work, an expansion of Florence Nightingale's original dual aims of curative care and preventative education, that added variety and interest to a post while enabling the nurse to offer comprehensive care to the community in which she worked. However, in Boston, for each new development of the work, an *additional* nurse was employed in a specialist role, and by 1910 the IDNA staff had grown to 33 nurses. The potential then existed for neighbors in the same tenement house, or even members of the same family, to be visited by several different district nurses at home, work, and school. This arrangement was already causing concern in 1906, when, in an address at the Annual

Meeting, one doctor stressed that he believed home nursing "to be the chief mission of your society. *'Caring for the sick poor at their homes'* is the phrase used in your act of incorporation. Other lines of work may appear attractive, but I beg you cling to your first mission."[87]

In addition, Stark's ability to supervise such an extensive and diverse staff was questioned in 1908, when IDNA president Cordner sought the advice of Dr. Hugh Cabot, a Boston physician. In a detailed five-page reply, Cabot stressed that "careful, constant supervision is essential to the best work," and that he could find "no evidence to show that anything of the kind has been done during the past few years." He considered the role of the managers to be ineffective, as meeting the nurses to discuss cases known only by name did not constitute the searching, semimedical inquiry essential to good work, while he found Stark more interested in "other parts of the work which she finds more congenial."[88]

By 1910, relations with the Boston Dispensary had so deteriorated that the doctors were planning to employ their own nurses, independent of the IDNA. The Executive Committee requested a meeting to discuss whether the plan "would be for the general good of the city," but nothing further was heard and no action was taken by the doctors.[89] However, concern remained, and in 1911 Michael Davis, director of the Boston Dispensary, voiced his opinion in a letter to Katherine Codman, wife of a prominent Boston surgeon and Cordner's successor as president of the IDNA from 1908 to 1922. Davis believed that specialization resulted in "the highest efficiency only when specialized workers are under a strong, broad and intelligent supervision" and the specialists have "a good background of training behind their particular skill. Otherwise, the result is a number of sets of specialists working more or less independently or else without the proper correlation." This led to "not only waste of effort but failure to effect the desired results." District nursing in Boston, he concluded, needed a "more authoritative centralized organization ... [and] less specialization in the field."[90] Eventually, the managers admitted in a pamphlet that the system involved "much duplication, waste of time and money, and the public, which we are all trying to help, is in reality the sufferer."[91] Clearly, the time had come to rationalize and reorganize the work of the IDNA, and the decision was made to create a new position of Director, "one head for the whole association who should have the final responsibility for both Training School and staff, with Superintendents under her."[92]

It would appear that Stark applied for the post, but dissatisfaction with her abilities and her approach to the work had grown to such a degree that the Board of Managers voted not to nominate her for the new position. It was also noted that her formerly annual contract had been changed: "the appointment is from month to month." By October 1911 it was known that "Miss Stark is on the watch for a new position," and she resigned at the end of the year. She was presented with a silver salver and $200, and was diplomatically assured that she "carries with her the interest and good wishes of the Managers for her future."[93]

In the meantime, the Board made inquiries to find a suitable nurse for the new post. Four of the leading figures of American nursing at that time (Ida Cannon, Edna Foley, Ella Crandall, and Ellen LaMotte) all declined the offer before an approach was made to Mary Beard, who had graduated from the New York Hospital in 1903 and had five years' experience as Head Nurse of the Waterbury, Connecticut, VNA. Beard visited Boston in November 1911, to look into the work and to meet the Executive Committee, who found her "charming." She then visited Chicago, Cleveland, and New York to study the nursing associations there before taking up residence in the IDNA house on February 12, 1912.[94]

Neighborhood Nursing

Beard approached the problems of the IDNA with "a sympathetic understanding of the traditions of the past and a clear vision of the possibilities for the future."[95] Within two years, she had transformed the organizational structure and consolidated the work of the nurses by developing the idea of neighborhood nursing, whereby specialization was abandoned and each nurse performed general duties. To this end, branch stations were established in seven localities throughout the city. A head nurse was appointed for each station, responsible for supervising and advising a team of nurses, dealing with administration, and liaising with the doctors and other agencies. The managers were also grouped into small committees, one for each branch station, which reduced their personal influence on the nurses while maintaining their interest in the work.

Beard also emphasized the need for keeping "scientific and accurate records" and introduced an elaborate system of card indices. The details of each family were recorded on a social history card, and each patient had a medical history card. These were cross-referenced with indices for diagnosis, nationality, and address, designed to illustrate social conditions and highlight areas where particular health problems existed.[96]

The nurses continued to attend "many patients who can pay nothing, and we shall always do so and wish to do so," but Beard believed that the impression this created of so-called charity nurses for the poor greatly limited the scope and usefulness of the work. A new uniform was introduced to advertise the change to neighborhood nursing, and a scale of prices was "advertised and canvassed conscientiously" to publicize the availability of the nurses' services to the whole community.[97] As a result, the number of patients rose from 9,948 in 1911, the year before the reorganization, to 13,112 in 1914, an increase of 32%, while the number of visits rose from 111,820 to 123,065, an increase of 10%. Of these, 24.5% were fee-paying patients, and a further 20% were policyholders with Metropolitan Life Insurance.[98]

Beard acknowledged that it was not "easy for all the staff nurses to adjust themselves to these many changes," which involved "much shifting and changing of districts." Some nurses who had worked for years in a particular district found themselves moved to another part of the city, while others "who have been doing a special work have had to give it up." However, she was convinced that the future of district nursing in the United States lay in generalization as opposed to specialization: "One health nurse, and only one, in each family: this is the ideal."[99]

To further her aim of creating a staff of neighborhood health nurses, Beard also dispensed with temporary agency nurses and gradually replaced them with permanent nurses who had completed the IDNA training, now called the Post-Graduate Course. The original four-month course was still offered, but an advanced course lasting eight months was also introduced. Both courses, for which the students paid, covered the History, Principles, and Administration of Public Health Nursing. Lectures in Medical-Social Relations of Disease were also given in affiliation with the School for Social Workers at Simmons College. Theory was combined with practical training in one district, now called the Model District, and included working with other agencies to observe their methods. In this way, the graduate students learned "by doing, but in consultation with and under the constant supervision of experienced, expert workers." The rigors of such a course, Beard believed, would attract "women who want to do this sort of nursing more than any other work, are full of enthusiasm, and have made sacrifices to obtain a special education for it." By the end of 1913, the IDNA staff consisted of 49 salaried nurses, and 20 postgraduate students.[100]

In addition to upgrading the IDNA's own staff, the Post-Graduate Course also aimed to supply educated women suitable for supervisory positions and "to send them out over the country,"[101] thus creating nationally recognized standards and techniques in district nursing. By 1914, the graduates attending the IDNA training school included nurses from California, Colorado, Maryland, Montana, Ohio, North Dakota, Washington, and Wisconsin, who all intended "to return to the place whence they came, to carry back the knowledge gained here."[102]

By abandoning specialization and consolidating the work of the nurses, Beard's reorganization of the Boston scheme produced a more efficient, professional association, providing nursing care of a consistently high standard, supervised by head nurses, supported by lay managers, and financed partly by fees that subsidized patients who were too poor to pay. In emphasizing the importance of training, standards, and professional supervision, Beard's approach was more in keeping with the English system on which the IDNA of Boston was originally based, but, equally, it became more specific to the city's needs at that time. However, within a decade, demographic changes and medical advances would undermine her vision of establishing public health nursing as a distinct community welfare movement of social importance in the United States.

Reflection or Shadow?

In 1901, there were 53 associations in the United States employing 130 district nurses.[103] By 1913, there were more than 1,000 American VNAs employing an estimated 3,000 nurses.[104] In the 30 years since Abbie Howes had first traveled to Liverpool to observe the work of English district nurses, the visiting nurse movement had spread throughout the United States, and the IDNA of Boston was justifiably proud of the leading role it had played in this expansion. However, Howes and the original IDNA committee of philanthropic women did not set out to establish a national system—their aim was to provide home nursing suitable for the poor of Boston. They therefore adopted and adapted only the elements of the English system that they believed met their city's needs. In particular, they did not make use of Emma Gordon's training in England, in the belief that the lady managers were capable of running the association without a nurse supervisor and without consulting either the nurses themselves or the doctors with whom they worked. Even when a superintendent was eventually appointed, the lay committee continued to dominate both policy and administration.

Contact was maintained and ideas exchanged with other visiting nurse associations throughout the country, but there were marked regional variations in aims, methods, and sponsorship, with responsibilities for public health initiatives overlapping with those of government-funded agencies.[105] Although it was based on the English system, without a central governing body to set and maintain national standards, visiting nursing in the United States grew into a collection of independent, isolated schemes similar to the disorderly situation QVJI had been designed to replace in England in 1889. Experienced and respected leaders of the nursing profession, such as Nightingale and Craven, were closely involved with the planning, establishment, and ongoing development of the district nursing movement in England, and affiliation with QVJI offered each District Nursing Association the advantage of operational independence combined with the benefit of guidance and support through shared aims and principles, rules and regulations, standards and training, overseen by local superintendents and national inspectors.

In the United States there were no generally accepted standards, and the kind and degree of training depended on the skill and experience of an association's superintendent, with the majority of nurses learning on the job.[106] The fact that the Boston IDNA opened America's first training school for district nurses in 1906, with an English-trained house superintendent, not only highlights the prominent position the city's organization held, but also illustrates the growing awareness of the need for specialist training *before* a visiting nurse took up her post, a primary and fundamental element of district nursing in England.[107] The expansion to include public health work, which in England was added to district nurses' duties but in Boston resulted in diverse specialist roles, led to further calls for more scientifically based knowledge and statistical competence.[108] Furthermore, as this concern became more widespread, the need for the *nurses* themselves to agree and fix standards was recognized.[109]

Beard's reorganization of the IDNA and expansion of the training school reflected this recognized need for "more supervision, … more education, more co-operation" if America's specialist visiting nurses were to evolve into general public health nurses.[110] The rewards of working as a visiting nurse had long been recognized and recommended,[111] but Beard believed that the public health nurse benefited from the "variety in her work," while the individual patient gained from "the influence of one guide and philosopher" rather than "a scattered influence," and the community would see "the lessening of duplication … [and] an increase of efficiency of working and reporting."[112]

The reorganization of the IDNA coincided with the creation of the NOPHN in 1912, in which Beard played a prominent role both locally and nationally. This represented a concerted effort by leading nurses to establish a link between visiting nursing and public health, and to influence the development of their role. However, the wealthy philanthropists who had painstakingly founded and generously funded the visiting nurse associations in the United States resented being relegated to, as one expressed it, "a role where one's money is thought more useful and desirable than one's self." She warned of the danger that nurses and managers would grow apart, with the latter confined to committee work and fund-raising, and emphasized the need for professionals and laity to work together.[113] The NOPHN did offer the country's diverse, uncoordinated associations the opportunity to discuss standards, analyze past achievements, and determine future needs, but it lacked both QVJI's authority to translate those needs into action and its organizational hierarchy that combined administrators and nurses in clearly defined, complementary roles.

By 1925, district nursing in England, which combined locally funded home nursing with government-funded health work, was available to 75% of the population, and QVJI's organizational structure remained unchanged from its foundation in 1889 until it was absorbed into the National Health Service in 1948. Florence Nightingale's original dual aims of curative care and preventative education remained the motivating force behind QVJI's work, but, with the changing times, the approved method of achieving those aims gradually progressed from patronizing officiousness to friendly advice and support. In her 1889 *Guide,* Craven declared that "the very essence of district nursing is, that a nurse … will *do what is best for the patients,* even against their will."[114] By 1905, Loane was stressing that "The most successful district nurse is the woman … who knows what *ought* to be done, but can cheerfully reconcile herself to what is practicable in any given case," while always remembering that "she works by influence, not authority, and that real and lasting influence can only be in proportion to the respect and liking that her patients have for her."[115]

The translation of theory into practice was always affected by the realities and practicalities of working with the poor in their own homes, but it was in approach, not in ideals and essentials, that QVJI's work developed. In the United States, with a health care system consisting of disparate local and state boards of health, charities, public agencies, and private insurance companies, the role of public health nurses was becoming increasingly marginalized by the 1920s. This was mainly due to the fact that no consensus had been reached concerning the desired balance between curative care and preventative education in the nurses' duties, while the introduction of immigration quotas, and growth and improvement in hospital care, reduced the numbers of patients needing home nursing and health education.[116]

It is not the intention of this article to suggest that every aspect of the English system of district nursing was better than the Boston scheme, or that QVJI's organizational structure and methods would have met all the needs of a country as vast as the United States, where many states were larger than the entire United Kingdom and their systems of health care varied. Rather, I have tried to establish the fundamental differences between the two systems and to assess the effect of these differences on the progress and outcome of the work in Boston. Some of the distinctions made between the IDNA and the English model may appear unimportant, particularly when compared with major differences such as training and supervision of the nurses and specialization versus generalization. However, these details influenced the efficiency of the nurses' day-to-day work, and their long-term, cumulative effect eventually determined the need for radical reform. The IDNA of Boston, one of the earliest district or visiting nurse associations in the United States and the first to open a training school, was at the forefront of the development of the movement throughout the country. By adopting and adapting the English system, much was achieved both locally and nationally, but the organization of district nursing in America was less effective and, unlike QVJI, it failed to develop into a cohesive and influential agency, central to the country's health care system. Thus, it is clear that, while district nursing in America began as a reflection of England's light, it never managed to fully emerge from the mother country's shadow.

Carrie Howse, BEd (Hons), MA, PhD
External Member, University of Gloucestershire
30 Rothleigh
Up Hatherley
Cheltenham Glos GL51 3PS
United Kingdom
01242–224774
carrievcm@fsmail.net

Acknowledgments

This article was funded by the AAHN Postdoctoral Award, 2005. My thanks to Diane Gallagher and Alex Rankin of the History of Nursing Archives, at the Howard Gotlieb Archival Research Center, Boston University, for their help, advice, and kindness during my research trips; and to Dr. Paul Berman and Dr. Jessica Munns for their help in locating journal articles.

Notes

1. Instructive District Nursing Association (IDNA), 8th Annual Report, 33, Instructive District Nursing Association of Boston Collection, Howard Gotlieb Archival Research Center, Boston University (hereafter IDNA Collection), Box 13, Folder 4.

2. See Susan M. Reverby, *Ordered to Care: The Dilemma of American Nursing, 1850–1945* (New York: Cambridge University Press, 1987), 41–43, 109–10; Karen Buhler-Wilkerson, *No Place Like Home: A History of Nursing and Home Care in the United States* (Baltimore: John Hopkins University Press, 2001), 18–22.

3. Zachary Cope, "The Early History of District Nursing," *Nursing Times,* August 12, 1955, 885.

4. Rules for District Nursing Associations in Affiliation with the Queen's Institute, Gloucestershire Record Office (hereafter GRO), D4057/3.

5. See Carrie Howse, "'The Ultimate Destination of All Nursing': The Development of District Nursing in England, 1880–1925," *Nursing History Review* 15 (2007): 65–94; Carrie Howse, "The Development of Rural District Nursing in Gloucestershire, 1880–1925" (PhD diss., University of Gloucestershire, 2004).

6. Emily M. Mansel to Abbie Howes, December 12, 1885, IDNA Collection, Box 1, Folder 1.

7. W. H. H. Hastings to Abbie Howes, November 23, 1885, IDNA Collection, Box 1, Folder 1. The Boston Dispensary was established in 1796. The city was divided into 10 outpatient districts, each covered by a physician who provided free medical and surgical treatment to the poor.

8. Secretary's Notebook, January 19, 1886–January 25, 1887, IDNA Collection, Box 2, Folder 1.

9. 2nd, 3rd, and 4th Annual Reports, IDNA Collection, Box 13, Folder 4.

10. Audrey B. Davis, "With Love and Money: Visiting Nursing in Buffalo, New York, 1885–1915," *New York History* 71, no. 1 (January 1990): 45–67. My thanks to Evelyn Benson for this reference.

11. Minutes of Board of Managers Meeting (hereafter MBMM), March 8, 1887, IDNA Collection, Box 8, Envelope 1.

12. Secretary's Notebook, January 19, 1886–January 25, 1887, IDNA Collection, Box 2, Folder 1.

13. Florence Nightingale, letter to the *Times,* April 14, 1876, 6, British Library Document Supply Centre.

14. Mansel to Howes, December 12, 1885.

15. Emily Mansel, "District Nurses and Their Work," *Nursing Record,* 20 (December 1888): 540–41.

16. Florence Craven, *A Guide to District Nurses and Home Nursing* (1889; repr., London: Macmillan, 1894), 1–2, 5, 8. Craven was born Florence Sarah Lees in 1841 and grew up in comfortable circumstances in St. Leonards, Sussex. In 1866, she trained at the Nightingale School at St. Thomas's Hospital, then traveled throughout Europe, visiting hospitals and nursing in Germany, France, Holland, Belgium, Denmark, Austria, and Italy. During the Franco-Prussian War (1870–71), at the request of Crown Princess Frederick (eldest daughter of Queen Victoria), and on the recommendation of Nightingale, Lees organized the nursing in a military hospital in Prussia. In recognition of her war service, Lees became the first woman ever to receive the Prussian Order of the Iron Cross. In 1873, she visited hospitals in the United States and Canada, and on her return to England, she agreed to undertake the 1874 nursing survey that led to the formation of the MNA.

17. 5th Annual Report, 5, IDNA Collection, Box 13, Folder 4.

18. 9th Annual Report, 10, IDNA Collection, Box 13, Folder 5.

19. Nightingale to the *Times,* April 14, 1876, 6.

20. Craven, *Guide to District Nurses,* 1.

21. Florence Nightingale, "Sick-Nursing and Health-Nursing," in *Woman's Mission: A Series of Congress Papers on the Philanthropic Work of Women by Eminent Writers,* ed. Baroness Angela Burdett-Coutts (London: Sampson Low, Marston, 1893), 194.

22. 6th Annual Report, 8, IDNA Collection, Box 13, Folder 4.

23. 5th Annual Report, 7.

24. 9th Annual Report, 16.

25. MBMM, November 26, 1896, IDNA Collection, Box 8, Folder 1.

26. MBMM, January 25, 1893, IDNA Collection, Box 8, Envelope 1.

27. See Carrie Howse, "From Lady Bountiful to Lady Administrator: Women and the Administration of Rural District Nursing in England, 1880–1925," *Women's History Review* 15, no. 3 (July 2006): 423–41.

28. Nightingale, "Sick-Nursing and Health-Nursing," 200.

29. Emily Mansel to Abbie Howes, August 11, 1887, Box 1, Folder 1; MBMM, May 3, 1888, IDNA Collection, Box 8, Envelope 1.

30. GRO D4057/3.

31. Nightingale to the *Times,* April 14, 1876.

32. Craven, *Guide to District Nurses,* 4.

33. GRO D4057/3.

34. Secretary's Notebook, January 19, 1886–January 25, 1887, IDNA Collection, Box 2, Folder 1; 3rd Annual Report, 18, Box 13, Folder 4.

35. 13th Annual Report, 27, IDNA Collection, Box 13, Folder 6.

36. MBMM, November 27, 1888, IDNA Collection, Box 8, Envelope 1.

37. MBMM, June 25, 1889, October 30, 1889, January 29, 1890, March 26, 1890, October 8, 1890, Box 8, Envelope 1.

38. MBMM, February 20, 1891, Box 8, Envelope 1.

39. MBMM, December 30, 1891, March 30, 1892, Box 8, Envelope 1.

40. MBMM, October 26, 1892, Box 8, Envelope 1.

41. MBMM, April 28, 1897, Box 8, Envelope 2.

42. Dr. W. M. Banks, letter to *British Medical Journal* 2 (1896): 43.

43. Dr. Alex McCook Weir, letter to *British Medical Journal* 2 (1896): 1523.

44. MBMM, March 8, 1887.

45. 3rd Annual Report, 6, IDNA Collection, Box 13, Folder 4; MBMM, March 22, 1899, Box 8, Envelope 2.

46. MBMM, March 8, 1887.

47. MBMM, March 26, 1898, March 22, 1899, IDNA Collection, Box 8, Envelope 2.

48. 7th Annual Report, 10–11, IDNA Collection, Box 13, Folder 4.

49. MBMM, December 29, 1897, January 12, 1898, April 21, 1898, IDNA Collection, Box 8, Envelope 2.

50. 11th Annual Report, 12, IDNA Collection, Box 13, Folder 5.

51. Minutes of Committee on Nurses Meeting, November 4, 1898, IDNA Collection, Box 8, Envelope 3.

52. MBMM, November 30, 1898, IDNA Collection, Box 8, Envelope 2.

53. Minutes of Committee on Nurses Meeting, December 30, 1898, IDNA Collection, Box 8, Envelope 3.

54. 6th Annual Report, 26.

55. 7th Annual Report, 26–67.

56. 8th Annual Report, 38.

57. Margaret Loane, *Outlines of Routine in District Nursing* (London: Scientific Press, 1905), 146, 148, 150. The date of Loane's birth is unknown, but her father was a captain in the Royal Navy and she spent her early life in Portsmouth. She trained as a nurse at the Charing Cross Hospital in London and worked as a Sister both there and at the Salop Infirmary before training as a district nurse. She then worked both in rural and urban areas of England before returning to Portsmouth as Superintendent of District Nurses.

58. Amy Hughes, "Some Responsibilities of Queen's Nurses," *Queen's Nurses' Magazine* (hereafter *QNM*) 1, Part 1 (May 1904): 11–13.

59. 24th Annual Report, 14–15, IDNA Collection, Box 13, Folder 8.

60. 7th Annual Report, 26.

61. 11th Annual Report, 11.

62. MBMM, June 25, 1889, Box 8, Envelope 1; November 26, 1896, Box 8, Folder 1.

63. 4th Annual Report, 10–11; 6th Annual Report, 13–14.

64. 8th Annual Report, 38.

65. 8th Annual Report, 13.

66. MBMM, May 23, 1898, IDNA Collection, Box 8, Envelope 2.

67. For example, see William Rathbone to Board of Managers, May 8, 1894, IDNA Collection, Box 1, Folder 1.

68. 10th Annual Report, 1985, 16, IDNA Collection, Box 13, Folder 5. See also Abbie C. Howes, "Account of a morning spent with a District Nurse in London," IDNA Collection, Box 2, Folder 7.

69. MBMM, March 28, 1900, April 25, 1900, IDNA Collection, Box 8, Envelope 2.

70. MBMM, May 29, 1900, IDNA Collection, Box 8, Envelope 2.

71. "Articles of Agreement between IDNA and Annie Ethel Beer, singlewoman of Boston," May 12, 1900, IDNA Collection, Box 2, Folder 3.

72. Miss Beer's Report, November 20, 1900, IDNA Collection, Box 2, Folder 3.

73. Superintendent's Monthly Report, April 17, 1901, IDNA Collection, Box 9, Folder 40.

74. Minutes of Committee on Nurses Meeting, May 24, 1900, IDNA Collection, Box 8, Envelope 3.

75. Miss Beer's Report.

76. MBMM, January 30, 1901, IDNA Collection, Box 8, Envelope 4.

77. Articles of Agreement.

78. Miss Beer's Report.

79. MBMM, March 5, 1901, IDNA Collection, Box 8, Envelope 4.

80. Miss Beer's Report.

81. 21st Annual Report, 14, 18, IDNA Collection, Box 13, Folder 7.

82. Minutes of Executive Committee Meeting, May 8, 1906, IDNA Collection, Box 8, Folder 6.

83. Moses Williams to Elizabeth Cordner, June 20, 1906, IDNA Collection, Box 1, Folder 1.

84. Miss Beer's Report.

85. Superintendent's Monthly Report, November 1902.

86. Q.N., "Some Reminiscences—And a Moral," *QNM* 10, Part 4 (October 1913): 97–98.

87. 21st Annual Report, 50, IDNA Collection, Box 13, Folder 7.

88. Hugh Cabot to Elizabeth Cordner, February 25, 1908, IDNA Collection, Box 1, Folder 2. These "other parts of the work" included talks to promote the work of the IDNA throughout the city and visits to gain knowledge of similar schemes elsewhere. In 1903 Stark visited the Henry Street Settlement in New York; in 1907 she observed the work of district nurses in Philadelphia; and in 1909 she attended the Jubilee Congress of District Nursing in Liverpool, England, where she gave a 15-minute talk on the work of the IDNA. While in Liverpool, she visited the District Nurses' Home and accompanied a nurse on her rounds. She then toured the country, observing district nursing in Chester, Leamington, Stratford, and Oxford, before arriving in London at the invitation of Amy Hughes, Superintendent General of QVJI, whom she had met at the Congress. In the capital, she visited hospitals and districts in Shoreditch and Whitechapel, among the poorest areas not only in London, but in England. See Martha Stark, Report of Jubilee Congress of District Nursing, Liverpool, May 12–14, 1909, IDNA Collection, Box 11, Folder 8.

89. Minutes of Executive Committee Meetings, January 7, 1910, February 4, 1910, IDNA Collection, Box 8, Folder 6.

90. Michael Davis to Mrs. E. A. Codman, April 27, 1911, IDNA Collection, Box 1, Folder 3.

91. 27th Annual Report, 22, IDNA Collection, Box 13, Folder 10.

92. MBMM, January 11, 1911, IDNA Collection, Box 8, Folder 2.

93. MBMM, February 8, 1911, March 1, 1911, October 18, 1911, December 13, 1911, IDNA Collection, Box 8, Folder 2. See also "Reasons for Miss Stark not being asked to accept position of Head of Whole Work," IDNA Collection, Box 1, Folder 3. This undated document, filed with correspondence from 1911, consists of a page of rough notes, each in a different handwriting, which suggests that the paper was passed around at a Board of Managers meeting with each member asked to add her opinion. The unequivocal comments include, "No true administrative power"; "Suspicious nature"; "Tremendously quick temper"; "Does not get along with other workers well"; and "Tampers with the truth."

94. MBMM, March 1, 1911, October 18, 1911, December 13, 1911, Box 8, Folder 2; 26th Annual Report, 9, IDNA Collection, Box 13, Folder 9. See also Ida Cannon to Mrs. E. A. Codman, February 15, 1911; Edna Foley to Mrs. E. A. Codman, June 28, 1911; Ella Crandall to Mrs. E. A. Codman, August 25, 1911; Ellen LaMotte to Mrs. E. A. Codman, September 26, 1911 and October 3, 1911; Ella Crandall to Mrs. E. A. Codman, November 9, 1911, November 21, 1911, IDNA Collection, Box 1, Folder 3.

95. 27th Annual Report, 16, IDNA Collection, Box 13, Folder 9.

96. 27th Annual Report, 16, 26–27.

97. 27th Annual Report, 16, 28, 25–26.

98. 26th Annual Report, 10; 29th Annual Report, 19, IDNA Collection, Box 13, Folder 10.

99. 27th Annual Report, 29; 29th Annual Report, 18.

100. 27th Annual Report, 42–43; 28th Annual Report, 21–22, IDNA Collection, Box 13, Folder 10.

101. 26th Annual Report, 13.

102. 29th Annual Report, 26.

103. Harriet Fulmer, "History of Visiting Nurse Work in America," *American Journal of Nursing* (hereafter *AJN*) 11 (March 1902): 415.

104. 28th Annual Report, June 24, 1918, 20–21; Report of Atlantic City Convention for Public Health Nursing, June 1913, IDNA Collection, Box 2, Folder 6.

105. Fulmer, "History," 424; Mary Sewall Gardner, "Twenty-Five Years Ago," *Public Health Nurse Quarterly* (hereafter *PHN*) 29 (March 1937): 142.

106. Gardner, "Twenty-Five Years Ago," 142; Isabel W. Lowman, "The Need of a Standard for Visiting Nursing," *Visiting Nurse Quarterly* 4 (January 1912): 9.

107. Fulmer, "History," 412–13.

108. Mary E. Lent, "Report of the Committee on Visiting Nursing," *AJN* 10 (June 1910): 868; Annie W. Goodrich, "The Need of Orientation," *AJN* 13 (February 1913): 340.

109. Lowman, "Standard," 9, 15, 16.

110. Mary Beard, "Generalization in Public Health Nursing," *PHN* 5 (October 1913): 47.

111. Eliza J. Moore, "Visiting Nursing," *AJN* 1 (October 1900): 21; Mayanna B. Tomlinson, "Compensation in Visiting Nursing," *PHN* 6 (January 1914): 77–78.

112. Beard, "Generalization," 45–46.

113. One of the Older Women, "A Decade of Change," *PHN* 5 (January 1913): 66–69.

114. Craven, *Guide to District Nurses,* 8–9.

115. Loane, *Outlines of Routine,* vii, 150.

116. Karen Buhler-Wilkerson, "False Dawn: The Rise and Decline of Public Health Nursing in America, 1900–1930," in *Nursing History: New Perspectives, New Possibilities,* ed. Ellen Condliffe Lagemann (New York: Teachers College Press, 1983), 99–100. See also Diane Hamilton, "The Cost of Caring: The Metropolitan Life Insurance Company's Visiting Nurse Service, 1909–1953," *Bulletin of the History of Medicine* 63 (Fall 1989): 414–34.

Nuns and Nurses: Debates on New Nursing Programs and Improving the Training of "Secondary Hospital Personnel" in France, 1890–1910

Daniel Hickey
Emeritus Professor, Département d'histoire et de géographie
Université de Moncton

Abstract. A major controversy in French medicine at the turn of the 20th century was how to improve the training and education of hospital nurses. In 1899 the new government agency responsible for health and social services, the Conseil Supérieur de l'Assistance, encouraged setting up new nursing schools and imposing a curriculum to be followed by all. The Conseil discussion concerning these steps was very heated. Some councilors demanded the dismissal of all the religious nursing orders as a first step toward improving nursing services. Others favored efforts to educate all the nurses possible, be they religious or lay, leaving it to the municipalities to decide on the internal organization of their hospitals. To examine the issues faced by both choices, the article analyzes two cases of hospitals that went on to adopt each of the different orientations discussed: Le Havre, which set up a nursing school and kept its nuns, and Valence, which sent off its religious congregation and tried to set up a nursing school.

At the turn of the 20th century, hospitals in France were at the cutting edge of a major debate over how to improve the education and training of their nurses. A corollary of this debate was the relative merit of the care provided to patients by religious nursing orders compared to that by the newer lay nurses. This debate fitted into a larger national discussion revolving around two poles. The first was the long-term effort by French medicine to improve the quality of health care in the hospitals of the country. Beginning with the Paris clinic movement in the late 18th and early 19th centuries and continuing with the aseptic discoveries of Louis Pasteur after 1878, doctors and surgeons tried to reform hospital practices and operations to improve the treatment and care given to patients.[1]

Nursing History Review 17 (2009): 80–100. A Publication of the American Association for the History of Nursing.
DOI: 10.1891/1062-8061.17.80

The second national debate over hospital organization was an essentially political one in which partisans and opponents of the new Third Republic confronted each other. Created in 1870, in the aftermath of the Franco-Prussian War and the fall of the Second Empire, the government of the Third Republic unleashed a wave of pent-up anticlericalism. Its supporters saw the Roman Catholic Church as the source of opposition to the new government, menacing both the state and the French nation. A determined cohort of politicians, elected in the republican victories in 1876 and 1879, took it upon themselves to begin dismantling church "privileges": school programs were secularized, normal schools were set up to laicize the teaching profession, religious congregations were expelled, divorce was recognized, and the presence of religious orders in French hospitals came under close scrutiny.[2]

The first part of this article examines these cleavages as they emerged in 1898 and 1899 during a national debate over how to reform the training and performance of the nursing staff, referred to as "secondary hospital personnel." The two camps clearly staked out their positions on the question. One favored better education and training for all nurses, both religious and lay, while the other made laicization of hospital services and the nursing profession a priority to any reform effort. The second part of the article examines local implementation of the eventual recommendations. It considers the hospitals of Le Havre in Normandy in northwestern France and Valence on the opposite side of the country, in the southeast along the Rhône valley in the Département of the Drôme. The strategies adopted by the two towns to improve their nursing services are typical of the divergent approaches of the camps in the national debate.

The Conseil Supérieur de l'Assistance and the Napias Report

The Conseil Supérieur de l'Assistance was founded in 1888 by the French government to oversee distribution of social and health services to the population. The minutes of its meetings allow us to follow the positions taken by the councilors in the debate over how far to go in laicizing nursing. One side, led by the outspoken Désiré Magloire Bourneville, a Paris neurologist and politician, argued for total laicization of the profession and the rapid training of young women to replace the nuns; the other side, represented by doctors from Lyon and most of the municipalities outside Paris, wanted to leave to local hospitals whether to continue to be served by nuns or hire young laywomen.

Bourneville had conducted a major campaign to improve nursing in Paris by hiring lay nurses to replace the nursing nuns in the city hospitals. Surrounded by collaborators, he founded and directed a Paris publishing house, Le Progrès Médical, and a major medical review by the same name, in which he and his supporters campaigned for a new, reformed health service, notably for laicization of hospitals and their nursing staff. The movement argued that the nuns were more interested in saving the souls than the lives of their patients, and that they lacked instruction and training, notably in the newer fields of hygiene and asepsis. It was noted that the sisters generally occupied the positions of direction in the hospitals, leaving the wards, kitchens, and cleaning to ignorant and underpaid help. Finally, a frequent reproach was their outdated woolen habits, difficult to disinfect and antihygienic.

As early as 1878, three nursing schools had been opened up in Paris hospitals, and the first edition of Bourneville's *Manuel pratique de la garde-malade et de l'infirmière* was published by Progrès Médical.[3] But Katrin Schultheiss has shown in her recent work on 19th-century nursing reforms in France that the schools did not attract anywhere near the number of students needed to replace the nuns, and that the quality of the training left much to be desired.[4]

This was the context in which the members of the Conseil Supérieur de l'Assistance met to try to upgrade hospital services in France. From their first meetings the Conseil members were especially preoccupied with the lack of formal education and training for nurses, the "secondary personnel" of the hospital system. In January 1889, this problem was underlined in an important report by Dr. Henri Monod, director of public assistance (assistance et hygiène publiques). He wrote that, if the self-denial and devotion of the secondary hospital personnel are worthy of praise,

> this is not the case, in general, for their technical instruction. Their knowledge is purely empirical; there is no sign of the most elementary scientific know how, the simplest notions of hygiene are absent or even worse they confront deeply rooted prejudices. . . . This flawed aspect of hospital organization becomes more and more evident with the progress made by medicine and surgery. It becomes increasingly detrimental with the development of antiseptic methods that require that those who aid the practitioner be aware and conscious of the importance of the minutest details of this question, taking the necessary precautions and being aware of the danger that the slightest neglect could pose to the patient.[5]

The two sides in the debate over laicization agreed that it was imperative to upgrade the education and training of nurses, be they nuns or laywomen. As early as 1878, Bourneville had set up courses in Paris for lay nurses and *gardes-malades.*[6] The question of establishing obligatory national courses was one of the principal concerns of the new Conseil Supérieur. In 1897, this body commissioned Dr. Henri Napias, inspecteur général de l'assistance publique and member of the Academy of Medicine, to prepare a detailed report on the subject.

The report was based on Napias's research and on studies prepared by Dr. Henri Monod and by Dr. Hermann Sabran of Lyon. It noted that hospital "secondary personnel" in England, Germany, and Switzerland were all better educated and trained than were nurses in France. Sabran studied the functioning of "secondary personnel" in French hospitals and concluded that "we cannot continue to care for the sick as we did in the past; good will and devotion are important qualities for a nurse, but they are not enough."[7] Napias went from there to elaborate on the functioning of nursing elsewhere.

Napias abundantly cited the work of Florence Nightingale, arguing that she had revolutionized nursing in England. From 1859 on, according to Napias, Nightingale had traveled to France and Germany to observe their systems, and had begun to apply the best elements of these systems in her small London hospital when the Crimean War broke out. It was there, in a wartime context, that minister of war Sidney Herbert had asked her to organize hospital services for the soldiers in Scutari.[8] From her experience there she came back to England a heroine of the war effort, immortalized in a poem by Longfellow.

After the war, Napias wrote, Nightingale's popularity led to a public subscription that became the Nightingale Fund, raising more than 1,250,000 francs to create a school of nursing. He argued that her work at the Saint Thomas's Hospital school set an example for other hospitals to attain Nightingale's major goals: furnishing bursaries to student nurses, having them selected by the matrons of nursing, and training them in organized courses for one year with a second year of apprenticeship. This model was adopted in hospital after hospital as Nightingale's nurses were sent to towns in England, Wales, and Scotland, and then to Bombay, Colombo, Philadelphia, and Montreal. The Nightingale Fund was transformed into a foundation to ensure the continuation of her work.[9]

The Napias report studied briefly the functioning of a similar nursing service in Switzerland, where an École Normale Évangélique de Gardes-malades had been founded in Lausanne in 1859. It then provided notes on the actual state of nursing and nursing training in French hospitals, highlighting Bourneville's pioneering role in the Paris region and noting a number of regional initiatives, like the École des Infirmières in Le Havre.

The Napias report was submitted to the Conseil Supérieur de l'Assistance in 1898, and led to long debates over what courses to set up and to whom to teach them.[10] The councilors finally created a commission to propose a standardized curriculum for nursing education. Under the direction of Dr. Henri Monod, Dr. Maurice Letulle, and Dr. Élie Faivre, the Commission was made up of a dozen doctors, surgeons, and health care specialists. They too confronted the problem of which model to adopt. Should they propose a program like that in the laicized Paris institutions or like that in the religious hospitals of Lyon and the many smaller hospitals scattered throughout the country?

The program presented to the Conseil on May 17, 1899, was a compromise, leaving it to each institution to select the proper institutional structure and organization for its courses. However, the commissioners did order that nursing education in all institutions should follow a standardized teaching program. They argued that the program should not be too theoretical or overloaded with unnecessary content. They recommended beginning with a course on elementary notions of anatomy (6 lessons), physiology (6 lessons), and general hygiene and asepsis (12 lessons). The second section was to deal with the nurse's role in minor operations and emergency care, both always to be supervised by doctors (19 lessons). It continued with the treatment of typhoid fever, how to use cold baths, and how to aid in childbirth (4 lessons). It was also to teach elementary notions of pharmacology (10 lessons). Courses on care to the mentally handicapped were reserved exclusively to nurses training to serve in asylums, and the lessons were to be accompanied by theoretical notions of neurology.[11]

The Commission wanted to recruit better-educated students as candidates for the new courses, with at least a school diploma or *certificat d'études,* but a compromise was reached leaving the door open to take in practicing nurses who did not possess *certificats.* The report cited precedents in England and the United States that women should be preferred over men except for certain specialized services like venereal wards, mental asylums, and surgical wards, where the commissioners felt that men were indispensable.[12] They recommended that the courses for nurses be given over a minimum period of one year, recognizing that in most cases it would take two years to complete the training.[13] Just as with the Paris clinic, it was recommended that nurses be integrated into hospital services and given on-the-job training in the wards as part and parcel of their education.[14]

When this program was presented to the Conseil in 1899, Bourneville openly contested the recommended curriculum and the time frame proposed for the courses. He argued that the commissioners had overly simplified the material to be taught, and he was particularly vexed that they had brushed aside the program and courses in the Paris schools as too theoretical and scientific. He argued that it was inexcusable to restrict courses on the mentally ill to nurses who were to work in an asylum. Finally, he objected to the one-year time frame, arguing that it would take at least two years to transmit the knowledge and training necessary to form good nurses. In all these cases, Bourneville defended the structure as adopted in Paris and resented the fact that the Conseil had chosen another approach.

Napias, Letulle, and Faivre, who had participated in writing up the program, replied to Bourneville's criticism. Napias stated that the Commission "received the mandate to elaborate a minimum programme that could be given not just in Paris or Lyon, but in all of France."[15] He noted that Bourneville had been absent from the meeting that had unanimously approved the mandate. Bourneville replied that the composition of the Commission had been stacked in favor of Lyon. None of the Paris doctors who collaborated with him had been chosen, and he argued that Drs. Sabian, Mouisset, and Nové-Josserand, all attached to Lyon, had had considerable influence on drawing up the curriculum. He particularly regretted that the Commission had allowed hospitals to set their own norms for the proposed courses. Examinations could vary under this system, with one hospital requiring two compositions to meet the requirements of a section and another requiring three or four. They could also differ on the criteria for admission with some schools abusing the possibility of taking in candidates without the *certificat d'études.* For him there had to be uniformity.

On this point, Dr. Henriot, former mayor of Reims, replied forcefully that

> It would be regrettable to impose an identical program on all the cities of France. Instead a model should be proposed in which each community can adopt all the elements possible. It is not easy to operate a nursing school in a small French town.[16]

The proposed program was eventually put to a vote and adopted by the Conseil Supérieur. The new resolutions were then passed on to the government and voted in the National Assembly. The directives issued on October 28, 1902, by the minister of the interior ordered that every hospital was to be served by nurses with the new technical education.

Implementing the New Programs

How were these directives received? How were they implemented? To reply to these questions, two cases will be examined in detail: Le Havre, a port city at the mouth of the Seine in Normandy that took in sailors from the French navy, and Valence, a small departmental capital with an army garrison located along the Rhône valley.[17] The national decree of October 7, 1796, had left it to municipal councils to name five-member Administrative Commissions to govern local hospitals. Subsequent changes reduced direct municipal control, and a decree on March 2, 1805, ordered that one-fifth of the commissioners be renewed every year, although a commissioner whose term was ending could seek renewal. Nominations for vacant positions were to be made by the prefect of the department from a list of five names proposed by the existing board.[18] A year later, Napoleon's minister of the interior ordered that the mayor of the municipality should preside over the commission with the right to vote in cases of tied votes.

The statutes were again modified in 1879, further clarifying the composition of the Administrative Commissions. Municipal governments were again given a more direct role; the commissions were to be presided over by the mayor, aided by two delegates from the municipal council, with the remaining four members to be named by the prefect. So in 1902 it was essentially the mayors and members of the municipal councils who decided how to interpret the ministerial decree, where to find financing for schools of nursing, and how best to implement the teaching program. In adopting the required nursing reforms, Le Havre and Valence demonstrate the cleavages that had surfaced in the national debate. Since mayors and administrative councils had the final word on the reforms, the key to their differences lay in the way local people and local politics interpreted the national decrees.

Le Havre

Le Havre, situated in Upper Normandy at the mouth of the Seine River, was the major French port during the 19th century. In 1879 the city had a population of 100,000 people. Serving the local population, the French navy, and the merchant fleet, the hospital at Le Havre was an important and respected institution. In 1880 the town contributed more than 600,000 francs to the construction of new hospital buildings and reorganization of existing hospital services. After this expansion, there were usually 14 doctors and surgeons and about 15 interns serving the institution with its 1,409 available beds.[19] By 1891 the personnel of the hospital comprised 325 people. Beside the revenues from its considerable real estate holdings the institution received annual grants from the city to aid in paying expenses.

Historically, the hospital at Le Havre had been very much influenced by its service to the French navy. Of a total of 660 patients in 1796, 37% were military men.[20] In 1847, when new internal rules for the hospital were adopted, 90 beds were reserved for injured and sick soldiers and sailors, almost 30% of the 359 beds for the injured and sick. Another 200 places were set aside to take in orphans and abandoned children (100 boys and 100 girls), and 196 were for the elderly (98 for men and 98 for women).[21] By 1873, admission statistics show that the hospital received only 75 sick and injured military men, about 10% of the 596 sick and injured civilians. The institution received 149 orphans and abandoned children and 264 elderly. The gradual reductions in beds reserved for the military seem to have been due to numerous complaints in 1879 that with 1,034 patients, hospital resources were stretched to the limit and plans had to be made to build a new hospital.[22] With the opening of the new Hôpital Pasteur in 1885, service to the military seems to have been abandoned and health services in the town updated: the new hospital was to receive the sick and injured, while a maternity section and a hospice for the elderly were to be maintained. The new Pasteur buildings were eventually able to take in 1,103 patients in addition to the approximately 350 places in the hospice and 22 beds in the maternity section.[23]

One reason for Le Havre's initiatives and active involvement in ensuring health services to its population was the presence of one very dynamic medical man. Several doctors at the Le Havre hospital were at the forefront of French discussion and debate over medicine and health services. The most remarkable was the surgeon Robert Sorel. Born in 1862, Sorel did his internship in Paris after passing the 1888 competitive exams.[24] He taught in the École Municipal d'Infirmières in Paris in 1891–93, after which he received his medical degree and accepted the position of assistant surgeon at Le Havre. There he became very involved in upgrading hospital services. He served as municipal councilor and as a member of the Administrative Commission for the hospitals. Under his direction a new section for aseptic operations was set up in 1897; thereafter surgical polyclinics were created at both the old and the new hospitals, with services for consultations, an operating room, laboratories, and so on. Sorel received a silver medal at the 1897 Brussels International Exposition for his contributions to upgrading hospital services.[25]

At the same time Sorel continued his research and contributions to medical and health studies. From 1893 to 1910 he served as collaborator to *Le Progrès Médical,* the very influential medical journal published under Bourneville's direction. Sorel wrote reviews of major medical works, comments on professional conferences, and articles on his own operations and research.

Sorel and his physician colleague François Chauvel, a member of the Administrative Commission, first approached the Commissioners in 1895 with the proposal to create a school of nursing attached to the hospitals of Le Havre.[26] They proposed to set up the school under the auspices of the municipal government and the Commission. Professors were to be named by the vice-president of the Commission and confirmed by the mayor. Students were to be between 18 and 40 years of age, holders of a *brevet* or *certificat d'études primaires* or having successfully passed an entrance exam. An inquiry would also be made concerning their morality. The normal length of the program would be two years, one year of courses and a second of practical training combined with courses. The program would be financed by the Administrative Commission with a provisional budget of 2,000 francs a year. A committee would be named to preside over the school and organize its courses. It would be made up of nine members: the president (the mayor or one of his assistants), two municipal councilors, two of the school's professors, two doctors or surgeons, one hospital administrator, and the director of the hospitals.[27] In September 1897, two years after the initial presentation of the project, the Commission and city council approved the creation of the new school. It began courses a full two years before the Napias report recommended establishing schools of nursing, and five years before the 1902 circular from the minister of the interior ordered hospitals to hire only nurses who had graduated from the new programs.

Sorel and his colleagues from Le Havre were certainly well informed of the Conseil Supérieur debate and the forthcoming ministerial decree. In May 1902, five months before the decree was published, Sorel and his colleague, Edouard Deronde, along with a doctor from Brest visited and studied hospital services and structures in the United States. Their mission visited hospitals in New York, Boston, Chicago, Baltimore, and Philadelphia. In a 1902 article in *Revue médical de Normandie,* Deronde praised the private enterprise system in American hospitals, particularly the nursing structure in Roosevelt Hospital in New York.[28]

Deronde described in detail the application procedures for admission to American schools of nursing and the hospital requirements for new candidates. He noted that the admission system was very competitive, and that at Saint Luke's Hospital in New York in 1901 only 199 of 2,054 applicants were admitted.[29] As for the curriculum, he gave details of the three-year program, noting that American nurses learned the details of illnesses, diseases, and operating procedures. There were courses on anesthesia, on diseases of the digestive and respiratory systems, on ear, nose, and throat disorders, and on eye problems. Nurses had courses on urine analysis and on pathology. Deronde noted that even the proposed new French nursing program was far removed from the detail and scientific nature of the American curriculum. He concluded, "The Americans have outdistanced us, it's up to us to catch up."

A year later, in 1903, Sorel published an article in the *Revue médical de Normandie* in which he came back to this question and strongly supported the 1902 decree, explaining how Le Havre had benefited considerably from its new school. He argued that the ministerial demand for schools of nursing was totally justified, adding advice and details on how municipalities should organize such programs and even appealing to the Le Havre administrators to go beyond the ministerial requirements. At the same time he replied to a number of criticisms of the new initiative. He argued that nurses trained in schools like that of Le Havre were "absolutely different" from the "servants" employed in hospital kitchens and laundries who were mistakenly called *nurses.* At the Pasteur hospital the nurses were what were formally called supervisors (*surveillants*) and assistant supervisors (*sous-surveillants*):

> this type of nurse is reserved for direct contact with the patients, she is the disciplined collaborator of the doctor and the surgeon; in addition to her personal honor, that must be protected, she should possess a legitimate pride in a profession that has at the same time both a philanthropic and a scientific character.[30]

One of his principal points was that the new organization would add qualified, trained personnel to the hospital team. He noted an 1899 study by one of his predecessors on the need for trained nurses in the region of Le Havre. It argued that the region should try to attain the level of one nurse for every six to eight patients. Sorel noted that his 52-bed surgical ward had only two nurses, and to treat his patients properly he should have at least four. He added that just as in the United States, the new Le Havre School of Nursing with the year of in-house practical training for students would add significantly to the number of student nurses available at little or no cost to the hospitals.

On adopting American methods and training, Sorel frequently cited Deronde's article on U.S. schools of nursing.[31] Both Deronde and Sorel had been impressed by the training, particularly by the practical training given in the wards to future nurses. He wrote that their course lasted three years compared to the two asked for by the Conseil Supérieur. That meant that American hospitals provided two years of practical training, during which student nurses represented additional personnel that cost next to nothing.[32]

The second major point in the Sorel article concerned the details of supervising and training student nurses. He argued strongly in favor of a boarding school approach and pointed to the example of the "Nurses Homes" in the United States. He contended that it was only through living in the hospital and with colleagues from the hospital that nurses could be brought to understand the importance of night duty and the necessity of remaining close to their sick and dying patients.[33] For Sorel, this regime of internship training should take place in the best possible circumstances. Each student nurse should have her own room, "furnished without luxury, but with good taste." Each room should have a bed, a wardrobe, a commode, a table and chairs, a radiator, electric lamps, and an electric alarm system to notify nurses when they were needed in the wards. There should be a refectory, a common room to receive guests and family, and clean and inviting washrooms. For Sorel, the supervisors' house at the Le Havre hospital would be an ideal location for such a Nurses Home. In such surroundings they would best learn the principles of hygiene and diet that should be applied in their wards.

Sorel's final point treated the general lack of consultation of doctors and surgeons concerning the work of the nurses in their wards:

> I want to attract the attention of the Administrators to this fact: it is very strange that the doctor, who every day sees the work accomplished by the hospital personnel, who alone is competent to judge their professional worth, it is strange, I say, that he is never consulted concerning the salary increases, promotions, rewards that are granted to supervisors and nurses.[34]

He argued that in the 10 years he had served in the hospitals, he had never been consulted concerning nursing, though doctors and surgeons were an indispensable element in setting up the future schools of nursing. Although hospital administrators often opposed such schools, citing the cost of setting up and maintaining them, at Le Havre the hospital doctors had given their time and energy without compensation to set up and to teach the courses in the School of Nursing. For him, this demonstrated the importance that doctors and surgeons gave to the establishment of such schools.

Specifically addressing the Administrative Commission of the Le Havre hospitals, Sorel concluded,

> this is an important step, a work for the future that I invite you to undertake and which in the last analysis will provide, on the one hand, a well equipped health service and on the other, important new work opportunities for women. . . . We can no longer tolerate entrusting the sick to the care of those who have no formal instruction . . . because despite the advances of the society and of medical science, ignorance can cause the death of those unfortunate enough to have to come to our hospitals to seek a cure.[35]

Sorel, although closely attached to Bourneville and his team of researchers at *Progrès Médical,* was not so determined that the first step in renewing hospital operations should be laicization. Nowhere in Sorel's writings do we find insistence that the Le Havre hospitals dismiss the 54 Sisters of Saint Thomas de Villeneuve before setting up a school of nursing, as Bourneville had done in Paris.[36] On the contrary, the nuns remained active in the hospitals, and most of the sisters working in the hospitals enrolled in the new courses (see Table 1). There were 14 nuns among the student nurses auditing the courses in 1898–99, and 13 actually took the course in 1900–1901. In 1901–2, 12 others took the course. They were joined by other nurses and male nurses, including the cohort of 15 nurses who had been enrolled as auditors in 1898–99. A good number of girls and women always signed up for the courses, although frequently they had difficulty passing the exams. Often, like the nuns, they spent one year as auditors before taking the course a year or two later.[37]

As is obvious from the statistics in Table 1, most of the practicing nurses at the hospitals enrolled in the new courses just to protect their jobs. Since

Table 1. Students and Auditors Enrolled at the School of Nursing of the Le Havre Hospitals, 1897–1902

Students	1897–1898	1898–1899	1899–1900	1900–1901	1901–1902
Men	5		2	1	4
Women	16	4	14	1	6
Nurses	2	15	2	12	10
Male nurses	5	9		5	4
Hospital workers			4		
Supervisors			16	6	4
Religious				13	12
Total	28	28	38	38	40
Auditors					
Men	28	7		9	1
Women	30	18		3	1
Nurses		9		7	
Male nurses		4		2	
Religious		14		2	
Total	58	52	19*	23	2

* for 1899–1900 the statistical breakdown for auditors is not given

the 1902 ministerial circular had ordered that future nurses hold a certificate or diploma from a school of nursing, it was clear that even practicing nurses would eventually be obliged to obtain such diplomas. There was, in fact, little change in the employment structure of the hospital. The nuns with their new diplomas retained their employment as supervisors or ward nurses and most of the practicing lay nurses also remained in their previous jobs.

Valence

Valence was a much smaller town than Le Havre and less strategically important. Located along the Rhône River between Lyon and Avignon, it was the *chef-lieu* of the Département of the Drôme and the seat of a major army garrison. Historically, it had been more important, and in the Early Modern period it had even possessed a major university with a medical faculty. By 1851, however, the population was only 14,000 and the local hospital with its six doctors and surgeons was hard pressed to balance its budget. With an annual grant of only 5,000 francs from the municipal government, it was very dependent on the extra revenues from its military patients.

In the aftermath of the French Revolution, the Administrative Commission of the hospital had reinstalled the Sisters of the Holy Sacrament in the Hôpital Général and the Trinitarian Sisters in the Hôtel-Dieu. Facing chronic deficits, the municipality merged the two hospitals in 1818, selecting the Sisters of the Holy Sacrament to oversee the new institution in the buildings of the Hôpital Général.[38] The deficits continued, however, and the municipal council regularly pressured the nuns to reduce staff and try to cut costs.

The military was the principal lifeline for the institution. From 1842 on the army paid 1.75 francs a day for the treatment of an officer and 1 franc for a simple soldier and the navy allowed for 1.50 francs a day for sailors.[39] Military men made up 80% of the 1,181 patients treated in the institution in 1807, and it was only around 1842 that civilian patients began to outnumber military ones. In that year 726 civilians and 667 military men were admitted. Through the 1870s, the hospital generally took in about an equivalent number of civilians and soldiers.[40] As with most such institutions, the number of sick and injured varied greatly from decade to decade, often doubling during epidemics or periods of war. The fact that ill and injured soldiers occupied such a predominant place meant that military officials kept a close watch over the institution. They regularly sent inspectors who complained about service.

However, one of the most important critiques of the hospital came in 1895, when the Ministry of the Interior carried out a general inspection. The report contended that the hospital "left much to be desired": the corridors and floors were not always clean; on the first floor a toilet near the staircase was terribly dirty and stank up the corridor. This, the inspector noted, was caused by the natural humidity of the nearby river and the lack of domestics to do the cleaning. The personnel comprised 16 sisters, but in fact there were 21, counting the lay nuns and novices who carried out the domestic work. For the inspector, these lay nuns were not simple domestics. They were exempted from the heavy work carried out by lay servants in other hospitals; in Valence this work was reserved to the older patients of both sexes. He argued that there were too many chiefs in the administration and the hospital would be better served with more lay servants, strong women used to doing domestic work, women who could be dismissed if the corridors were not swept and the toilets not cleaned. A second problem was that a quarter of the population of Valence were Protestant. The inspector argued that it would be better if the nurses who worked with the sick and dying were not all Catholic nuns.

The negative conclusions of the 1895 report concerning the hospital staffing must have added to the anticlerical perceptions of a good percentage of the city population. In Valence, as in many French towns at the turn of the century, the debate over church and state power dominated municipal politics, especially after the Third Republic accorded direct voting rights to the municipal electorate. Antireligious sentiment came to a head after the 1903 ministerial directive ordered that religious orders had to justify their rights to dispense services (education, nursing, welfare) or be replaced. In the 1904 municipal elections, the anticlerical party in Valence won a majority and, among other measures, the resulting municipal government appointed a commission headed by Councilor Dumont to examine laicizing the hospital staff. Dumont wrote in the first pages of the report that in fact the Commission "had only one goal, that of carrying out the idea of laicization that had been the dominating principle behind the last municipal elections."[41]

The report submitted to the Council in 1905 had a double orientation. First, it considered the objections to laicization: moral issues, recruitment of new nurses, and financial implications of the decision. Second, it compared the budget of the present system of religious staffing with a similar budget using lay nurses. The first part of the report used testimony from Toulon and Beziers, two towns that had laicized their hospitals. Both were very positive concerning the change. The letter from the administrators of Beziers noted that

> The results obtained from the point of view of health services were remarkably satisfactory and the doctors who had feared the consequences of the change marveled

> at the competence and devotion of the laywomen. . . . Order and discipline reign in the institution, a situation that was impossible to attain with the nuns who were outside the control of the administration.[42]

It was noted that the principal obstacle to laicization lay in recruiting the new personnel. To resolve this problem Toulon and Beziers had opened or proposed to open nursing schools attached to their hospitals in order to dispense the new technical and practical instruction.

The Valence administrators argued that such a school could be set up in their hospital and that their doctors would be pleased to offer the courses. A commission of doctors from the hospital and members of the administration would make up the written and oral exams the future nurses would take after serving for a year in the hospital as aides. The new "titulaires" could be integrated into the staff as vacancies appeared. In all this debate the doctors and surgeons attached to the hospital were noticeably absent. They had been solicited by the mayor and the town council in 1904 to prepare a report on how to reorganize the town's health services, defining those who had the right to be treated free of charge and fixing rates for doctors, midwives, and pharmacists, setting up an external polyclinic, and extending consultations to the schools, dispensary, and house calls.[43] In the entire document, there was no mention of nurses and the role they should play and the doctors never seem to have been consulted by the town council before adopting the new policy.

Comparing the two budgets in the second part of the report, the Commission argued that 14 laywomen could easily replace the 20 nuns presently serving the hospital. It noted that only 10 nuns were actually serving the sick and that 6 lay nurses would be sufficient to replace them. All told, the report stated that the new system would cost the hospital administrators an additional 3,000 francs a year. Dumont argued that the benefits far outweighed the additional cost, and his commission advised the municipal council to take the initiative to cancel the 1839 contract with the Sisters of the Holy Sacrament.

The 1895 inspection and the Dumont report allow us to identify the reasoning behind the two divergent positions regarding nursing and patient care. The arguments both for and against the nuns had been present a century earlier in a major confrontation at the Hôtel-Dieu in Paris. In that conflict, just as in Valence, the sisters held to their long tradition of bedside care, treating their patients in the image of Christ, taking in the poor and disabled as well as the sick and dying, keeping patients in their wards longer than doctors deemed necessary, overfeeding them, and refusing them access to medications and treatments deemed unnecessary. The administration position aimed at streamlining hospital services, taking in only the sick and injured, treating and operating on them in order to discharge them as soon as possible.[44] The Dumont Commission argued that this latter approach would allow administrators to reduce personnel and yet provide the same or even better services.

Valence did follow the recommendations of the Commission, but the administrators ran into more problems than had been anticipated. The most immediate difficulty came in recruiting the few trained nurses available and financing the training of new ones. The Commission had argued that the administrators should set up a school of nursing. But who would pay for the school and for training? Even before receiving the Dumont report, the municipal council had begun negotiations with the Prefect of the Drôme to try to convince departmental officials to fund training of the new lay personnel and eventually to set up a school for nurses in Valence. On December 9, 1903, the hospital administrators also turned to the city of Valence, asking municipal officials to contribute to a fund to aid in the formation of new lay nurses, noting that hospitals in most towns of comparable size possessed considerably superior financial resources.[45]

The correspondence between the mayor of Valence and the Prefect of the Drôme on January 15 and 20, 1904, reveals that a departmental commission had rejected the financial request by Valence to set up a school of nursing.[46] As an alternative, the mayor had entered into discussions to try to convince the prefect to fund bursaries to send young girls to Lyon or Grenoble for training. The two finally decided that bursaries would be set up for girls from Valence at the École des Infirmières in Lyon.[47]

In Valence, the questions of laicization and better-trained nurses did, in fact, conflict. At the same time that Bourneville and his disciples enthusiastically supported combining laicization of a hospital with the establishment of a school of nursing, it is clear that budgetary problems frequently compromised the efforts to move toward both. Municipalities like Valence often had to choose one direction or the other.

Gerard Carrière, a doctor in the hospital of Alès, not far from Nîmes in the Département du Gard, commented on the laicization movement in his 1902 inaugural address to the students of the new school of nursing set up in his hospital. He was clearly in favor of creating new schools and encouraging training of new nurses, but he was opposed to the all-out laicization movement in Valence. He noted that

> One disturbing element has precipitated and troubled this evolution [toward improving nursing training]: it is politics. It has created in one camp the all-out la-

icization movement—while in the opposing camp the proponents of the religious orders' monopoly blindly fight back—and in both camps, the sick and the dying are forgotten … [among the first group] administrators have replaced the nuns who possessed unquestionable moral qualities albeit with certain weaknesses, with a personnel recruited hastily among the retarded and untrained—the handicapped, the indolent, drunkards, even criminals. … . Before laicizing, it is necessary to prepare lay personnel, well chosen and sufficiently qualified: we must first organize, everywhere possible, nursing schools along the models of those that are in operation.[48]

Conclusion

As the 1899 debate in the Conseil Supérieur demonstrated, the country was divided over the question of laicizing hospital care. If Valence followed Beziers, Toulon, Saumur, Lille, Reims, Amiens, Evreux, and others on the route toward laicization proposed by Bourneville, others were less eager to toss out their nuns. Hospitals in major French cities like Le Havre, Rouen, Lyon, Grenoble, Avignon, and Marseille accepted the project to set up schools of nursing, but continued to be served by nursing sisters.

There were several reasons for the reticence of the major hospitals to laicize their nursing personnel. The first was economic. Following the 1905 decree on "separation" of church and state, the cities of Amiens and Evreux did laicize their hospitals in 1909. The mayor of Le Havre feared that he would be forced to follow suit and eliminate the 54 nuns serving the hospital. He evaluated the cost of such a measure at 150,000 francs. Eventually, he was able to avoid laicization by treating the grant given to the nuns as a salary and having the nuns pay part of their personal expenses.[49]

Second, as was seen in Le Havre, the religious orders accepted the necessity of upgrading the training of their nursing sisters and apparently encouraged them to enroll in the new courses to earn diplomas as trained nurses. As can be seen from the success rates at the Le Havre school of nursing, it was apparently very difficult to educate and train new lay nurses. The women who enrolled in the courses frequently dropped out during the first year or failed to pass the exams for the diploma. Generally the success rate among nuns and men was higher than was that of young women. This is probably a reflection of the lack of primary school education of French girls.[50]

Despite the problems in recruiting and integrating new lay nurses, the rhetoric on the laicization of hospital services repeated by reformers like Bourneville was accepted in places like Valence where the anticlerical movement was deep-rooted. For Bourneville and his disciples, hospitals had first and foremost to eliminate all religious elements, including the nursing sisters, in order to have a clean slate to laicize services and train lay nurses. Towns like Valence followed this advice and turned the page on religious nurses essentially for ideological and political reasons. But this was not the case everywhere. As both Jacques Léonard and Olivier Faure have argued, both the medical community and the general population apparently accepted and supported the work of the nursing sisters.[51] They were seen as devoted and conscientious women who had served the hospitals and their patients well over the last century. Doctors were accustomed to dealing with them, had trained them to assist in operations, and often were not ready to upset routines and practices to integrate a new corps of untrained and untested lay nurses.

In fact, the most radical long-term change was carried out in towns like Le Havre where a competent, devoted medical man like Sorel was engaged in upgrading the local hospital. For him the improvement of nurses' training was part and parcel of improving medical services. Paying little attention to the national debate over laicizing nursing, he founded the Le Havre École des Infirmières and worked to improve its teaching, internship programs, and dormitory facilities. Both religious and lay nurses received theoretical and practical training in the Le Havre school, which implemented the directives of the Napias report and the 1902 and 1905 ministerial decrees. Most other provincial schools of nursing eventually followed this pattern.

Throughout the late 19th and early 20th centuries the lack of scientific knowledge and training of what the early reformers called the "secondary personnel" in French hospitals had become obvious to all. At the end of the 19th century, the members of the new Conseil Supérieur de l'Assistance began taking action to improve the situation. In 1899 they opened discussion over how best to reorganize nurses' training, but in so doing they provoked a major debate over the need to reform hospital services and eliminate all religious elements from French health care. The best intentions of tackling the need for schools of nursing, educational programs, and hospital training thus became entangled in the political, religious, or medical rhetoric of the different interest groups who sought a major reform of French health care. With the directives published by the central government and the actions taken by the local hospitals between 1902 and the 1920s, a step was taken toward improving the education and training of nurses, but the terms of the larger debate over the place of religion in hospital services continued to divide the French population well into the 20th century.

Daniel Hickey, PhD
Emeritus Professor, Département d'histoire et de géographie
Université de Moncton
Moncton, New Brunswick, Canada
236 rue de la Renaissance
Blainville, Québec J7B 1S7
Canada
daniel.hickey@umoncton.ca

Acknowledgments

The author would like to thank Mlle Jacqueline Roubert, former archivist of the Hospices Civils de Lyon, for her aid in researching this article and the Associated Medical Services for its financial aid in carrying out the research.

Notes

1. Michel Foucault, *The Birth of the Clinic: An Archaeology of Medical Perception* (New York: Vintage, 1994), 64–87; Erwin Ackerknecht, *Medicine at the Paris Hospital, 1794–1848* (Baltimore: Johns Hopkins University Press, 1967); Bruno Latour, *The Pasteurization of France* (Cambridge, Mass.: Harvard University Press, 1988).

2. On this question see René Rémond, *L'anticléricalisme en France de 1815 à nos jours* (Paris: Fayard, 1976), 17–44 and John McManners, *Church and State in France, 1870–1914* (New York: Harper and Row, 1973).

3. *Le Manuel pratique de la garde-malade et de l'infirmière,* 3 vols. (Paris: Progrès Médical, 1878).

4. Katrin Schultheiss, *Bodies and Souls: Politics and the Professionalization of Nursing in France, 1880–1922* (Cambridge, Mass.: Harvard University Press, 2001), 20–50. Schultheiss treats a series of reformers besides Bourneville; she has a chapter on Dr. Anna Hamilton and a major article, "La Véritable médecine des femmes: Anna Hamilton and the Politics of Nursing Reform in Bordeaux, 1900–1914," *French Historical Studies* 19, no. 1 (Spring 1995): 183–214.

5. Henri Napias, "Rapport sur le recruitement du personnel secondaire des établissements hospitaliers," 1897 (hereafter Napias report), Conseil Supérieur de l'Assistance, fasc. 64 (1897), Archives des Hospices Civils de Lyon (hereafter AHCL).

6. The term *garde-malade* is a traditional French expression for nurse (*infirmière*). Hamilton preferred *garde-malade* to designate hospital nurses in her thesis on the new nursing programs; see Schultheiss, "La Véritable médecine des femmes," 189; Schultheiss, *Bodies and Souls,* 31–33.

7. Napias report, 10–11. Napias's information on Nightingale reflected the widespread positive publicity diffused by the Nightingale Training School and was not always an accurate portrayal. For a more objective look at Nightingale's work see Monica Baly, *Florence Nightingale and the Nursing Legacy* (London: Croom Helm, 1986); Carol Helmstadter, "Building a New Nursing Service: Respectability and Efficiency in Victorian England," *Albion* 35, no. 4 (Winter 2004): 590–621; "Old Nurses and New: Nursing in the London Teaching Hospitals Before and After the Mid-Nineteenth-Century Reforms," *Nursing History Review* 1 (1993): 43–70.

8. Sidney Herbert, who recruited Nightingale, was not a minister but one of the secretaries of state.

9. Napias report, 15–21.

10. Napias report, 32–36.

11. AHCL, Conseil Supérieur de l'Assistance (hereafter CSA), fasc. 66 (1889), 18–19.

12. AHCL, CSA, 23.

13. AHCL, CSA, 23, 29.

14. AHCL, CSA, 27.

15. AHCL, CSA, 30.

16. AHCL, CSA, 33.

17. Many municipalities and hospitals did not act on the ministerial decree. In Poitiers, only in 1939 did the Administrative Commission finally set up an École du Service Hospitalière et Social. The vice-president of the school wrote on February 1, 1939, asking the departmental Conseil Général for a grant of 20,000 francs to operate the school, which would have the double goal of forming nurses and social workers. Archives Départementales de la Vienne, Rapport du Dr. Veluet, February 1, 1939, 86, 1X 88.

18. Archives Départementales de la Vienne, Rapport du Dr. Veluet, 10.

19. Philippe Manneville, *Regards sur quatre siècles de vie hospitalière au Havre* (Le Havre: Centre Hospitalière du Havre, 1994), 46, 48–49.

20. Manneville, *Regards sur quatre siècles,* 34.

21. Archives municipales du Havre (hereafter AMLH), Hôpital du Havre, Déliberations, October 19, 1847, L 2, 9.

22. Manneville, *Regards sur quatre siècles,* 70.

23. Manneville, *Regards sur quatre siècles,* 70–75.

24. "Robert Sorel," *Index-Catalogue of the Surgeon-General's Office, Authors and Subjects,* 2nd ser. (Washington, D.C.: U.S. Army, 1911), xvi, 181.

25. "Robert Sorel," *Archives provinciales de la chirurgie* (Paris: Institut international de bibliographie scientifique) 8 (1899): 575–78. Robert Sorel and O. Widmaier, "L'organisation d'une clinique chirurgical privée au Havre," *Archives provinciales de la chirurgie* 4 (1895).

26. AMLH, Hôpital du Havre, Déliberations, July 23, 1895, L 47, 154, 97–116.

27. Hôpital du Havre, Déliberations, 155.

28. Edouard Deronde, "Les Écoles d'infirmières aux Etats-Unis," *Revue médical de Normandie* 3 (1902): 359–65.

29. Deronde, "Écoles d'infirmières," 365.

30. Robert Sorel, *École d'Infirmières: Lettre à MM. Les Membres de la Commission Administrative des Hôpitaux du Havre* (Rouen: J. Le Cerf fils, 1903), 3–4, 7, reprinted from *Revue médical de Normandie* 4 (1903), 78–92.

31. Deronde, "Écoles d'infirmières," 359–65; Robert Sorel, "Écoles d'infirmières au Havre et en Amérique," *Progrès Médical,* October 4, 1902, 213–214 and December 6, 1902, 444–447.

32. Sorel, "Écoles d'infirmières," 6.

33. Sorel, "Écoles d'infirmières," 7.

34. Sorel, "Écoles d'infirmières," 9.

35. Sorel, "Écoles d'infirmières," 9–10.

36. Manneville, *Regards sur quatre siècles,* 51.

37. École des gardes-malades, 1897–1902, Hôpital du Havre, AMLH, K8. In Rouen, there were 32 nuns among the 37 student nurses in 1900–1901 and 12 among the 17 in 1901–2. Creation d'Écoles d'infirmières conformement à la circulaire ministerial du 28 Oct. 1902, Archives Départementales de la Seine Maritime, 5M 46.

38. Jean-Sébastien Gauthier, "L'Hôpital de Valence dans la 1ère moitié du XIXe siècle (1802–1850)," mémoire de maîtrise, Université Pierre Mendès-France (Grenoble, 1996), 87.

39. Gauthier, "L'Hôpital de Valence," 88.

40. Médiathèque de Valence, Archives de l'Hôpital de Valence, Registres, Comptes moraux 1807, 1842, 1870.

41. Archives départementales de la Drôme (hereafter ADD), 26X/1 Rapport de M. Dumont, Valence, Conseil municipal, meeting of May 26, 1905.

42. ADD, 4.

43. Médiathèque de Valence, Dr. Calvet, "Rapport présenté a MM les members du conseil municipal par les médecins de Valence sur l'organisation de service de santé de la ville," November 3, 1904, A3202–7.

44. Louis S. Greenbaum, "Nurses and Doctors in Conflict: Piety and Medicine in the Paris Hôtel-Dieu on the Eve of the French Revolution," *Clio Medica* 13, nos. 3–4 (1978): 247–67. Also on the same question, see Toby Gelfand, "A Confrontation Over Clinical Instruction at the Hôtel-Dieu of Paris During the French Revolution," *Journal of the History of Medicine and Allied Sciences* 28 (1973): 268–82.

45. ADD, Commission administrative, Déliberations, Valence Hospital, December 9, 1903, 6T5/3.

46. ADD, Prefect of the Drôme to President of the Administrative Commission of the Valence hospices, January 15, 1904, ADD 6T5/3 and Déliberations, Administrative Commission, December 9, 1903, 6T5/3.

47. ADD, Mayor of Valence to Prefect of the Drôme, January 20, 1903, 6T5/3.

48. AHCL, Dr. G. Carrière, *La Garde-malade et l'infirmière: role professionnel et programme d'enseignement* (Paris: Baillière et fils, 1903), 8–9, HA 435.

49. Manneville, *Regards sur quatre siècles,* 51.

50. Françoise Meyeur, *L'Éducation des filles en France au XIXe siècle* (Paris: Hachette, 1979), 167–168, 178–179.

51. Jacques Léonard, "Religieuses et médecins au XIXe siècle," *Annales ESC* (1972): 32, 901; Olivier Faure, "Des médecins aux maladies: tendencies récentes en histoire social de la santé," in *Pour l'histoire de la médecine, autour de l'œuvre de Jacques Léonard,* ed. Michel Lagrée and François Lebrun (Rennes: Presses Universitaires de Rennes, 1994), 62–63.

Russian Romances: Emotionalism and Spirituality in the Writings of "Eastern Front" Nurses, 1914–1918

Christine Hallett
School of Nursing, Midwifery and Social Work, University of Manchester

Abstract. The nursing work of the First World War is usually associated with the trench warfare of the Western Front. Nurses were based within fairly permanent casualty clearing stations and field hospitals, and patients were moved "down the line" to base hospitals, and then to convalescent hospitals "at home." The nurses and volunteers who worked on the Eastern Front and offered their services to the *letuchka* or "flying columns" of the Russian medical services had a very different experience. They worked with highly mobile units, following a rapidly moving "front line." The diaries of three British (one Anglo-Russian) nurses who worked alongside Russian nursing sisterhoods in three different flying columns—Violetta Thurstan (*Field Hospital and Flying Column*), Florence Farmborough (*With the Armies of the Tsar*) and Mary Britnieva (*One Woman's Story*)—stand as an important corpus of nursing writing. Written in a highly romantic style, they take up similar themes around their work on the Eastern Front as a heroic journey through a dreamlike landscape. Each nurse offers a portrayal of the Russian character as fine and noble. The most important themes deal with the *romance* of nursing itself, in which nursing work is portrayed as both character-testing and a highly spiritual pursuit.

The Great War of 1914–1918 conjures images in most Western European minds of the fixed, unmoving warfare of the Western Front, of months spent holding down a devastated strip of land, followed by the occasional push forward and the acquisition of a few square miles in exchange for hundreds of casualties.[1] People in England and the United States through the 20th century were educated and acculturated to view the war in terms of the relentless boredom and inconsequentiality of trench warfare.[2] In other parts of the world the war has a different image. In Australia and New Zealand the annihilation of thousands of men on the rugged cliffs behind Anzac Cove is part of a national

Nursing History Review 17 (2009): 101–128. A Publication of the American Association for the History of Nursing.
DOI: 10.1891/1062–8061.17.101

mythology. There, in 1915, troops moving into the Gallipoli Peninsula met fierce Turkish resistance and were unable to advance. Stories about the courage and tenacity of these troops fighting in an untenable situation have done much to fuel myths of the First World War as a conflict in which heroic troops were led by callous and inadequate generals. In Southern Europe, it is the heroic Serbian retreat of 1915 and the grueling travel through the Italian Alps that has captured the imagination.[3] The troops of Germany and its allies had advanced so rapidly into Serbia that British and Serbian forces were forced to flee, along with a large section of the populace, across the Alps in winter, with many dying of starvation and exposure. The advance through the Italian Alps toward the end of the war was seen as a dramatic reversal of fortune.

The Russians experienced a Great War that was very different from any other. Theirs was a mobile war that ranged over thousands of miles, with massive, rapid advances, and precipitous retreats.[4] The nurses who participated in the Eastern campaigns had a very different experience from those who nursed in the fixed casualty clearing stations and base hospitals of the Western Front. Although Russia had military hospitals, they were often many hundreds of miles from a rapidly moving front. Much of the immediate and urgent medical and nursing care was undertaken by staff attached to *letuchka,* or "flying columns": mobile hospitals housed in makeshift accommodation or tents, carried on cumbersome wooden horsedrawn wagons, but often moving almost as rapidly as an army.[5]

The experience of nurses in these settings has been captured by the writings of three women—two English and one Anglo-Russian. Violetta Thurstan was a fully trained British professional nurse who offered her services to the Russian Red Cross, and was taken on by a flying column that left Moscow in 1914.[6] Thurstan had already experienced a perilous adventure. After working for several months in a field hospital in Belgium, she had experienced the bombardment of Antwerp and been taken prisoner, along with a number of colleagues, by the German army. Allowed to travel to neutral Denmark but unable to get back to England easily, she contacted the Red Cross and negotiated a posting in Russia.[7] After a long and arduous journey via Sweden and Finland, which she describes in minute detail, Thurstan arrived in Moscow, where she worked in a base hospital run by a sisterhood for a while before being posted, first to a hospital in Warsaw, and then to a flying column, in which she worked for several months. In 1915, Thurstan was obliged to leave Russia due to ill health.[8]

Florence Farmborough was a governess teaching the two daughters of a Russian nobleman in Moscow when war broke out. Like many women in combatant countries at the time, she experienced a strong desire to participate in the

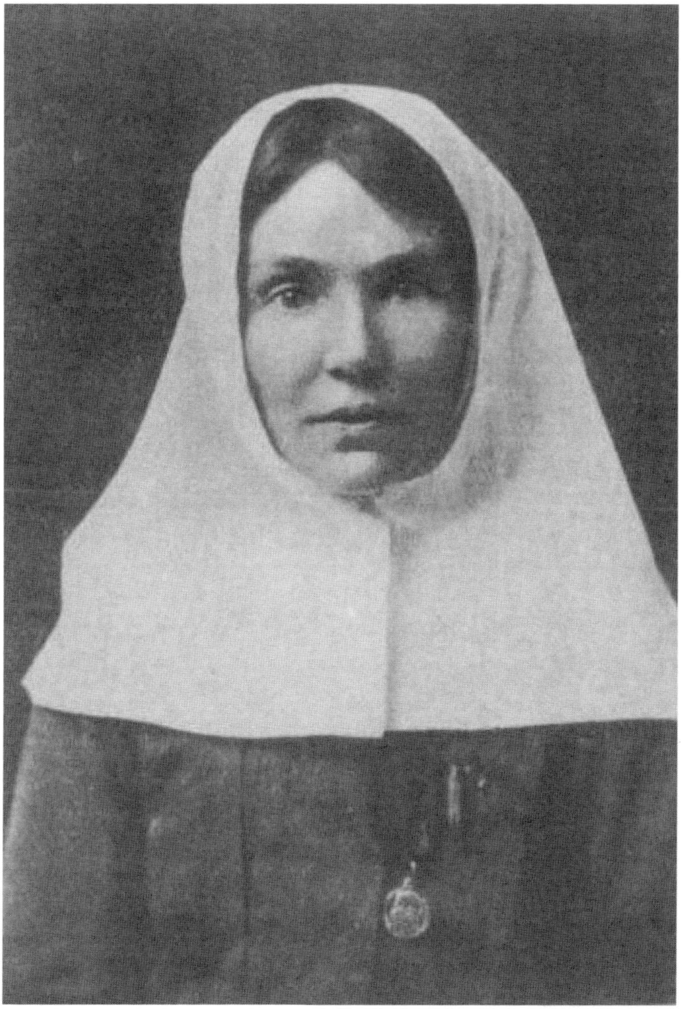

Figure 1. Violetta Thurstan, frontispiece to her book *Field Hospital and Flying Column.*

conflict on behalf of her adoptive country; she joined the Red Cross, received six months training, and worked as a volunteer nurse for the remaining years of the war—until the Revolution forced Russia to withdraw from the conflict.[9]

Farmborough had lived in Russia for years before the outbreak of war. Happily placed, she was very unlike the governesses of English Victorian novels. She was close to her employers, treated as a member of the family, and very attached to Russia, which she saw as her adoptive homeland. Farmborough's experiences in a flying column are recounted in dramatic style. The retreat of

1915 is given particular emphasis and pathos, and an episode in which the heroine and her colleagues have to flee for their lives from a rapid German advance in Poland is particularly gripping.[10] Farmborough, like Thurstan, writes in a highly novelistic style; her work is not only a romance but a thriller. When the Revolution began, she attempted to stay in Russia for a time, but

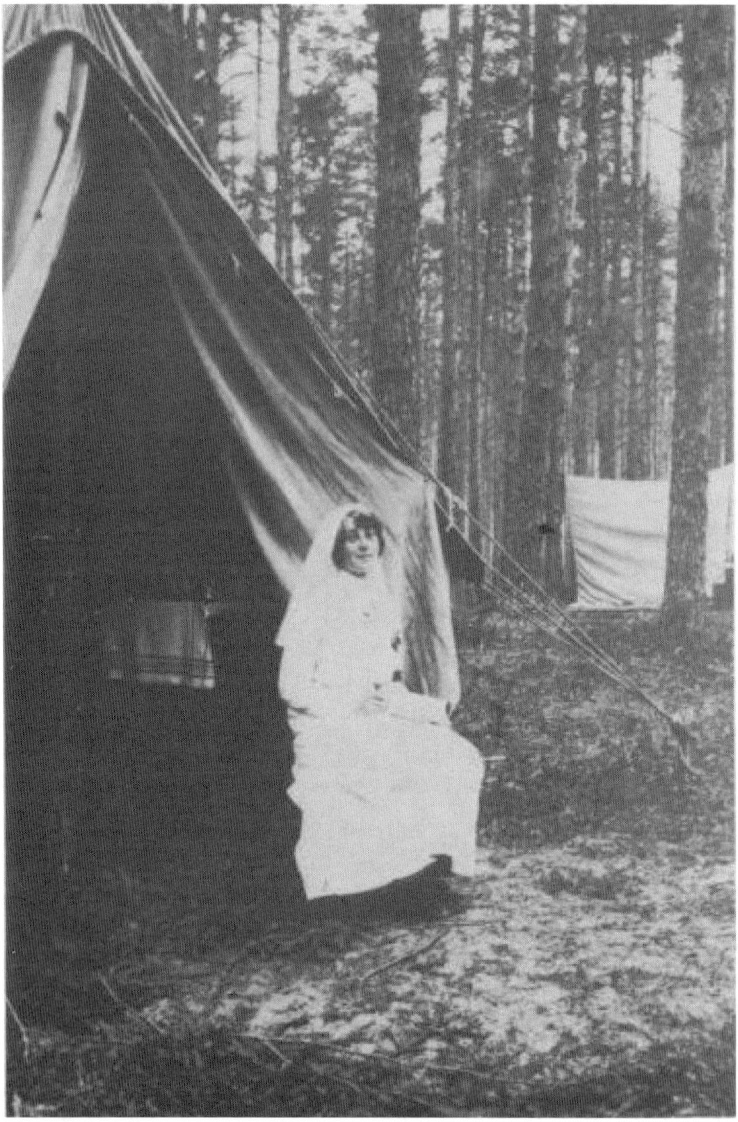

Figure 2. Florence Farmborough, frontispiece to her book *Russian Album, 1908–1918.*

eventually undertook a dramatic train journey that carried her the length of Russia to Vladivostok, whence she embarked for the United States.

Mary Britnieva was perhaps the most unusual of the three. An Anglo-Russian living in St. Petersburg, she, like Farmborough, trained as a Red Cross nurse at the beginning of the war, and then was able to obtain one of the much-coveted positions as a member of the flying column funded by the Russian Council of State.[11] Britnieva's story is particularly poignant. After working for two years in the flying column, she married the head doctor and they returned to St. Petersburg, where they stayed for three years under Bolshevik rule. Interestingly, Britnieva's husband is described in terms suitable for a romantic hero. Although, "strict as a disciplinarian," he was also charming, with a "really remarkable personality." We are informed that "to his deep sense of duty and boundless devotion were added a great love of justice and a sense of humour which, blended with his natural kindness, quickly endeared him to

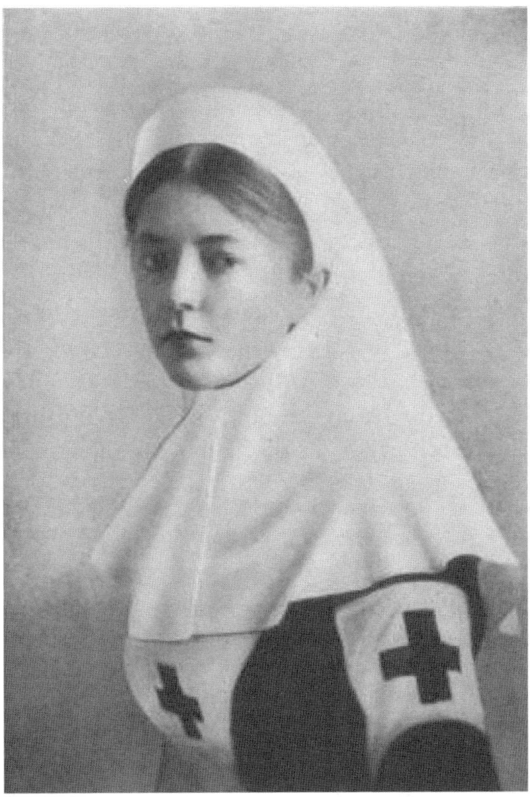

Figure 3. Mary Britnieva, frontispiece to her book *One Woman's Story.*

all hearts, patients and staff alike."[12] Britnieva married, had two children, lived in extreme poverty, faced starvation, and eventually negotiated her way out of Russia, with her children, via Finland, to stay with her family in England. Upon reaching England, she was pronounced three months from death, yet managed to survive and regain her health.

The three women published memoirs of their experiences as Eastern Front nurses. All three wrote in English. Their works are readily available to modern Western audiences and provide one particular perspective on the experiences of nurses during the war. I am unaware of any similar works by Russian nurses. It is highly likely that they also wrote diaries and memoirs; yet they were unlikely to have published these works, which were then either lost or destroyed. Trained nurses in Russia at the outset of the First World War were members of religious orders; they were much less likely than secular nurses to write about their experiences. The mobile flying columns in which Thurstan, Farmborough, and Britnieva worked, although apparently staffed largely by secular nurses from several European countries, were run under the auspices of these Russian nursing sisterhoods alongside a small number of Russian "civil nurses".[13]

Russia was drawn into the First World War by its involvement in early 20th-century diplomacy, as a member of the Triple Entente along with Britain and France. It withdrew in 1917, unable to sustain its war effort as its state and populace became engulfed by revolution. As Adele Lindenmeyer points out, very little has been written about what she labels the "charitable activities" of Russian women, including nurses, during this time. Lindenmeyer explains this gap in the literature in terms of the tendency for Russian historians to focus on radical, feminist, and revolutionary figures, dismissing what were seen as the more traditional feminine drives of the Russian nursing sisterhoods.[14] It may be that many of the records and writings of the Russian nursing sisterhoods were destroyed during the Revolution of 1917. Russian nursing in the first few decades of the 20th century was, in fact, built on a long-standing tradition that predated the Crimean War.[15]

"Dreams in Words": Western Romanticism Translated Into Eastern Epic Romance

The writings of British nurses based in Russia are interesting for three reasons. First, they offer a British perspective on Russia's involvement in the war and on the Eastern Front campaigns. Second, their authors appear to have taken on, very readily, the cultural perspectives and preoccupations of their adoptive country. Their views, ideas, and, indeed, ideals come across to the reader very differently from those of Western Front diarists such as Mary Borden, Rebecca West, or Ellen la Motte, with their cynical undertones, and bleak portrayals of reality.[16] The Eastern Front diaries considered here are very different from their Western Front counterparts. For Thurstan, Farmborough, and Britnieva Russia's involvement in the war was easily portrayed as an epic romance, a spiritual journey in which Russian life and honor prevailed even in the midst of despair and disaster. Thus, thirdly, these works are couched in peculiarly *romantic* terms. There is a sense of adventure, of journeying, both physically and spiritually, across an extraordinary landscape. These works are unique in their combination of both Western Romanticism and Eastern romance.

The quality of these works as romantic texts is offered as the primary focus of this article. They can, however, also be viewed as examples of a particular type of travel writing. They provide clear expositions of Western Europe's fascination with Russian exoticism. Stephanie Lin has emphasized the importance of the role of "exotic othering" in creating a sense of one's own national identity. In her discussion of 19th-century French travel narratives, Lin argues in a way that has relevance for British writings (particularly the three texts discussed here) that there was a tendency for writers to contrast Western European freedom and enlightenment with Russian enslavement. Yet this comparison was not one that denigrated the Russian people. Quite the opposite: although Russia's populace was seen as oppressed, and its society backward, the Russian character was celebrated as noble and fine.[17]

Alison Sinclair similarly examined what she saw as Spain's love affair with the East, observing that Russia was often symbolized in Spanish writings as "the exotic woman."[18] A number of Western texts of the 19th and early 20th centuries took up the theme of Russian culture as a source of something enriching and sustaining to the West. Steven Marks explores the tendency of Western writers and musicians to see the Russian soul as the antithesis of Western imperialism and capitalism.[19] The three nurses' memoirs presented here can be seen as part of this corpus of texts. Yet the quality of these nurses' writings that seems most powerful is their romanticism. Thurstan, Farmborough, and Britnieva fuse Russian exoticism with Western Romanticism in a way that demonstrates how deeply they themselves are immersed in both cultures.

Romanticism had been particularly current in British culture in the late 18th and early 19th centuries, and had found its strongest voice in the works of Romantic poets such as Wordsworth, Coleridge, Keats, and Blake.[20] These poems have been defined as "dreams in words."[21] This dreamlike quality characterizes Romanticism: the sense that the truth behind anything lies in its spiritual reality rather than its superficial appearances, just as dreams may appear more real than actual experiences, even when they are incomprehensible. In Romanticism everything possesses a spirit—even nature itself. There is a link to deism in which all elements of nature have a divine component. The other side to this reality is, however, a dark side. Romanticism permits the existence of evil as well as goodness; demons are present as well as gods. In epic romance, the audience is invited to witness the journeying, the travails, and the "great deeds" of a hero or heroine, whose innermost nature is tested. This central figure's success in overcoming the trials before him or her is inextricably linked to the endurance of human values themselves, and these epics can be seen as allegories for the spiritual survival of the world and of humanity.[22]

Romanticism as a philosophy rests, therefore, on a strong sense of the spirituality in human nature, and in the universe as a whole. As a cultural perspective, it could be seen, in a debased form, as mere emotionalism—emotion devoid of spiritual depth. The archetypically pragmatic and sensible novelist Jane Austen famously parodied the romanticism she saw around her in Regency England in her novel *Northanger Abbey,* in which the heroine, Catherine Morland, identifies too closely with the characters in her gothic romantic novel and loses her own grip on reality.[23] Romanticism could therefore be seen, throughout the 19th century and into the 20th, as a potentially dangerous cultural medium. *True* Romanticism expressed the depths of human nature, yet it could easily be portrayed as merely empty-headed emotionalism. It has also, at times, been seen as a potentially radical cultural medium, which identified Enlightenment rationality as a prop and justification for social injustice. The Romantics therefore saw their work as being "of the people." As Paul Keen emphasizes, they "championed the spontaneous power of inspired intuition over critical enquiry, and of poetry over rational explication."[24]

Romanticism as a cultural form survived throughout the Victorian era, and remained a strong element of the emotional inner lives of the young people of Western Europe—both male and female—who participated in the war.[25] Fussell's famous text *The Great War and Modern Memory* engages with the, until recently, widely accepted theory that young men went willingly to war, seeing their involvement in the conflict in terms of duty, honor, and also adventure, only to become rapidly disenchanted by the horrors of the Western Front.[26] Women's historians have argued that, although not direct participants in the fighting, women who had some indirect encounters with war trauma—particularly nurses—had a similar experience of disenchantment.[27] What is interesting about the texts written by British women in Russia is that not only did they, from the start, express a different, peculiarly Eastern form of Romanticism, they also retained that Romanticism, even in the face of multiple war casualties and the collapse of discipline and humanity during the Revolution. Their works never slip into cynicism; the sense that honor, right, and the human spirit will eventually prevail—that an essentially *good* world will ultimately right itself, through the heroic endeavors of human beings—endures throughout. The correspondences between the three writings are remarkable, and the thesis of this article is that the strongly and uniformly romantic element in their writings derives from their similar backgrounds and experiences as middle-class, genteel women of the early 20th century who were gripped by the emotionalism and spirituality of the Russian culture they encountered, which to them seemed both dark and noble.[28]

The approach to analysis of the texts adopted in this article was an essentially hermeneutic one. My own prejudices and preconceptions as a trained nurse and historian intersected with the intentions and perspectives of the three authors whose works I considered. I adopted some of the techniques of discourse analysis, searching these texts for their underlying influences. Overall, the process was an interpretive one: a search for meanings conveyed both intentionally and unintentionally.[29]

The Nurse as Romantic Heroine

Thurstan, Farmborough, and Britnieva all published their memoirs. Using diary entries written contemporaneously with events, then adding later from memory, they compiled autobiographies that read like epic romances. Their stories would be heroic even without the medium of the romantic style in which they were written. These women were clearly tough, extraordinary, and committed. The novelistic style in which they tell their stories, however, makes them even more compelling, and these women emerge from their respective texts as they probably wished to be remembered: courageous, humane, and with the depth of character of true heroines.[30] Their intention was not merely to promote themselves, however. They appear to have genuinely valued their experiences on the Russian front, and wanted to bring both the sufferings and the brave endurance of the Russian people to a wider audience, particularly after Communism had shut the doors of the Russian empire to the West, transforming what had always been a remote place into an unknown and mysterious land.

These "authorial intentions" clearly had an important influence on the texts that were produced. Violetta Thurstan's was the only diary that went to press while the war was still in progress. Britnieva's text was published in

1934, during a prolific period of outputs relating to and reflecting on the war. It was during this time that many of the most famous First World War memoirs were produced, including those of Vera Brittain, Edmund Blunden, and Siegfried Sassoon.[31] It was a time of emotional outpouring. Farmborough's work was published much later than the other two, at a time when so-called second-wave feminism was flourishing, but the war was, perhaps, a more distant memory.

The photographs of the three nurses enhance our image of them as romantic heroines: they have ethereal looks and personae. All are small and slight but with apparent inner strength; our impression is of outward, apparent fragility with underlying toughness. Their perspectives on their nursing work, and on the strong moral code underlying it, are simple, clear, and uncompromising. All express gratitude that they were allowed to participate in the work of the Russian flying columns, which were clearly regarded as the elite units of Russian military health care during the war. Thurstan describes her excitement at the prospect of "going right into the thick of things," and her hope that "we should rise to the occasion and do the utmost that was expected of us."[32] In one episode of her diary, she describes her work in a forward field dressing station on a railway line, close to the trenches of Radzivilow during the 1915 retreat from Poland. The nurses were caring for their patients in total darkness, to avoid being seen by enemy artillery, and were using small torches to guide their work. Working for many hours without a break, they clearly demonstrated grit and toughness. Although Thurstan expresses excitement and the pleasure of being able to do what she sees as such important work, it is clear that working under such conditions for prolonged periods of time took great courage.[33] She describes a typical meal break in the dressing station:

> About four in the morning there was a little lull and some one made tea. I wonder what people in England would have thought if they had seen us at that meal. We had it in the stuffy dressing-room where we had been working without a stop for sixteen hours with tightly closed windows, and every smell that can be imagined pervading it, the floor covered with mud, blood and debris of dressings wherever there were not stretchers on which were men who had just been operated upon . . . Two dead soldiers lay at our feet—it was not safe just at that moment to take them out and bury them. People would probably ask how we *could* eat under those conditions. I don't know how we could either, but we *did* and were thankful for it—for immediately after another rush began.[34]

Nursing in a Russian flying column was clearly no place for the faint-hearted. Yet the authors of all three texts also viewed their role as a peculiarly feminine one. Britnieva describes how, during her dedication as a Red Cross volunteer nurse, Senator Koni, a member of the Russian Council of State, made a "brilliant and moving" speech in which he expressed the view that "a woman's calling in life was sometimes to heal, often to alleviate and always to comfort."[35] All three writers appear to have recognized these feminine elements of nurse's persona easily and without any sense of conflict. They saw their nursing work as, appropriately, women's work. They also saw it as divinely inspired. When Farmborough describes her first encounters with gruesome wounds in the Russian hospital where she trains, she explains that, at first, she and her fellow volunteers flinched from the horrors they saw. However, they quickly became tough, though she stresses that they did so without becoming hard:

> We are very raw recruits, and it is not surprising that we sometimes wince, even shrink into the background, when an unusually ugly wound is bared for dressing, or when a man's cry of anguish follows an awkward attempt to alleviate an excruciating pain. It is, however, astonishing how quickly even a raw recruit can grow accustomed, though never hardened, to the sight and sound of constant suffering. It is a special and merciful dispensation of God that, in time of great stress, both mental and physical, extra strength is given, with the ability *to do* and *to bear.*[36]

Eventually, she explains, she began to feel the "exultation" of active service, in which she believed herself to be in touch with "the intensity of life," experiencing "the urge to grapple with destiny, or to pit one's strength against a thousand ills."[37]

Farmborough perhaps more than Thurstan or Britnieva devotes a considerable amount of space in her published diary to subjects that form the very core of romantic philosophy: the nature of suffering, emotion, and the human spirit. In one evocative passage she describes a conversation with an army officer, who is in a state of despair:

> "No wonder," he said with a painful laugh, "no wonder that you don't recognise me, for I am not the same person that I was. I am not even I! The someone who was I has been rooted out for ever; I feel it, I feel the immense void. I cannot recognise myself, so how can I expect others to recognise me?" His voice broke. He was quite unnerved, I could see, and very near a collapse. I pitied him with all my heart. Gently, I led him into the yard. "No, Stephan Grigoriyevich," I said. "You must not despair; believe me, not one of us but is changed by this violent, abnormal life; it could not be otherwise. But behind it all, deep down within us, in perfect safety, is our true self—which can never change."[38]

Eventually, during the Russian advance of 1916, Florence's diary begins to express fear that she, too, will succumb to exhaustion and despair. She describes an episode in July 1916 in which she encounters in stark and gruesome terms the consequences of war:

> There are no on-duty or off-duty regulations now; all hands are needed. Amputations of arms and legs have been many; one leg was so heavy that I could not lift it from the table and, the orderlies being occupied, a Brother helped me carry it to the tiny shed where a stack of amputated limbs awaited burial. I had not been in that shed before and I turned away hastily; I went to our room, drank some water and swallowed two aspirins; the choking feeling disappeared and I was myself again. But my thoughts would not adjust themselves so easily: after the war, what would happen to these limbless men.... I began to wonder how long my physical strength would hold out under the heavy burden of these never-ending sorrows. And there seemed no end to these tragic days.[39]

Endurance, then, is seen as one of the most important qualities of the romantic nurse-heroine. Eventually, in August 1916, Farmborough succumbed to fever, fell dangerously ill and was transferred to a sanatorium in the Crimea, before returning to the front in December.[40] By September 1917 she was expressing disillusionment with her work, becoming "sick of wounds, illness, dirt and filth."[41] It came as a relief to her when she heard that the unit was soon to be disbanded.

Thurstan's perspective on nursing contains many similarities to Farmborough's. There is also, however, one important difference in her outlook. There is a greater pragmatism to her style, and a greater tendency to relate facts and insights as well as emotions. As a fully trained nurse, she is very interested in the differences between British nurses, Russian nurses, and volunteers. She comments that, although many of the Russian Sisters of Mercy she encountered were excellent nurses, their approach to their work was rather haphazard by comparison with that of British nurses.[42] Thurstan's comments on the work of Russian Nursing Sisters can be found mainly in chapter 7 of her diary, where she comments, in particular, that she was shocked at the way these nurses administered unprescribed medications without consulting or informing the doctors.[43] She can at times be scathing about the limitations of the semitrained or "war-trained" volunteers.[44] Her values and perspectives on war nursing are, nevertheless, very similar to those of Farmborough and Britnieva. One of the most compelling chapters in her book is her description of the retreat from Lodz, one of the many Polish cities that were overrun by the rapid German advance of 1915. She describes her own efforts, and those of her colleagues, to nurse patients in a squalid, run-down temporary hospital under enemy bombardment, capturing the courage and capacity for endurance of both staff and patients.[45]

The Romantic Epic Journey and the Romance of Russia

Among the most important qualities of 20th-century romantic fiction were its epic and folkloric elements. Extraordinary journeys take place, and these often act as allegorical mirrors for the *journey* of the human spirit through darkness and light.[46] Thurstan, Farmborough, and Britnieva all experienced such journeys, and the message is conveyed clearly in each memoir that the geographical journey mirrors the journey of the soul. The vast terrains of the Russian steppes and the mountainous regions and forests of Eastern Europe provide the backdrop to the horrors of war and the renewal—both physical and spiritual—of the flying columns' healing work.

There are times when all three memoirs read like travelogues. Britnieva's unit sets up hospital for a time in a palace belonging to a Polish prince. Teresino Palace, we are informed, was

> A real fairy palace with turrets and galleries, gleaming white and dazzling in the moonlight.... It appeared huge but was beautifully proportioned and seemed unreal in its sheer beauty amidst the perfect stillness and calm of the night. We stood spellbound.[47]

The language here is important in creating an effect: the idea of a "fairy palace" before which the nurses stand "spellbound" evokes a feeling of unreality, and convinces us that Britnieva and her colleagues have been transported by their nursing experience into a different world and a different life from their previous "ordinary" existence. The reader, too, has been invited to enter this world of spiritual archetypes: of emotions and experiences that are "beyond reality." In one episode, Britnieva's English friend Nelly has a dream in which a group of officer-friends are seriously gassed, with many fatalities. The dream is later identified as a premonition, when the nurses find themselves caring for their friends, helpless against the "fiendish" poisonous gas.[48]

Britnieva describes the beauty of the Eastern European and Russian countryside in summer: the "magnificent orchard [at Teresino] ... that yielded cherries and apricots in profusion ... the strawberries and the lovely roses."[49] During the retreat from Poland, in the summer of 1915, we are told,

> It was a beautiful sunny summer with an unchanging blue sky overhead and soft breezes moderating the heat; the fields were full of flowers, the dark forests cool and refreshing. On and on we went through the lovely smiling country, and when the time came for a halt a bonfire would be lit and our cooking would commence.

> How delicious were those meals in the open air! How we enjoyed every minute of our "campaign" retreat, often forgetting its tragic meaning.[50]

Both Farmborough and Britnieva describe in some detail the "moleben or Te Deum service,"[51] in which, having completed their Red Cross training with one of the Russian sisterhoods, volunteer nurses were presented with their insignia—a Red Cross badge worn on the chest and a brassard. Britnieva explains how the remarkable spirituality and aesthetic beauty of the Catholic ceremony evoked deep feelings in those participating:

> The simple service was very beautiful. . . . The lighted candles and the magnificent singing accentuated the solemnity of the service; tears of emotion dimmed the eyes of the Sisters and their relations and parents alike. I am quite certain that not one of us young women had ever before experienced such profound feelings of reverence, patriotism and enthusiasm, all in perfect harmony, as were evoked in us by this memorable service.[52]

Farmborough similarly describes the sense of awe and devotion with which the Red Cross trainees receive their insignia. She herself experiences "great contentment in mind and spirit." Later she receives a chain with a small cross and an icon from her "adoptive mother," and reflects, "I too was a soldier, going to war, for thus did all Russian mothers to their soldier sons."[53]

The religiosity of the Russian and Eastern European people is an important element in the three authors' descriptions of the spirituality they encountered. Thurstan describes a midnight mass she attended on Christmas Eve, 1914:

> Soon a young priest got up into the pulpit and gave them a little sermon. It was in Polish, but though I could not understand the words, I could tell from the people's faces what it was about. When he spoke of the horrors of war, the losses and the deaths and the suffering that had come to so many of them, one woman put her apron to her face and sobbed aloud in the tense silence. And in a moment the whole congregation began sobbing and moaning and swaying themselves to and fro. The young priest stopped and left them alone a moment or two, and then began to speak in a low persuasive voice. I do not know what he said, but he gradually soothed them and made them happy. And then the organ began pealing out triumphantly, and while the guns crashed and thundered outside, the choir within sang of peace and goodwill to all men.[54]

This sense of the innate spirituality of the Russian people is conveyed by Farmborough in another of her works—her *Russian Album*—when she describes one of the simple but reverent funeral ceremonies for the soldiers who died while under the care of the *letuchka*:

> The ceremony was simple: a coffin was made and the soldier laid to rest wrapped in a sheet and strewn with flowers. Our chaplain ... recites the beautiful old Slavonic prayers and the men reverently intone the ancient funeral dirge.[55]

Britnieva's own focus is, if anything, more spiritual—and more inherently Russian—than those of the other two writers. Her emphasis is on the spirituality of her patients, and one of her purposes in writing appears to be to convey to her readership an almost otherworldly sense of their engagement with trauma and death.[56]

Farmborough's published diary, more than any of the others, reads like an epic, romantic journey. In the Preface, she writes:

> I always knew that I should have to travel. The longing was strong within me from my earliest years.... My feet were restless with the urge to wander and my eyes strained after the veiled ways ahead, eager to behold all that wide, wonderful world held in store for me.... When I am asked: "Which land did you love most?" unhesitatingly, I answer: "Russia; because she taught me the meaning of the word 'suffering'."[57]

At the end of her story, Farmborough is obliged to travel by train across Siberia to escape the persecutions of the revolutionaries. Her description of the journey contains all the qualities of romance—epic adventure, survival of the human spirit, and a sense of connectedness with nature:

> As we gradually made our way across this mighty land of Siberia so, gradually, do my overwrought feelings find solace.... And strange though it may sound—Siberia is for me the greatest tonic of all. I begin to love this immense spacious land, with its wealth of weird and rare lineaments. I know that its very name conjures up torment for thousands of Russians but, I tell myself, that misery comes from the harassed people, not from the land; these wide, changeless spaces can bring only comfort and peace.... So it has come to pass that Siberia herself, the soothing saunter of our lazy locomotive and the slowly passing days and nights spent in the wide, open spaces, far from human habitations, have reacted upon me as a wholesome, bracing stimulus. There is an openness, a wideness, an emptiness about these immense stretches of flat land which make an instant appeal. I came immediately under their gentle influence. I can sense the marvellous undercurrent of peace which pervades earth and sky.[58]

The commonalities in the experiences of the three nurses are striking. All three experience adventure and danger, and their escapes are narrow. They face death; they also witness death. These elements of their writings form one important element of the epic journey—the encounter with death is the ultimate heroic encounter. All three visit the trenches. Britnieva sees the trenches near Wirballen at the invitation of doctors from a nearby field hospital. She and her fellow nurses experience the horror of war when they come across a number of corpses:

> There were five frozen bodies, they lay in their trench-coats, but the boots had been stolen by marauders. They were all in different crouching positions and it looked as if they had all crawled into one place. They were terrible to behold. Field-mice had made a nest in the head of one and they scuttled away under our feet.[59]

Thurstan describes how a Siberian captain took her and some colleagues to the front line trenches in Radzivilow. The visit, during an enemy action, is fraught with danger:

> We went through the wood silently in single file, taking care that if possible not even a twig should crackle under out feet, till we came to the very front trenches at the edge of the wood. We crouched down and watched for some time. Everything was brilliantly illuminated by the moonlight, and we had to be very careful not to show ourselves. A very fierce German attack was going on, and the bullets were pattering like hail on the trees all round us. We could see nothing for some time but the smoke of the rifles.... We stayed a while talking, and then crawled along to visit one of the men's dugouts, a German bullet just missing us as we passed, and burying itself in a tree.[60]

A feature common to all three memoirs is the writers' sense of the somewhat old-fashioned heroism and courtesy of the Russian soldiers, which is conveyed as a survival from a different era. Both Farmborough and Britnieva describe the "dog-like" devotion of some men for their officers: "blindly devoted ... ready for any sacrifice."[61] Thurstan describes the dedication of an officer's Cossack servant:

> The officer was quite a young, delicate-looking boy, who had been shot through the chest. His servant was a huge, rough Cossack, who would hardly let any of us touch his master if he could help it, and stayed by his bed night and day till the end, when, his great frame heaving with sobs and tears streaming down the seamed and rugged face, he threw himself over the officer's body and implored God to let him die too.[62]

This quality, Farmborough informs us, soon seems to disappear with the Revolution, as if the men are waking out of a dreamlike existence that had held them in feudal servility. Unfortunately, to Farmborough's dismay, this servile devotion is replaced by base opportunism. We are nevertheless left with the impression these writers have created of "splendid men, bronzed and stalwart ... unfailingly courteous and charming to us nurses."[63] We also have the sense that an old world is dying, and it is the older patients among those who are nursed who cling to its values. Thurstan describes one of her most aged patients:

> Another poor old fellow was brought in with nine wounds in the abdomen. He looked quite a patriarch with a long flowing beard—quite the oldest man I have seen in the Russian army. Poor Ivan, he had only just been called up to the front and this was his first battle. He was beautifully dressed, and so clean; his wife had prepared everything for him with such loving care, a warm knitted vest, and a white linen shirt most beautifully embroidered with scarlet in a [sic] intricate key-pattern. Ivan was almost more unhappy at his wife's beautiful work having to be cut than at his own terrible wounds. He was quite conscious and not in much pain, and did so long to live, even a week or two longer, so that he might see his wife once again. But it was not to be, and he died early the next morning—one of the dearest old men one could ever meet, and so pathetically grateful for the very little we could do for him.[64]

For these writers, Russia is an extraordinary and remarkable place, so different from the world they had previously known that it almost takes on the quality of a dreamworld. The women's adventurous lives also take on a dreamlike quality, as expressed in the following passage of Farmborough's:

> What an extraordinary world I was in! What a distorted side of life was teeming about me! What a monstrous scene enveloped me! Could it be I who, barely a year ago, was loitering along the tranquil, leafy lanes of the English countryside? But here, indeed, I was; walking in the darkness, at dead of night, down an unending, dusty road, trying to keep pace with the muffled tread of innumerable exhausted and footsore men, while behind us the cannon boomed and shrapnel crackled and exploded in the keen night air. From the great stretches of plain on either hand came the hoarse cry of some night-bird. The inflamed heavens told their pitiful story. One could sense the complete desolation of those burning towns, and villages. I saw them all and felt their weight.[65]

Thurstan also wrote of feeling that she was living in a dream world, far removed from reality:

> A shell burst quite close to us in the street, but no-one was hurt. These shells make a most horrible scream before bursting, like an animal in pain. Ordinarily I am the most dreadful coward in the world about loud noises—I even hate a sham thunderstorm in a theatre—but here somehow the shells were so part of the whole

> thing that one did not realize that all this was happening to *us,* one felt rather like a disinterested spectator at a far-off dream. It was probably partly due to want of sleep; one's hands did the work, but one's mind was mercifully numbed.[66]

Thurstan describes the hardships encountered by her flying column during the retreat from Warsaw. Having nursed the wounded in a makeshift hospital in an old theater at Skiernevice, the flying column was transported down the line by hospital train to Zyradow. Arriving at three o'clock in the morning during a heavy downpour, they wandered from place to place searching for accommodation. Eventually, they slept on the floor, all crowded into a single room at the Red Cross Bureau.[67]

Hardship, heroism, adventure, and romance fill the pages of these nurses' diaries, which are so extreme in their intensity, and so far removed from normal day-to-day life, that the authors themselves comment that they resemble dreams.[68]

The Romance of Nursing

Thurstan, Farmborough, and Britnieva portray their own stories as epic romances, yet their writings are at their most emotional and spiritual when they are talking about their nursing work. Nursing itself—certainly nursing in a theater of war—takes on a heroic quality. One of Thurstan's most emotional experiences appears to have been the retreat from Warsaw. For Farmborough, retreat and the necessity of leaving behind injured men is also agonizing.[69] Both Farmborough and Britnieva offer strikingly horrific descriptions of the difficulties and dilemmas they encountered with particular patients. One of Britnieva's most compelling passages describes the battle against death of one of her patients, Vassili, who had wounds in both legs and "septic poisoning." Amputation fails to arrest the sepsis, and the patient's condition deteriorates. Britnieva states that she will never forget this patient: "he fought so frantically with death, he so ardently wanted to live."[70] She describes his suffering in detail, along with his courage and patience in enduring it.

An important element of these memoirs is the way in which nursing is identified as a "heroic pursuit." All three authors probably achieve this impression largely unconsciously. None of them deliberately indulge in self-promotion. Nevertheless, the impression is conveyed that they are all extraordinary women with heroic qualities. Often, they describe how they are faced with "rushes" of injured men, who come to them straight from the battlefield, following a particularly fierce engagement, and have to cope for many hours with an unremitting workload:

> They came in groups, singly, on stretchers, in vans, battered and mutilated. We cared for them as best we could; God knows that our hearts were in our work, for we felt their agony, endured their despair and shared their misery.[71]

Thurstan describes a front-line hospital her flying column worked in briefly in Lodz, Poland as an "inferno." Her description is emotional yet precise:

> It was more like hell than anything I can imagine. The never-ending processions of groaning men being brought in on those horrible blood-soaked stretchers, suffering unimagined tortures, the filth, the cold, the stench, the hunger, the vermin, and the squalor of it all, added to one's utter helplessness to do more than a very little to relieve their misery, was almost enough to make even Satan weep.[72]

Although they never directly attribute heroic qualities to themselves (these are conveyed to the reader by inference) all three authors frequently describe their patients as "heroes," as in the following passage by Farmborough:

> Here was a man with half-a-dozen fatal wounds on his body and his strength of will is such that he can ask the time of day, the exact location of our Red Cross unit, even the latest news from his sector of the Front. And having received the answers, he turns his face to the wall and quietly surrenders his wounded body to Death. Is there in our language no greater, more laudatory word than "hero" for a man of this calibre?[73]

Farmborough's style seems at times to be consciously romantic. She skillfully juxtaposes passages in which the beauty of nature is contrasted with the horrors of the war:

> I went into the garden for half-an-hour this morning. It was a brief respite, but in those thirty minutes I had seen something which steadied my nerves and refreshed my mind. . . . It was the flowering beauty of the Austrian countryside. How strange that men should want to kill each other in springtime! . . . How monstrous that war can exist when all the world is in blossom! . . . More wounded had arrived. One look at them lying on the stretchers or on the grass, was sufficient to tell one that they were suffering intolerably and that many of them were dying. Doctors, Brothers and hospital orderlies gathered in full force and we worked hard and steadily for some hours. Fatal injuries to head, lungs or stomach predominated; several were dying on arrival.[74]

All three diarists attach a particular significance to their deathbed roles. Being with a patient as he dies is particularly important to them. Britnieva's patient Vassili, already mentioned, experiences a slow, tortured death from septicemia. She describes his experiences, and her witnessing of them, in terms of a morality tale. We are invited to admire the courage and spiritual purity displayed by both nurse and patient. Britnieva informs us that the patient's suffering was "almost intolerable," but that he bore it with "amazing patience, trying even to suppress his groans." Once he realized that he was dying, "an utter change came over him," and he expressed himself with "meekness" and "resignation," asking for paper to permit him to write a farewell letter to his wife, and for a priest to confess him.[75] After this,

> Vassili lay back on his pillows, his face radiant with joy. But soon his agony commenced. He became terribly restless as all septic patients do, tossing about from side to side, his twitching fingers clutching at the sheets and pillows, now praying aloud, now talking deliriously. "Put me down on the floor, Sestritza," he kept imploring me, "we are sinners and we must die on the ground." Greater and greater grew his agony. I had never seen anyone dying before and the feeling of my utter helplessness was terrible. . . . Suddenly he raised himself: "Hold me, Sestritza," he said in a frightened voice, "hold me tight, it is coming!" I put my arms around him, holding him up with all my strength. "Now kiss me, Sestritza," he said. I kissed him. Then slowly he made the sign of the cross, and in a few moments he was dead.[76]

There was an interesting sequel to this episode. The story takes a further romantic twist: Britnieva informs the reader that the head doctor of the unit, eventually to be her husband, fell in love with her because of the tearful emotion she showed during and after this episode.[77]

The quality of Eastern Front nursing that we are invited to admire most is the courage with which it is practiced. These nurses display an ability to continue working in the face of unimaginable horror. Farmborough more than the other writers is keen to bring those horrors to her readership, even as she emphasizes the importance of the nurses' stoicism and endurance:

> As we continued our journey, we passed more than one battlefield. . . . And there were lacerated, crushed bodies lying on darkly-stained patches of earth. There was one Austrian without a leg and with blackened, swollen face; another with a smashed face, terrible to look at; a Russian soldier, with legs doubled under him, leaning against the barbed wire. And on more than one open wound flies were crawling and there were other moving, thread-like things. . . . Those "heaps" were once human beings: men who were young, strong and vigorous; now they lay lifeless and inert; shapeless forms of what had been living flesh and bone. What a frail and fragile thing is human life! A bullet passes through the living flesh and it ceases to live. But a bullet cannot kill

> the soul; one knows, most assuredly, that the Spirit—God's breath in man—returns to God Who gave it. Oh! one *must* believe and trust in God's mercy, otherwise these frightful sights would work havoc with one's brain; and one's heart would faint with the depth of despair.[78]

The romantic battle of the soul against despair is significant here, as is the religious emphasis, probably at its strongest in the work of Farmborough. Her work is steeped in the culture of Russian Orthodox Christianity. Her religiosity intersects with her romanticism, enhancing its spiritual emphasis.[79] She frequently expresses love of the Russian temperament and spirit, yet she also comments on her own English qualities—particularly the ability to keep her feelings under control.[80] At the end of her diary she sums up her feelings about her work on the Eastern Front:

> As I pondered on all that had happened, in that great suffering Russia, my heart contracted with pain, and I felt that I could weep . . . and weep. . . . I prayed that those bitter-sweet wartime experiences of mine had not been in vain. And because sorrow and suffering teach great truths, I prayed too that I had learnt from them never to grumble; to be compassionate and merciful; and to recognise always, and try to alleviate, the sorrow in another human heart.[81]

Thurstan offers us a perspective that views participation in war on the Eastern Front as "High Adventure."[82] Her experience is altogether more pragmatic and secular than Farmborough's, yet it is still a Romance:

> War would be the most glorious game in the world if it were not for the killing and wounding. In it one tastes the joy of comradeship to the full, the taking and giving and helping and being helped in a way that would be impossible to conceive in the ordinary world. One has to die some time and the Russian peasants esteem it a high honour to die for their "little Mother" as they call their country. The vision of the High Adventure is not often vouchsafed to one, but it is a good thing to have had it—it carries one through many a night at the shambles.[83]

The diaries of Violetta Thurstan, Florence Farmborough, and Mary Britnieva contain all the qualities of epic romance. The life of the Eastern Front nurse, as it has been identified here, contains the characteristics of the romantic tradition of the West, infused with the religiosity and spirituality of early 20th-century Russia. Romance is to be found in the characters of the women themselves, with their capacities for heroism and humanity. It is also to be found in the vast splendors of the Russian and Eastern European landscapes. Above all, though, it is to be found in the practice of nursing. The romantic ideal is, for these writers, a core quality of nursing work, in which the practitioner displays courage, endurance, and virtue, not only through the hard physical work of caring for her patients but also in the capacity to stay with them on their bleakest, darkest, and most arduous spiritual journeys, even to the point of death.

The Eastern Front: Nursing as Epic Romance

Violetta Thurstan, Florence Farmborough, and Mary Britnieva saw nursing as a romantic pursuit in a way that went beyond the perceptions of other nurse-diarists—particularly those based on the Western Front. One important element of these writings is the existence of a powerful and markedly uncontrived moral code. All three authors appear to be adhering to what they see as a set of peculiarly Russian values. A modern audience may find some of what they write discomfiting. To modern Western eyes, these values seem at times to be naïve, possibly even deluded. Yet they are also compelling, representing, as they do, a lost era. Nursing appears to these writers to be a perfect expression of these values—humane, virtuous, and at times heroically dangerous.

All three diarists thus saw their lives during the war in terms of "High Adventure." Thurstan speaks for them all when she writes of "the life on the open road—with its joys and sorrows, its comradeship, its pain and its inexplicable happiness."[84] Yet the writings of all three—but particularly Farmborough and Britnieva—express deeper sentiments than these. They speak of the character and capacity for endurance of the nurses, and of their inherent spirituality.

Thurstan, Farmborough, and Britnieva were the heroines of their own stories. They lived epic adventures, the like of which most individuals—particularly early 20th-century women—only expected to encounter in romantic novels. And when they recounted their adventures they did so in romantic style, emphasizing the emotional and spiritual content of their experiences. They were justly proud of the way they had behaved; by their own standards, they had been hard-working, courageous, humane, and honorable. They often encountered despair, but never gave in to it. As far as I am aware, they never met, yet their stories, and their perspectives on those stories, are so remarkably similar that one is tempted to wonder if they were typical of the nurses and volunteers who served in the flying columns of the Russian army medical services. Whether typical or not, these women come across to a modern audience, via the media of their own published diaries, as extraordinary human beings—20th-century "romantic heroines."

Christine Hallett, PhD, BNurs, BA Hons, RGN, DN Cert, HV Cert
School of Nursing, Midwifery and Social Work
Coupland 3 Building
University of Manchester
Oxford Road
Manchester, M13 9PL
United Kingdom
00441612755577
Christine.Hallett@manchester.ac.uk

Notes

1. Marc Ferro, *The Great War,* trans. Nicole Stone (London: Routledge, 1973); A. J. P. Taylor, *The First World War* (1963; repr., Harmondsworth, UK: Penguin, 1966); Michael Howard, *The First World War* (Oxford: Oxford University Press, 2003); John Keegan, *The First World War* (London: Hutchinson, 1998), esp. chaps. 4 and 6; David Stevenson, *1914–1918: The History of the First World War* (London: Allen Lane, 2004). But see also the revisionist perspective of Gary Sheffield, *Forgotten Victory: The First World War: Myths and Realities* (London: Headline Books, 2002).

2. The classic text on the lasting impact of trench warfare on British culture is Paul Fussell, *The Great War and Modern Memory* (1975; repr., Oxford: Oxford University Press, 2000). One of the most evocative recent portrayals of trench warfare can be found in Richard van Emden, *The Trench: Experiencing Life on the Front Line, 1916* (London: Corgi Books, 2002). See also Taylor, *First World War.*

3. Keegan, *First World War,* 223–76; Howard, *First World War,* 49–58; on the Anzac campaign, particularly as it related to the work of nurses, see Ruth Rae, *Scarlet Poppies: The Army Experience of Australian Nurses During World War One* (Burwood, NSW: College of Nursing, 2004).

4. Keegan, *First World War,* chap. 5, 151–87.

5. The flying column and its purpose are described in Violetta Thurstan's published diary: Violetta Thurstan, *Field Hospital and Flying Column: Being the Journal of an English Nursing Sister in Belgium and Russia* (New York: G. P. Putnam's Sons, 1915), 125–27. It should be noted that the flying column Thurstan worked with appeared to be better-funded than most, and used automobiles rather than horsedrawn carts. This meant that there were limitations on where the column could go; there was a need to avoid rough terrain. For an overview of Western Front nursing, as a comparison, see Yvonne McEwen, *"It's a Long Way to Tipperary": British and Irish Nurses in the Great War* (Dunfermline, UK: Cualann Press, 2006). For army medical services on the Western Front, see Jeffrey Reznick, *Healing the Nation: Soldiers and the Culture of Caregiving in Britain During the Great War* (Manchester, UK: Manchester University Press, 2004).

6. Thurstan, *Field Hospital and Flying Column.*

7. Thurstan, *Field Hospital and Flying Column.* The passages describing Thurstan's work in Belgium can be found in chaps. 2, 3, and 4. Her capture by the Germans, and her subsequent journey to Denmark, and then via Sweden and Lapland to Russia, are recounted in chaps. 5 and 6.

8. On her work in Moscow and Warsaw, and her comments on Russian Sisterhoods, see Thurstan, *Field Hospital and Flying Column,* chaps. 6 and 7.

9. There are two editions of Farmborough's published diary: Florence Farmborough, *Nurse at the Russian Front: A Diary, 1914–1918* (London: Constable, 1974); Florence Farmborough, *With the Armies of the Tsar: A Nurse at the Russian Front in War and Revolution, 1914–1918* (New York: Cooper Square Press, 2000). The latter edition has been used for all citations in this article. Farmborough also publicized a heavily illustrated précis of her story, Florence Farmborough, *Russian Album, 1908–1918,* ed. John Jolliffe (Salisbury, UK: Michael Russell, 1988).

10. Farmborough, *With the Armies of the Tsar,* 40–45.

11. Mary Britnieva, *One Woman's Story* (London: Arthur Baker, 1934).

12. Britnieva, *One Woman's Story,* 10.

13. There are also unpublished diaries by British women who nursed in Russia. Perhaps because they were never reworked for publication, these diaries have a more pragmatic style than the published works this article focuses on. See The TS Diary of Miss K. Hodges, Imperial War Museum, 1974, 92/22/1; The MS Diary and Letters of Dorothy Cotton, Canadian Nursing Sister based in Petrograd, Library and Archives, Canada, http://www.collectionscanada.ca/nursing-sisters/025013–2200-e.html (accessed May 30, 2008).

14. Adele Lindenmeyer, "Public Life, Private Virtues: Women in Russian Charity, 1762–1914," *SIGNS: Journal of Women in Culture and Society* 38, no. 31 (1993): 362–72.

15. Tatiana S. Sorokina, "Russian Nursing in the Crimean War," *Journal of the Royal College of Physicians* 29, no. 1 (1995): 57–63; Evelyn R. Benson, "On the Other Side of the Battle: Russian Nurses in the Crimean War," *Image: Journal of Nursing Scholarship* 24, no. 1 (1992): 65–68; J. S. Blair, "The Russian Florence Nightingale," *Journal of the Royal Army Medical Corps* 149, no. 1 (2003): 79–80.

16. Mary Borden, *The Forbidden Zone* (London: William Heinemann, 1929); Rebecca West, *War Nurse: The True Story of a Woman Who Lived, Loved and Suffered on the Western Front* (New York: Cosmopolitan, 1930); Ellen la Motte, *The Backwash of War: The Human Wreckage of the Battlefield as Witnessed by an American Hospital Nurse* (New York: G. P. Putnam's Sons, 1916). See also Margaret Higonnet, ed., *Nurses at the Front: Writing the Wounds of the Great War* (Boston: Northeastern University Press, 2001). Other classic Western Front diaries include Vera Brittain, *Testament of Youth* (1933; repr., Glasgow: Fontana, 1978); Irene Rathbone, *We That Were Young* (1932; repr., London: Virago Press, 1988); Susan Mann, ed., *The War Diary of Clare Gass, 1915* (Montreal: McGill-Queen's University Press, 2000); Enid Bagnold, *A Diary Without Dates* (1918; repr., London: Virago Press, 1978). There were exceptions to these somewhat bleak portrayals. The Western Front diary of Olive Dent, for example, contains some of the romantic influences here attributed to Eastern Front nurses: Olive Dent, *A VAD in France* (London: Grant Richards, 1917). For a more general overview of British military nursing, see Ian Hay, *One Hundred Years of Army Nursing* (London: Cassell, 1953); Anne Summers, *Angels and Citizens: British Women as Military Nurses, 1854–1914,* rev. ed. (1988; repr., Newbury, UK: Threshold Press, 2000); Eric Taylor, *Wartime Nurse: One Hundred Years From the Crimea to Korea, 1854–1954* (London: Robert Hale, 2001).

17. Stephanie Lin, "Image (and) Nation: The Russian Exotic in 19th-Century French Travel Narratives," *Dialectical Anthropology* 27, no. 2 (2003): 121–39.

18. Alison Sinclair, "Spain's Love Affair With Russia: The Attraction of the Exotic (Br)others," *European Review of History: Revue Européenne d'Histoire* 11, no. 2 (2004): 207–24.

19. Steven Gary Marks, *How Russia Shaped the Modern World: From Art to Anti-Semitism, Ballet to Bolshevism* (Princeton, N.J.: Princeton University Press, 2003). See also Susan Layton, "The Search for the Primitive in Russian Literature: From Tolstoy to Pasternak," *Dialectical Anthropology* 4, no. 3 (1979): 179–203.

20. Classic examples would be William Blake's "The Tiger" (483); William Wordsworth's "Intimations of Immortality From Recollections of Early Childhood" (495–513); Samuel Taylor Coleridge's "Frost at Midnight" (524–25); and John Keats's "Ode to a Nightingale" (605–7). All page numbers are taken from Helen Gardner, ed., *The New Oxford Book of English Verse* (Oxford: Oxford University Press, 1972).

21. Keith Brindle, personal communication, May 2007.

22. Paul Keen, ed., *Revolutions in Romantic Literature: An Anthology of Print Culture, 1780–1832* (Toronto: Broadview Press, 2004); the author refers to the "profound mysteries of the human psyche" as these are portrayed in romantic philosophy (171). See also Heather Glen and Paul Hamilton, eds., *Repossessing the Romantic Past* (Cambridge: Cambridge University Press, 2006); Deborah Forbes, *Sincerity's Shadow: Self-Consciousness in British Romantic and Mid-Twentieth-Century American Poetry* (Cambridge, Mass.: Harvard University Press, 2004); Leon Chai, *Romantic Theory: Forms of Reflexivity in the Revolutionary Era* (Baltimore: Johns Hopkins University Press, 2006). These themes remain current in Western culture and have been taken up most recently by novelist Philip Pullman in the *His Dark Materials* trilogy, *Northern Lights, The Subtle Knife, The Amber Spyglass* (London: Scholastic, 2001). For commentary, see Millicent Lenz with Carole Scott, *His Dark Materials Illuminated: Critical Essays on Philip Pullman's Trilogy* (Detroit: Wayne State University Press, 2005).

23. Jane Austen, *Northanger Abbey* and *Persuasion* (1817; repr., London: Collins, 1980).

24. Keen, ed., *Revolutions in Romantic Literature,* 171; see also Keen's discussion of the influence of *bardic* and folkloric elements in Romanticism: "it implied a preference for primitive energy over refined elegance; and it suggested a concern with a popular rather than an elite cultural history" (171), and his interpretation of the rejoinders of writers such as Mary Wollstonecroft, who saw these perspectives as "artificial sentiment" (172). See also Jerome J. McGann, *The Scholar's Art: Literary Studies in a Managed World* (Chicago: University of Chicago Press, 2006). On the folkloric elements in Western culture, see also Jill Terry Rudy, with Diane Coll, eds., *William Albert Wilson: The Marrow of Human Experience: Essays on Folklore* (Logan: Utah State University Press, 2006).

25. As mentioned in note 22 romanticism can still be seen as an important and influential cultural medium, recent expressions being the 20th-century novels of C. S. Lewis, J. R. R. Tolkien, and Philip Pullman.

26. Fussell, *Great War*; Samuel Hynes, *A War Imagined: The Great War and English Culture* (London: Bodley Head, 1991); Jay Winter, *Sites of Memory, Sites of Mourning: The Great War in European Cultural History* (Cambridge: Cambridge University Press, 1995), esp. 2–8; Janet Watson, *Fighting Different Wars: Experience, Memory, and the First World War in Britain* (Cambridge: Cambridge University Press, 2004), esp. 1–13.

27. Claire Tylee, *The Great War and Women's Consciousness: Images of Militarism and Womanhood in Women's Writings, 1914–64* (Houndsmills, UK: Macmillan, 1990); Sharon Ouditt, *Fighting Forces, Writing Women: Ideology and Identity in the First World War* (London: Routledge, 1994); Angela Smith, *The Second Battlefield: Women, Modernism and the First World War* (Manchester, UK: Manchester University Press, 2000); Angela Smith, ed., *Women's Writing of the First World War* (Manchester, UK: Manchester University Press, 2000); M. R. Higonnet, J. Jensen, S. Michel, and M. C. Weitz, *Behind the Lines: Gender and the Two World Wars* (New Haven, Conn.: Yale University Press, 1987); Margaret Higonnet, *Lines of Fire: Women Writers of World War I* (Harmondsworth,UK: Penguin, 1999); Miriam Cooke and Angela Woollacott, *Gendering War Talk* (Princeton, N.J.: Princeton University Press, 1993); Ariela Freedman, "Mary Borden's 'Forbidden Zone': Women's Writing From No-Man's Land," *Modernism/Modernity* 9, no. 1 (2002): 109–24.

28. On women and romantic philosophy, see Roxanne Eberle, *Woman and Romanticism, 1790–1830* (London: Routledge, 2006); Bridget Fowler, *The Alienated Reader: Women and Popular Romantic Literature in the Twentieth Century* (Hempstead, UK: Harvester Wheatsheaf, 1991).

29. On hermeneutic approaches to interpretation, see H. G. Gadamer, *Truth and Method* (London: Sage, 1975); Tina Koch, "Implementation of a Hermeneutic Inquiry," *Journal of Advanced Nursing* 24 (1996): 174–84; Christine Hallett, "Historical Texts: Factors Affecting Their Interpretation," *Nurse Researcher* 5 (1997): 61–71. On discourse analysis, see Stefan Titscher, Michael Meyer, R. Wodak, and Eva Vetler, *Methods of Text and Discourse Analysis* (London: Sage, 2000); Michael Traynor, "Looking at Discourse in a Literature Review of Nursing Texts," *Journal of Advanced Nursing* 26 (2006): 1155–61.

30. On the debate whether the *sublime* quality in the romantic *hero* is viewed as exclusively male or related to female character, see Stephen Hancock, *The Romantic Sublime and Middle-Class Subjectivity in the Victorian Novel* (London: Routledge, 2005). On heroism and masculinity, see Graham Dawson, *Soldier Heroes: British Adventure, Empire and the Imagining of Masculinities* (London: Routledge, 1994).

31. Brittain, *Testament of Youth*; Edmund Blunden, *Undertones of War* (1928; repr., Harmondsworth, UK: Penguin, 1982); Siegfried Sassoon, *The Complete Memoirs of George Sherston* (1937; repr., London: Faber and Faber, 1952); Ernest Hemingway, *A Farewell to Arms* (1929; repr., London: Vintage, 1999); Richard Aldington, *Death of a Hero* (London: Chatto and Windus, 1930).

32. Thurstan, *Field Hospital and Flying Column,* 125.

33. Thurstan, *Field Hospital and Flying Column,* chap. 10, 161–67.

34. Thurstan, *Field Hospital and Flying Column,* 165–66.

35. Britnieva, *One Woman's Story,* 12.

36. Farmborough, *With the Armies of the Tsar,* 22.

37. Farmborough, *With the Armies of the Tsar,* 59.

38. Farmborough, *With the Armies of the Tsar,* 98.

39. Farmborough, *With the Armies of the Tsar,* 220.

40. Farmborough, *With the Armies of the Tsar,* 238–46.

41. Farmborough, *With the Armies of the Tsar,* 316.

42. Thurstan, *Field Hospital and Flying Column,* chap. 7.

43. Thurstan, *Field Hospital and Flying Column,* chap. 7, esp. 117–18. Thurstan also comments, however, on the remarkable dedication of the Russian nurses (118–19).

44. Thurstan commented, in particular, on the tendency for "war-trained" volunteers to fail to recognize the limitations of their own skill and knowledge: *Field Hospital and Flying Column,* 4–5, 23–24, 47, 120–21. On the tensions between trained nurses and VADs on the Western Front, see Janet Watson, "Wars in the Wards: The Social Construction of Medical Work in First World War Britain," *Journal of British Studies* 41 (2002): 484–510; Margaret Vining and Barton Hacker, "From Camp Follower to Lady in Uniform: Women, Social Class and Military Institutions Before 1920," *Contemporary European History* 10, no. 3 (2001): 353–73.

45. Thurstan, *Field Hospital and Flying Column,* chap. 8, "The Bombardment of Lodz," 128–43.

46. The folkloric elements in romantic fiction have been mentioned earlier; see note 24.

47. Britnieva, *One Woman's Story,* 27.

48. Britnieva, *One Woman's Story,* 33–36.

49. Britnieva, *One Woman's Story,* 34.

50. Britnieva, *One Woman's Story,* 40–41.

51. Britnieva, *One Woman's Story,* 9.

52. Britnieva, *One Woman's Story,* 9–10.

53. Farmborough, *With the Armies of the Tsar,* 28–30.

54. Thurstan, *Field Hospital and Flying Column,* 168–69.

55. Florence Farmborough, *Russian Album, 1908–1918,* ed. John Joliffe (Salisbury, UK: Michael Russell, 1979), 32.

56. This is particularly marked in the passage presented later in this article, in which Britnieva describes the death of her patient, Vassili; Britnieva, *One Woman's Story,* 18–20.

57. Farmborough, *With the Armies of the Tsar,* Preface.

58. Farmborough, *With the Armies of the Tsar,* 396–97.

59. Britnieva, *One Woman's Story,* 22.

60. Thurstan, *Field Hospital and Flying Column,* 172–74.

61. Britnieva, *One Woman's Story,* 32.

62. Thurstan, *Field Hospital and Flying Column,* 123.

63. Britnieva, *One Woman's Story,* 33.

64. Thurstan, *Field Hospital and Flying Column,* 162–63.

65. Farmborough, *With the Armies of the Tsar,* 56.

66. Thurstan, *Field Hospital and Flying Column,* 136.

67. Thurstan, *Field Hospital and Flying Column,* chap. 9, 144–60.

68. This dreamlike quality is a classic element of Western romantic fiction. See Anita O'Connell, *A Place of Vision: Romantic Dream Poetry and the Creative Imagination* (Durham, UK: University of Durham, 2006), passim.

69. Farmborough, *With the Armies of the Tsar,* 40–45.

70. Britnieva, *One Woman's Story,* 17.

71. Farmborough, *With the Armies of the Tsar,* 49. On the trauma encountered by nurses and others during the First World War, see Joanna Bourke, *Dismembering the Male: Men's Bodies, Britain and the Great War* (London: Reaktion Books, 1996); Santanu Das, *Touch and Intimacy in First World War Literature* (Cambridge: Cambridge University Press, 2005).

72. Thurstan, *Field Hospital and Flying Column,* 136–37.

73. Farmborough, *With the Armies of the Tsar,* 191.

74. Farmborough, *With the Armies of the Tsar,* 198.

75. Britnieva, *One Woman's Story,* 18.

76. Britnieva, *One Woman's Story,* 18–19.

77. Britnieva, *One Woman's Story,* 19–20.

78. Farmborough, *With the Armies of the Tsar,* 222.

79. For a further example of Farmborough's tendency to describe the suffering of patients, followed by a comment on the strength she draws from religious faith, see Farmborough, *With the Armies of the Tsar,* 277–79.

80. Farmborough, *With the Armies of the Tsar,* 327.

81. Farmborough, *With the Armies of the Tsar,* 408–9.

82. Thurstan, *Field Hospital and Flying Column,* 174.

83. Thurstan, *Field Hospital and Flying Column,* 174–75.

84. Thurstan, *Field Hospital and Flying Column,* 177.

Beyond the Glass Wall: Black Canadian Nurses, 1940–1970

Karen Flynn
African American Studies and Research Program, University of Illinois Urbana-Champaign

Abstract. Until the mid-1940s, young Black women who wanted to train as nurses in Canada were prohibited from doing so. The first cohort of Black Canadian registered nurses integrated Canadian nursing schools beginning in the early 1950s. I argue that despite entering an occupation that defined itself around Victorian ideals of "true womanhood," an archetype that excluded Black women, these nurses were able to negotiate and secure a place in the profession. This research not only contributes to Canadian nursing, it also situates Canada, with respect to scholarly discussions about the Black Diaspora.

> Back in the 1950s, they were not really accepting Black girls in nursing. I got into nursing because one of the principals was so kind and nice to me, and I had very good marks. When I got into nursing, I had no idea who my roommate would be, but there she was, another Black girl. I just felt that they didn't ask us who we wanted to room with. They just put us together because we were two Black girls. And I think that kind of set the tone for our whole three years. My roommate—her mother was White and her father was Black, so she had issues coming into nursing—but we got along fantastic. But she was always favored. She was fair, [had] long beautiful hair and you know my colour (laughs). It didn't matter to me. In the last year of nursing, they put another Black girl with us. The other Black girl definitely did not want to be there with us. She would dress in the closet . . . she didn't want to be with us. Other girls would have faded away, but I wasn't of that caliber. Nursing wasn't hard . . . there was some amount of segregation but nothing held me back.
>
> Agnes (Scott) Ellesworth[1]

In 1953, Agnes Scott and her roommate Dorothy Richards graduated from St. Joseph's School of Nursing at the Hotel Dieu in Windsor, Ontario. Prior to Scott and Campbell, only six Black nurses had graduated from the school. The fact that Dorothy (Richards) Scott was only the seventh Black nurse in the

Nursing History Review 17 (2009): 129–152. A Publication of the American Association for the History of Nursing.
DOI: 10.1891/1062–8061.17.129

history of the hospital was not coincidental. Canadian nursing schools had a history of excluding Black women from obtaining nurse training. Indeed, compared to other Canadian hospitals, Hotel Dieu stood out with respect to the number of Black students it admitted during the post-Second World War era. Between 1948 and 1961, 13 Black students graduated from its nursing program.

This article explores the complex subjectivities of the first cohort of Black Canadian registered nurses embodied in Agnes Scott Ellesworth's quote at the beginning. Relying primarily on oral interviews, a magazine short story, and nursing and nonnursing texts, I explore how Black Canadian-born nurses negotiated and secured a place in an occupation that defined itself around Victorian ideals of "true womanhood," an archetype that excluded Black women. I argue that Black Canadian nurses nevertheless capitalized on the opportunities nursing offered to carve out a satisfactory professional and personal life. Their ability to negotiate and secure a place in nursing was a result of several related factors: their commitment to and investment in the professional ideals of the occupation; their childhood experiences growing up in Canada; their awareness of the exclusionary practice of nursing; and a tacit acceptance of their role as trailblazers in tandem with their ancestral legacy.

The research presented here is part of a larger project in which I conducted interviews with Black Canadian and Caribbean nurses who trained in Britain, various Caribbean islands, and Canada. Born between 1929 and 1950 in Ontario, Nova Scotia, and Manitoba, all but two of the Black Canadian nurses I interviewed were trained in religious-based nursing schools.[2] The majority of the nurses found employment in Ontario hospitals. Three chose to work in the United States; the others all ultimately lived, worked, and retired in Canada. Keenly aware that they were among the first Black nurses, these young women entered an occupation that was organized on principles and ideals that reinforced White Canadian nurses' cultural hegemony. They trained and worked in homogeneous environments of White nurses, doctors, students, and administrators whose encounters and interactions with Blacks had been limited.

I chose to focus on this group of nurses partly to remedy the paucity of available scholarship,[3] but also because of the valuable information in their oral testimonies. Black Canadian nurses provide a unique perspective on constructions of race and gender. As a group, they disrupt the commonly held perception of Blacks as a monolithic category whose experiences are determined primarily by race. They also challenge the notion that because they are in a predominantly female occupation, they automatically share a commonality regardless of social location. Equally important is what Black

Canadian nurses reveal about nursing and the wider Canadian society. Their ancestors' struggle for justice and their own presence in Canada allow them to make claims to a form of national liberalism about their rightful place as both nurses and Canadians. Finally, excavating Black Canadian nurses' subjugated knowledge,[4] while highlighting the specificity of their experiences, not only complicates the category *nurse,* but also reveals much about claims to professionalism, social space, and place.

The Development of Canadian Nursing

The development of nursing as a profession for middle-class White women was inextricably linked to Victorian ideals of respectability and femininity that culminated in an occupational hierarchy based on gender, socioeconomic status, and racial difference.[5] Black women were not the only group of women excluded from nursing. Other women of color and White working-class women also did not fit the image of the "proper" nurse that nursing leaders promoted for the profession. Working-class White women, however, could possibly be assimilated into middle-class respectability; Black women and women of color had a more difficult time. Bolstering the professional image of the occupation was more important to nursing administrators than addressing its discriminatory legacy. Indeed, nursing administrators were hardly the vanguard of fighting against discrimination in nursing. Many were unable to extend the "ethic of care," purported to be one of the core values of nursing, to their non-White sisters. This position was most reflected in some nursing administrators' inability to advocate for young Black women who wanted to train as nurses.

Nursing leaders had a strong investment in maintaining White privilege in the occupation, including defending the exclusionary policy maintained by nursing schools. A 1940 letter by Arthur C. Moore to Mr. G. Roberts, president of the Toronto Coloured Liberal Association, is quite telling.[6] Moore's daughter wrote Toronto General Hospital (TGH), told them she was "coloured," and requested an application. According to Moore, his daughter received a letter stating there were no vacancies at TGH, and she never received the application. According to Moore, "She wrote them again using another name, [her own name in Spanish] and another address. They replied saying call at the hospital for an interview." It is unlikely that the young woman contacted the hospital, given that the Association president wrote a letter to Minister of Health Harold Kirby on behalf of her father.

No response from Kirby exists, but a letter from Miss A. M. Munn, director of nurses' registration, to Dr. B. T. McGhie, deputy minister of health, objected to a proposal to establish a separate nurses' training school for Black women. Munn stated that "the Negro population of Toronto would hardly justify the establishment of a separate training school."[7] She neither advocated separate training schools for Black nurses nor supported their working in hospitals with White nurses, patients, and doctors. According to her, "The Superintendent of any general hospital must keep in mind the reaction of patients to nurses in training, and there would no doubt be many protests from patients and doctors if coloured nurses were introduced into the wards."[8] She further asserted that "training schools were established in the United States for this reason." White nurses' racism and their relentless campaign for professionalization through standardizing the curriculum and controlling admission requirements and state licensing,[9] all of which had an adverse impact on Black nurses in the United States, were never mentioned. Mann's refusal to admit Black women to train as nurses was couched in the need to serve the interests of White doctors and patients.

Unfortunately, such attitudes were common, as is reflected in archival documents regarding the migration of Anglo-Caribbean and Haitian nurses to Canada. The postwar era was turbulent for the Canadian health care system, and that turbulence was intensified by the shortage of nurses that persisted through the 1950s and 1960s. Ignoring urgent demands for hospital staff nurses, immigration officials relied on century-old stereotypes of Blacks as lazy and dishonest to deny entry to Caribbean and Haitian nurses.[10] Regrettably, these decisions were often supported by nursing administrators who shared similar attitudes. At the same time, while nursing leaders were reticent about Black nurses working alongside doctors and caring for patients, they did not all reject outright Black women's desires to train as nurses. Even Mann believed that Black nurses could train in Canada as long as they returned to their "land."[11] She was obviously not referring to native-born Black Canadian nurses. Other nursing administrators accepted Caribbean migrant nurses and students on the condition that their qualifications were above average. In Quebec a nursing administrator in a memorandum to immigration officials explained that "if a coloured nurse or nursing assistant succeeds and graduates, she usually has outstanding qualifications which make them very recommendable."[12]

Contemplating the thought of a disproportionate number of Black women working in hospitals perturbed nursing personnel such as Miss Weir, director for Mount Sinai Hospital. In dialogues with immigration officials about Caribbean nurses, Weir echoed the Canadian Nursing Association proclamation "that there is no discrimination whatsoever, and if the person is acceptable she is registered without regard to race or creed."[13] Yet the officials reported that "Miss Weir confidentially stated the hospitals desire to maintain a considerable majority of white nurses on staff."[14] Indeed, Black female bodies on the wards working alongside White doctors and nurses simultaneously threatened the homogeneity of the occupation, White privilege, and whiteness.

Whether as loyalists, free people, and fugitive slaves who escaped to Canada from the United States before, during, and after slavery, or later as migrants in the mid-20th century, Black people's lives were circumscribed and dictated by institutional, systemic, and everyday forms of racism. Black and Caribbean people, regardless of the time period, chose resistance over acquiescence as they responded to the myriad forms of oppression that affected them individually and collectively. Individuals such as Pearline Oliver in Halifax, Nova Scotia, who wanted to be a nurse but feared rejection, and organizations such as the Nova Scotia Association for the Advancement of Coloured People (NSAACP) and Canadian Negro Citizenship, campaigned tirelessly, quietly, and eventually challenged the racially exclusionary policies of nursing schools, as well as those of Citizenship and Immigration Canada. Individual Caribbean nurses and potential students whose applications were rejected by Citizenship and Immigration Canada also appealed to the state and Black organizations hoping to get their rejections reversed.[15] The Canadian Nursing Association declared in 1944 "that there be no discrimination in nursing,"[16] but this formal elimination of racist barriers did not erase the structures of White privilege that were embedded in the occupation. Through the 1960s, nursing as a site of White privilege continued to be acknowledged in various media.

Nursing Image, Whiteness, and Representation

Popular culture scholar Julia Hallam contends that "White middle-class images of femininity that represent[ed] nursing and nurses in popular fiction and recruitment literature throughout the postwar period were not only representative of professional ideals and practices but also constitutive of those ideals and practices."[17] As Black women entered the profession, concerns about professional image and identity registered in popular cultural forums. In 1964, Sheila Mackay Russell published a short piece of fiction in *Chatelaine* called "The Glass Wall," which captured the imagined anxiety that administrators, staff, and students felt around hiring a Black nurse "for a key post on the faculty of nursing" at the fictional Civic General Hospital.[18] After much debate, the protagonist Lydia Sanford was reluctantly hired, much to the delight of her friend Julie Matthews, who chose to emphasize Sanford's qualifications rather than her skin color. Despite Sanford's impeccable qualifications, she found Civic General an uncomfortable environment, in which her colleagues avoided her or pretended she was invisible. The students made jokes that portrayed Blacks as barbaric, even as they admitted that Sanford was the best instructor they had ever had.

Russell's story aptly summarizes the central anxieties of White colleagues and administrators. In discussing whether Sanford will fit in, one instructor sums up her feelings to a colleague in the following manner: "Being brilliant isn't enough for the job she'll be stepping into. You know how students tend to regard the senior employees of the faculty as the ultimate in the professional image. Well I don't see how they can identify with Lydia Sanford. She just doesn't fit the image."[19] This image of the professional nurse, however fluid, contested, and historically specific, encompassed the characteristics of White femininity and womanhood, and was connected to middle-class White women's complicity in the domination of non-White women. It drew on the gender ideology of the 19th century that reserved the title *ladies* for White women, a status that was impossible to attain for Black women, even if they tried. Indeed, in the 20th century, the question was not about Black nurses' respectability but about their leadership capabilities. As I discuss later in this article, some Black Canadian nurses attested that a similar discourse resonated in nursing, that, regardless of qualifications, their ability to teach or provide care was, and to some extent still is, scrutinized by peers, patients, students, and administrators.

The image of the "Other" exemplified by Russell's fictional heroine has perpetually preoccupied White scientists, academics, journalists, and reporters in both Canada and the United States.[20] Nursing was no exception from this deep concern about image—its own and that of the "Other." A short news piece in *Canadian Nurse* by Suzanne Lego, entitled "White Nurse Can Help Negro Change Self-Image," referred to conditions in the United States, but it must have struck the editors as appropriate and valuable for a Canadian publication.[21] The article focused on a 1966 presentation to the American Nurses Association by Lego, a well-known and respected instructor in the Advanced Program in Psychiatric Nursing at Rutgers University, who positioned herself as an authority on the genetic composition and psyche of Blacks, and as well versed in Black culture and family. These institutions, she asserted, "[give the Negro] a self-image ... [of] feelings of inferiority and dependency." White nurses had a special calling in addition to administering patient care—they could also assist Blacks with their inferiority complex. For Lego, "the White nurse taking care of a Negro patient might have been able to give him more than valuable nursing care—[she] might have helped him improve his self image." The White nurse demonstrating to the Black patient that she had high expectations of him "allowed room for growth or development of potential." Lego further urged White nurses to "consider the Negro as an equal with the same capabilities for growth and development of potential as any other human being."

Lego's seemingly benign gesture spoke to White liberalism, which did not reflect the fear and contagion generally associated with Black male bodies. Missing from her assessment, however, was the way ideological, systemic, and institutionalized forces of racism operated to circumscribe Black lives. For her, Black culture and family, not White supremacy, was the culprit for Black patients' negative self-image. In the end, the Black patient was viewed as childlike, docile, and dependent, the very same racist images against which Black Canadians lobbied. Furthermore, the tone of the article reflected the paternalistic and maternalistic attitudes typical of some White men and women, which were extended toward Blacks in general, not just those who were sick. Indeed, Lego's explanation cannot be considered only an American phenomenon, as historian Kathryn McPherson explains in reference to White Canadian nurses, who were expected to "serve as role models for their social 'inferiors,' such as immigrants and non-Whites."[22] Taken together with Russell's story, Lego's analysis speaks to issues connected to identity formation and representation in nursing.

A closer examination of the article and Lego's presentation gestures to the formation of White racial identity and the privileging of Whiteness in nursing. Beginning in the late 19th century, nursing leaders in North America and Britain lobbied tirelessly to establish nursing as a White, middle-class, female occupation associated with respectability and gentility.[23] Additionally, nurses relied on images of "White femininity with its cultural associations to chastity [and] purity," which were often linked to Christian virtues and morals.[24] Victorian notions of femininity were used, on the one hand, to exclude some women from nursing, but, on the other hand, also to legitimize the occupation within the medical field and as a response to medical doctors' hegemony. The 19th-century racialist discourse of non-Whites as dirty and contaminated also reverberated in nursing, and was reworked to fit the context of later periods. Unlike the category of *Blackness, Whiteness* for Lego was universalized, normative, and legitimate. By using the social marker *White* to identify particular nursing groups, Lego and others like her participated in privileging *Whiteness* and all that it embodies. In theory, only White nurses possessed the capacity not only to cure, care, and heal, but also to serve as mentors to Black patients. With the White nurse serving as the epitome of *White* values, the Black patient was then supposed to emulate Whiteness and all that it signified. British professor of film studies Richard Dyer notes in his provocative article "White":

> Power in contemporary society passes itself off as embodied in the normal as opposed to the superior. This is common to all forms of power, but it works in a particularly seductive way with Whiteness, because of the way it is rooted in common sense thought ... there are inevitable associations of White with light, and therefore with safety.... Socialized to believe the fantasy, that Whiteness represents goodness and all that is benign and non-threatening, many White people assume that is the way Black people conceptualize Whiteness.[25]

The idea that Black patients might reject being cared for by White nurses due to their racism exposes the normative and commonsense assumption about *Whiteness.* Equally significant is how Lego's indexing of Whiteness eclipsed Black nurses' own capacity to care, to cure, and, in the case of the fictional Lydia Sanford in Russell's story, to teach.

In his classic work *The Wages of Whiteness,* historian and critical Whiteness scholar David Roediger explores the investment White workers have in Whiteness, even though as a category it is historically specific and unstable. Roediger elucidates the implications of White workers' identification with Whiteness in relation to how they see themselves and those designated as "Others." He points out that "White workers could, and did, define and accept their class position by fashioning identities as 'not slaves' and as 'not Blacks.'"[26] Although Roediger focuses on the 19th century, his argument is useful in thinking about the development of Canadian nursing. Notwithstanding that White nurses were not always as explicit in claiming their White skin privilege as the working-class immigrant men Roediger discusses, their collusion in linking nursing identity to Whiteness is not negated. It is exemplified not only in fiction such as Russell's "The Glass Wall," but in the actual responses of nursing leaders. Whether intentionally or not, educators such as Lego and administrators like Mann, in different contexts, both privileged and reified Whiteness as the norm.

Nor were nursing leaders alone in maintaining and perpetuating such images of Whiteness and Blackness. Nursing students participated in their own popular forms of reinforcing White privilege through stereotyping Blacks. As shown the 1967 issue of *The Pulse,* the Atkinson School of Nursing yearbook, White nurses painted their faces black to perform in a minstrel show entitled "This Is Vaudeville."[27] This late 19-century American form of entertainment was presented despite the visible presence of Black nurses on staff. Minstrel shows were popular forms of entertainment in a number of Canadian churches during the mid-20th century, much to the consternation of community activists such as Stanley Grizzle, president of the Canadian Pacific Railway Division of the Brotherhood of Sleeping Car Porters, and Donald Moore, president of the Negro Citizenship Association. Whites in general viewed performances such as "This Is Vaudeville" merely as amusements.[28] As audiences sat passively absorbing blackface entertainment, they were being schooled about racial identity, including their own.

Hallam further asserts that "imaginary constructions have social implications; they are not only 'fictions' of the material world; they mediate dominant ideals and values, creating insecurity and doubt, and even fear."[29] For Grizzle, minstrel shows "perpetuated the stereotypes cherished in the minds of many White people."[30] The audiences, he continued, "have never suffered from prejudice and discrimination to understand the humiliation caused by childish forms of entertainment involving minority groups." The minstrel performance cannot be viewed as an isolated or innocent incident, but must be understood within the context of nursing and of how Black people were viewed in the larger Canadian society. Furthermore, the examples about White privilege and Whiteness illustrate the extent to which nursing leaders attempted to define nursing based on their own cultural values, beliefs, and practices. It is on this racialized terrain that Black Canadian nurses would subsequently enter nurse training and work.

Formation of Racialized Identity During Childhood

To understand how and why Black Canadian nurses positioned themselves within the nursing profession necessitates an exploration of their childhood experiences. The encounters with race and racism these women had growing up not only influenced how they navigated the racially hierarchical world of nursing, but contributed to the development of their subjectivities in relation to nurse training and work. As children, these nurses were subjected to legal ordinances that often created separate facilities for Blacks and Whites. White children were able to go to restaurants and movie theaters at will.[31] Black children were excluded from entering these spaces; moreover, some schools were also segregated. Marlene Watson, who grew up in Panuke, Nova Scotia, explained that "we had a White school for juniors from Kindergarten through to grade 8, and there was a Black school down in the plains from Kindergarten to grade 8."[32] She pointed out, however, that the town where she grew up was somewhat unique; despite the existence of separate general stores and other facilities for Whites and Blacks, it was a predominantly Black community with some White families. Moreover, some Blacks and Whites were willing to cross racial boundaries. As a child, Watson played with White children, but she explained that "in a sense it was terrible in that we played together after school, and before school, and when we got down to Panuke Road in the morning, I went right and they went left to our separate schools because that was the way things were at the time." Laura Tynes described Kentville, Nova Scotia, where she grew up, as a "poor rural area." Despite a shared socioeconomic status with Whites, Tynes pointed out "there was a good deal of prejudice in Nova Scotia, and we were restricted as to where we could go, like you couldn't go to certain restaurants."[33]

The recollections of Virginia Travis are even more salient. She recalled that her upbringing in Dresden, Ontario, was marred by a number of incidents common in a "White community that had racist attitudes."[34] In contrasting the contradictory nature of the public, which was sometimes hostile, with the supportive environment of home, church, and community, Travis pointed out that "it was difficult to assess how you were treated as a child, when you knew there was a difference in how you were treated publicly."[35] According to H. R. Burnett, secretary of the National Unity Association of Dresden, an interracial antiracist organization, "school children learn about Jim Crow before they learn to read and write."[36] They also learned, he continued, "that it [was] all right to go to the Girl Guides or Boy Scouts together, but it [was] not all right to go for ice cream or soda pop together." On one occasion, three children aged five to seven "went to a restaurant for ice cream and the waiters not only refused to serve them, they just stood there looking at them." Unfortunately, the Racial Discrimination Act adopted by Ontario in 1944, which "prohibits the publication or display, on lands, premises, by newspaper or radio, of any notice, sign, symbol, emblem, or other representation indicating racial discrimination,"[37] was not applicable to public spaces. As educators Ken Alexander and Avis Glaze pointed out, "most areas of concern to Blacks fell under provincial jurisdiction."[38]

While Black communities across Canada were embroiled in various battles concerning unequal treatment meted out toward Blacks, Dresden, Travis's hometown, was characterized as more racially segregated than most.[39] The extent to which Blacks experienced discrimination there led commentators to compare Dresden to *Dixie,* the colloquial term for the southern United States. Together with labor unions, local Blacks joined forces with the Joint

Committee for Human Rights, the Brotherhood of Sleeping Car Porters, the United Auto Workers, the Canadian Jewish Congress, and the Toronto Association for Civil Liberties, and took their case to the Ontario government. The efforts of these groups working toward social justice and equity resulted in the 1954 Fair Accommodation Practices Act to "protect the rights of citizens against discrimination in public places."[40] Despite obvious problems with the legislation, the Act was considered a victory, given that White Dresden residents in 1949 voted in a referendum against the issue of "non-discriminatory licensing . . . by a vote of 517 to 108." Of course, restaurants continued to refuse service to Blacks until one restaurateur was successfully charged under the Act. Still, Travis remembered the lobbying efforts of those who made the Act a reality and how the landmark decision was a proud moment for Dresden's Black residents. "I had an awareness of this all growing up; this was not unique to me," she stated.

Similarly, Frieda Steele, who grew up in Windsor, recalled always being aware of racism. "I remember going to a restaurant [with her family] on our main street with another couple and being refused. That was a horrible experience for me because I never experienced my father being powerless before."[41] Steele's father, Alton C. Parker, who later became Windsor's first Black uniformed officer and Canada's first Black detective, was active in fighting for racial justice. He was a member and was once Vice-President of the Central Citizens Association of Windsor, a group of citizens committed to advocating for full citizenship rights for Black people.[42] In fact, on a visit to Dresden, Travis's hometown, Parker arrived in time at a restaurant where "four or five Black men, who were refused service . . . decided to serve themselves. The Dresden police were called," but it was Parker who "managed to get things under control."[43]

There were, of course, some variations in the childhood experiences of these nurses. Born in Winnipeg during a period when formal discriminatory policies were slowly being eliminated, Darlene Barnes's experience of racism growing up was relegated to racist name-calling. She explained that her peers were afraid of her because she could "out-run, out-climb, and fight as well as any boy. I had a twin brother, and I was as tough as he was. We would smack someone if they called us a name, and they never called you nigger again."[44] Barnes's experiences with racism began mostly in elementary and high school. She went to a private Catholic school and left because she believed the nuns "were racist." During one class, Barnes claimed that she "kicked up a storm" because the teacher was unable to understand "why the slaves wanted their freedoms, because they had free medical care, free clothing, free housing and free food." Barnes attempted to explain to the teacher why freedom was important to the slaves, but the teacher felt she acted out of line. According to Barnes, "I caused a riot in the classroom; they were going to call my parents. I said, 'If you think I'm terrible to deal with, wait until my father gets here. He'd like to know what you are teaching.' "[45] Barnes was kicked out of class, and her parents enrolled her in public school. Overall, though, Barnes believed that her childhood was great.

In preparing Black children to survive the inequities they encountered, the institutions of the family and the church were crucial, even when they did not explicitly discuss the pernicious effects of racism. Some parents instilled a sense of racial pride in their children; others repeatedly affirmed to their children how unique and important they were as individuals. These strategies would become critical in helping children make the transition into adulthood. Barnes's father had migrated to Canada from the United States to escape racism, only to find that Canada was not the haven he had envisioned. As a result, Barnes maintained, "He talks about Canada as if Canada was no better than the United States, and it wasn't. They had the same Whites-only restaurants. Canada truly wants the world to believe that racism does not exist here, that it was an American thing. But guess what, it was blatant as hell in this country." Barnes's father was also a member of the Brotherhood of Sleeping Car Porters. "He was a union person and was very outspoken, very vocal. I learned a lot from him. I learned a lot about intolerance." These childhood memories were part of the formative years for Black Canadian girls. Barnes and her earlier predecessors drew on these early lessons to deal with inequities. These young Black Canadians brought these lessons along with their own coping mechanism, when they entered nurse training.

Once Black nurses entered training and the workplace, how did they negotiate their lives as students and workers? What bonds, if any, were forged between Black and White nurses? Here again, Russell's fictional narrative of Sanford's position as the only Black woman on the staff of "Civic General" is instructive. In trying to convince her colleagues why Sanford would not have any difficulty working at the Civic due to her race, Julie Matthews had offered the following explanation: "Difficulties are nothing new to Lydia Sanford.... To prove her equality; she has had to know more and work harder than everybody else all her life."[46] The nurses in this study would certainly concur with such an assessment. As children, their parents inculcated in them the idea that they would have to work harder than Whites. In addition, they entered training aware of the occupation's exclusionary history. Some had heard stories of young women who were denied training and had to go to the United States. One nurse pointed out that being admitted to nursing was contingent on having a family member admitted as well.

Even though they entered nursing school with memories of unequal treatment growing up and had an arsenal of strategies to deal with unpleasant encounters, some nurses were surprised and expressed disappointment that the residences were segregated. Drawing a parallel to the biblical story of Noah who boarded the ark with two of each kind of animal, they pointed to the "unofficial" policy of nursing schools that admitted only two Black nurses at a time. Tynes states, "There were only two Black nurses that went into training before my cousin and I went. You had to have another Black person to room with you. They wouldn't allow you to room with a White person. It was very bad."[47] Similarly, when Steele entered training at Hotel Dieu in Windsor in 1947, she observed that "there were two [Black] students in training when I entered."[48] Except for one, all Black students in residence had Black roommates. Some claimed this was a deliberate choice on the part of nursing administrators who feared that they might be isolated and shunned by their White counterparts. For Ellesworth, White administrators were more concerned with protecting White students. "They put us together, and we stayed in the dormitory. If there were any Blacks, they would put them by themselves. I could have lived with Whites, but they couldn't have lived with me."[49] Yet, this unfortunate reality did not deter the student nurses, as I have demonstrated above; their experiences growing up had prepared them to deal with any inequities they faced.

Equally significant is the nurses' own acceptance of, and belief in, the tenets of the profession. As I have argued elsewhere regarding Caribbean migrant nurses,[50] Black Canadian nurses were invested in both symbolic and real gender-specific ideals about nursing that were propagated by their communities, popular culture, and churches, as well as by the occupation once they entered it. They believed that nurses had a special calling to heal and care, and embraced the core principles of nursing explicated in the 1967 Atkinson School of Nursing yearbook:

> She is judged not by her race or religion, or social standards, she is measured by her professional yardstick that measures her ability to make a bed, apply a bandage, or sacrifice her time to ease the pain of a patient simply for the satisfaction of a job well done. She is a hardworking, determined young girl doing her best for her school and hospital.[51]

Although this statement was written more than two decades after the majority of the nurses in this project started training, these nurses believed in and espoused the core values it mentions. Perhaps as a result, they had few concerns about the structure and regimentation characteristic of nurse training.

Black Canadian nurses accepted the rigid hierarchy, discipline, long hours, and hard work that were endemic to the environment in which they trained, regardless of social identity and location. Nurses formed bonds based primarily on their status—first as probationers (the colloquial *probies*), then as juniors, and eventually as graduates. Throughout the three years, they learned the skills, with special emphasis on bedside care, that led them to realize their dreams to become full-fledged professional nurses.

Ellesworth began her training at Hotel Dieu in 1953. A typical day, she stated, began around 6:00 A.M., with prayers followed by breakfast. The trainees then proceeded to the wards. Ellesworth pointed out that "We worked very hard. We had to do a lot of the menial work. We did bedpans, we were really hands on. We were doing a lot of the work that nurses do not do today. We had to cook and serve the breakfast. We made the beds and served the medications. We were trained quite well."[52] She took pride in her training as it prepared her to provide optimal care for her patients. Nurses like Ellesworth lament the bedside and practical training missing from contemporary nursing.

Likewise, Travis began training at the Public General Hospital in Chatham, Ontario, in 1954. She summed up her three years of training in the following manner:

> As a student nurse you were up early. You went to breakfast, went to Chapel, and then you had to be on the unit at 7:00 A.M. It was hands-on experience integrated with classroom experience. The first few weeks were in class and we toured different sections of the hospital. Within a few months we were on the units doing clinical practice as a probationer. We took temperatures, made beds, baths, and monitored patients after surgery.[53]

These nurses were fully cognizant that students' unpaid labor contributed to the smooth functioning and maintenance of the hospitals. Commenting on the rigidity, strictness, and lack of remuneration, Tynes, who also began training in the 1950s, at the Isaac Walton Killam Hospital in Halifax, Nova Scotia, categorically stated that "[the hard work] didn't do us any harm; it made us into strong women."[54] However menial the tasks, the nurses found immense satisfaction in their capacity to do the work they were assigned.

Except for Barnes, who was the youngest of the nurses interviewed and who trained in Britain, none of the nurses recalled experiencing overt forms of racism from their colleagues during training. By and large, they attributed any hints of racist attitudes to limited knowledge about and lack of interaction with Blacks on the part of Whites. In their experience, when White nurses realized that they shared aspirations and goals with their Black counterparts, they were less likely to react in racist ways.

More common was patient-nurse racism, and again, the nurses attributed the problem to an absence of opportunity for cross-cultural relations. Patients' family members also expressed surprise when they encountered the few Black nurses working on the wards. Ellesworth noted that the typical reaction of parents when they met her on the obstetrics ward was to express surprise that there were any Black nurses working there. She simply responded "Here I am."[55] An occupational identity based on rigorous training and harsh discipline made the very few Black nurses who entered training in the late 1940s and 1950s feel included. This is not to say that notions about race and Whiteness failed to permeate the social organization and social relations of nursing. Still, the few Black nurses who worked alongside White nurses often subsumed any possible racial tensions to forge bonds that continue until the present. For these nurses, it appeared that their joint subjugated status as students partially superseded a focus on racial issues.

Indeed, Steele fondly remembered the nurses she trained with at Hotel Dieu:

> We encouraged and discouraged each other from quitting when the going got rough. We knew each other's families and boyfriends. I think our method of training melded us together. One girl told me that she would never talk to Blacks until she met us [Steele her roommate Cecile Wright]. She was ripped of all the stereotypes and rumors. She had no real experience to compare [all the rumors and stereotypes to]; we became fast friends and remain friends throughout.[56]

The friendship and camaraderie Steele discussed was visible in the reaction of her peers to an incident that took place on the night they graduated. Steele and Wright were asked by the proprietor of the banquet hall where the graduation party was being held to leave the premises. According to the reporter who interviewed Steele and Wright, "the request came after the party was in progress. No reason was given, they said, but they considered the reason obvious and departed without informing their 46 classmates as to the real cause."[57] Their classmates, oblivious to the fact that the only two Black students were not at the party, told reporters following the incident that, had they been privy to the details of why the nurses were asked to leave, "they would have staged a mass walkout."

Ironically, before graduation, the proprietor of the roadhouse and his daughter had been gravely ill, and it was Wright and Steele who had cared for them. "When those two girls nursed the proprietor, it was alright if they were colored, but Frieda and Cecile weren't wanted as guests at his roadhouse," one classmate explained. At their 50th anniversary celebration, in September 2000, Steele had to relive the experience for Marty Gervais, a *Windsor Star* columnist.[58] Steele recalled how painful and hurtful the experience had been. For her, though, it was important to move on. When Gervais wrote about the roadhouse experience, he explained "As Genie (Denomme) Van Hooren tells it, the cement of friendship, the loyalty, the camaraderie [was] born on the very day they met 50 years ago. It survives everything."

Ellesworth, too, continues to cherish the relationships that resulted from her training. Despite segregated residences and working in the United States, she added that "It's been a life long friendship" with the students she met in training. As American nurse historian Barbara Melosh points out, "the hospital was school, workplace, and home combined."[59] It is thus not surprising that these nurses were able to forge the ties they did. Tellingly, although they are currently retired, Ellesworth, Travis, and Steele remain active in nursing alumnae associations.

As the first group of Black Canadian nurses to enter the occupation, these nurses were committed to professional excellence. They believed that by doing extremely well they would open doors for other Black women. Coincidentally, the majority of the nurses interviewed entered the occupation at a time when the Canadian health care system was undergoing an immense transformation. In the aftermath of the war, the Canadian government developed a number of programs that led to state-funded hospitals, hospital insurance programs, and, by 1968, Medicare. Authors Pat and Hugh Armstrong contend that health care not only stimulated economic growth due to investments, but also created employment for a variety of people within institutions.[60]

During this period, permanent hospital-based employment engaged the majority of nurses, still mostly White. As hospitals expanded and new technical and surgical procedures were introduced, nursing leaders needed to make adjustments. They pushed for more education for graduate nurses and hired subsidiary workers, creating a hierarchy of nurse managers and nurse workers.[61] These changes gave Black Canadians an opportunity to prove their worth. As only one or two of the RNs on the ward, Black Canadian nurses excelled, not only in their areas of expertise, but also because they undertook various leadership roles throughout their careers. They epitomized professionalization, a concept often used to denote the occupational strategies of education and registration adopted to maintain control over nursing work.[62] Their personal and individual investment in professionalization was reflected in the positions they held as head nurses, supervisors, directors, and, in the case of Travis, nursing instructor. Throughout their careers, these nurses continued their education, whether, like Travis, by obtaining a Bachelor of Science degree, or by obtaining other kinds of certificates that would cement their roles as skilled professionals.

Even though the experiences of the nurses were not identical, there were similarities in their commitment to professionalism. When she graduated from Hotel Dieu, Ellesworth immediately found employment at Providence, a Catholic hospital in Southfield, Detroit, Michigan. She spent one year at Providence and returned to Hotel Dieu to start a family. In 1960, she found employment at Mercy General, a Black hospital in Detroit located at 688 Windmere. Ellesworth explained her decision to work in Detroit: "If I wanted to work, I was going to make the best of it. The things I wanted to do were there [Michigan], and I could have the best of both worlds. I work there and live here [Windsor]."[63] She did exceptionally well. In a short time, she became the director of the operating room at Mercy. At the same time she attended school to become a nurse anesthetist, something she had always wanted to do but which was not offered anywhere in Canada.

When Mercy General closed in the early 1970s, Ellesworth found employment at Sidney A. Sumby Memorial Hospital, located in River Rouge, Michigan, where she was director of anesthesia until that hospital closed its doors in the late 1980s. She added that she also worked at another hospital part-time to pay for her children's education. Stressing how much she enjoyed working with and among African American nurses, she explained that "They were highly respected and motivated, which in turn motivated me. We didn't have that in Windsor."

Besides wanting to obtain her license in anesthesia, Ellesworth also disclosed that her decision to "cross the border" was based on the lack of recognition that educated Blacks received in Windsor.

> In Michigan it was less about colour and more about your education. We [Blacks] have this background and foundation and I think we were a bit overlooked. I got good positions [in Michigan], I had four children to raise, and I was able to do that. That was done all because I was in the States. I would have worked and wouldn't have made that here.

Paradoxically, Ellesworth was able to find validation and employment in a country where her ancestors were unable to, and in hospitals that were created because of White racism.

Overall, the work experiences for Travis, Watson, and Steele were positive, and in some ways they followed similar patterns in terms of their professional positions. Upon graduation in 1957, Travis worked in the surgical unit at the Public General Hospital in Chatham. She then moved into the operating room, where she was assistant head nurse for two years and head nurse from 1962 to 1964. She took some time from nursing to teach operating room and postoperative care for three years at the school of nursing at Chatham General. Following her stint at teaching, she returned to the operating room as supervisor. Although the position was highly stressful, she enjoyed it, "which is why I worked there for 23 years." Along with nursing, teaching, and raising a family, Travis was active in the Registered Nurses Association of Ontario (RNAO), where she sat on the Complaints and Disciplinary Committee and a number of other committees. Similar to the other nurses in this study, during the 1970s, Travis voted for and supported collective bargaining for nurses, a group she feels was disadvantaged even though it was the largest group of health care workers in Ontario. Now retired, she pointed out that "I miss nursing, and I miss it tremendously."[64] Travis continues to be active in nursing initiatives and will be until she is no longer able.

After she graduated in 1950, Steele worked part-time at Hotel Dieu while raising a family. In 1970, she returned to the hospital full-time and took an administrative position that brought a great deal of responsibility and authority. According to Steele, it was sometimes difficult for patients and family members to accept a Black nurse in charge. She tells the story of a gentleman who had a complaint regarding the care his wife was receiving.

> He was directed to come down and see Mrs. Steele. One of our clerks said, "This is Mrs. Steele." He said he wanted to see Mrs. Steele. The clerk then pointed to me and I said, "I'm Mrs. Steele." He then said, "He wanted to see Mrs. Steele the person in charge." I said, "That's me." I directed him to the CEO's office and before long he returned very humbly and asked if "I had a minute for him." We discussed the problem and what we were prepared to do. He was very pleased and thanked me and left. I called the CEO and asked him what had been said to this gentleman. He said that "I told him that that's not my domain, it's Mrs. Steele's and you will have to discuss it [the problem] with her."[65]

While Steele's experience ended satisfactorily, this was not always the case for the other nurses. Like the fictional Sanford in "Glass Wall," who is tired of her skin color being seen as an impediment, Steele wanted more than anything else for her colleagues to realize that underneath her Black skin, she too wanted to be "just one of the girls."[66] Black Canadian nurses strove to prove themselves as qualified, capable, and professional nurses; they wanted to excel in order to open doors for other Blacks but also to prove to Whites that they were capable of excellence.

Throughout their careers, Black Canadian nurses defined their work experiences in terms of their identity as nurses rather than "Black nurses." Did this mean that these nurses were oblivious to the way they were sometimes perceived by their colleagues and patients? Steele pointed out that her interactions with Whites at times constituted a testing of the self. She maintained that "when you are Black Canadian, you are conscious of the racism in society. Very often, and most often, it's not blatant but every once in a while it rears its ugly head and you have to be ready to meet it."[67] Besides being equipped with determination and the tools to succeed, Black Canadian nurses also evoked their ancestors' 400-year presence in Canada and their history of struggle to claim a space in the larger Canadian society. This discourse of Canada as "home," and of their inherent right to "belong" even if the nation sought to exclude or marginalize them, was extended to nursing.

Certainly, the desire of Black Canadian nurses to succeed was based on an understanding of their role as "trailblazers" in conjunction with their ancestral legacy in Canada. For Travis, the reality that "my predecessor couldn't enter nursing influenced [me]."[68] Edna Black Searles, whose sister Ruth Bailey is reputed to be the second Black nurse to train in Canada, and whose father, Joe Bailey, once president of the United Negro Improvement Association (UNIA), wrote Prime Minister Mackenzie King after his daughter was refused training by a number of Toronto hospitals, illustrated how important it was that Bailey succeed. She explained that "they [Ruth and the other Black nurse] went and studied. She [Ruth] was an exceptionally good nurse. She said, 'I gotta blaze the trail for everybody else, so I'm gonna do a good job,' and she did."[69]

To use historian Darlene Clark Hine's term, these nurses essentially accepted "the burden of racial obligation."[70] As a result, there were certain responsibilities one had to undertake by virtue of being born Black and Canadian. When Bailey left Nova Scotia, she received a certificate in public health from the University of Toronto and went to Chatham, Ontario, to practice. Searles asserted that her sister's experiences were not always positive, but that like Ellesworth she did not chafe. Speaking on behalf of her sister, Searles explained:

> Once you were born in this country, we know that we are fighting our way, and while we talk about it, we try to do something about it. If you want something in any place, especially the country you were born into, you have to fight. That's why my father fought, that's why he wrote the letter. Nothing is impossible, you have to start someplace. So [Ruth] enjoyed [Chatham] whether it was one hundred percent to her liking, there is not a job that you get one hundred percent to your liking, but if you are blazing the trail for others, you accept the good and the bad, you accept some of the things or you get out.[71]

Given the racial climate in Canada and nursing, Bailey assumed she would have to participate in the role of racial uplift. For her, being a trailblazer and setting a good example were not a matter of choice, it was something that was necessary.

For the Black Canadian nurses studied in this project, Canada had represented for their ancestors a safe haven from the racism and violence of 19th-century United States. Contrary to what is suggested in positive nationalist narratives, however, Canada was not always hospitable. In Dresden, Windsor, Africville, Chatham, and Buxton, the descendants of African Americans struggled to build institutions and create communities. This legacy of struggle was passed down from generations to generation, and people continued to fight the various forms of oppression endemic to Canadian society. It was this history, then, coupled with their belief that they had a right to train as nurses that provided Black Canadian nurses the necessary affirmation to begin their training in the postwar era and to blaze a sometimes arduous trail for the generation of Black Canadian and Caribbean nurses who have followed.

Karen Flynn, PhD
African American Studies and Research Program
1201 W. Nevada Street, MC 143
University of Illinois, Urbana-Champaign
Urbana, Illinois
217–333–7781
kcflynn@uiuc.edu

Acknowledgment

The author would like to thank Jayne Elliot, Meryn Stuart, Sarah Clarke Kaplan, and the anonymous reviewers for their insightful comments.

A version of this article was presented at the Hannah 2005 Nursing History Conference at the University of Ottawa, Ottawa, Ontario.

Notes

1. Agnes Ellesworth, interview by author, tape recording, Windsor, Ontario, June 5, 2001. The interviews took place in the interviewees' homes and lasted from 1.5 to 3 hours. All interviewees signed written consent forms.

2. Of the nurses who began their training in the late 1940s and early 1950s, only one mentioned choosing to train in a public institution as opposed to a religious-based hospital; for the other women, their decisions were based on convenience and hospitals' willingness to accept them as students.

3. Overall, there is a paucity of research on Black women generally in Canada. Most studies on Black Canadian and Caribbean migrant nurses tend to focus on their experiences as waged laborers and racism in the workplace. See, for example, Agnes Calliste, "Women of 'Exceptional Merit': Immigration of Caribbean Nurses to Canada," *Canadian Journal of Women and the Law* 6 (1993): 85–103; Tania Das Gupta, *Racism and Paid Work* (Toronto: Garamond Press, 1996); Josephine Etowa, R. Thompson, and S. Sethi, "The Worklife Experiences of African Canadian Nurses," Virginia Henderson International Nursing Library, International Conference, Impact of Global Issues on Women and Children, Dhaka, Bangladesh, February 12–16, 2006, http://www.nursinglibrary.org/portal/main.aspx?pageid+4024&pid=8412, 2006 (accessed November 27, 2007); Karen Flynn, "Experience and Identity: Black Immigrant Nurses to Canada, 1950–1980," in *Sisters or Strangers: Immigrant, Ethnic, and Racialized Women in Canadian History,* ed. Marlene Epp, Franca Iacovetta, and Frances Swyripa (Toronto: University of Toronto Press, 2004), 381–97; Margaret Shkimba and Karen Flynn, "'In England We Did Nursing': The Experiences of Caribbean and British Nurses in Great Britain and Canada," in *New Directions in the History of Nursing: International Perspectives,* ed. Susan McGann and Barbara Mortimer (New York: Routledge, 2005), 141–57.

4. For Michael Foucault, "subjugated knowledge" refers to that which is delegitimized or excluded from what counts as "real knowledge." In this case, Black Canadian women's subjectivities are marginalized within nursing scholarship and Canadian history generally.

5. Kathryn McPherson, *Bedside Matters: The Transformation of Canadian Nursing, 1900–1990* (Toronto: Oxford University Press, 1990); Catherine Judd, *Bedside Seductions: Nursing and the Victorian Imagination, 1830–1880* (New York: Palgrave Macmillan, 1996).

6. Letter to G. Roberts, President, Toronto Coloured Liberal Association, July 14, 1940, Archives of Ontario (AO), RG 10–107–0-166, container 23, file #1 ("Nurses Training,) etc.," 1939–1940; McPherson, *Beside Matters,* 119; Karen Flynn, "'I'm Glad That Someone Is Telling the Nursing Story': Writing Black Canadian Women's History," *Journal of Black Studies* 3, no. 38 (January 2008): 445.

7. Miss A. M. Munn, RN, Director, Nurses' Registration, Letter to Dr. B. T. McGhie, Deputy Minister of Health, October 2, 1940, AO, RG 10–107–0-166, container 23, file #1 ("Nurses Training,) etc.," 1939–1940; McPherson, *Bedside Matters,* 119; Flynn, "I'm Glad That Someone Is Telling the Nursing Story," 446.

8. Munn, Letter to Dr. B. T. McGhie; McPherson, *Bedside Matters,* 119.

9. Darlene Clark Hine, *Black Women in White: Racial Conflict and Cooperation in the Nursing Profession 1890–1950* (Bloomington: Indiana University Press, 1989), xx.

10. Karen Flynn, "Race, the State and Caribbean Immigrant Nurses, 1950–1965," in *Women, Health, and Nation: Canada and the United States Since 1945,* ed. Georgina Feldberg, Molly Ladd-Taylor, Alison Li, and Kathryn McPherson (Montreal: McGill-Queen's University Press, 2003), 259.

11. Munn, Letter to Dr. B. T. McGhie; Flynn, "Race, the State, and Caribbean Immigrant Nurses," 259.

12. Library and Archives Canada Record Group, 76, vol. 553–110, pt. 2, to Director of Immigration; from Eastern District Superintendent, Montreal, Quebec, "Haitian Nurses Aides," June 9, 1958.

13. Flynn, "Race, the State and Caribbean Immigrant Nurses," 257.

14. Flynn, "Race, the State and Caribbean Immigrant Nurses," 257.

15. For Black Canadian and Caribbean organizations in Canada, see, for example, Calliste, "Women of Exceptional Merit"; Constance Backhouse, "'Bitterly Disappointed' at the Spread of 'Colour-Bar Tactics': Viola Desmond's Challenge to Racial Segregation, Nova Scotia, 1946," in Backhouse, *Colour-Coded: A Legal History of Racism in Canada, 1900–1950* (Toronto: University of Toronto Press, 1999), 226–71; Amoaba Gooden, "Community Organizing by African-Caribbeans in Toronto, Ontario," *Journal of Black Studies* 3, no. 38 (January 2008): 413–26; Peggy Bristow, "A Duty to the Past, A Promise to the Future: Black Organizing in Windsor—The Depression, World War II, and the Post-War Years," *New Dawn: Journal of Black Canadian Studies* 2, no. 1 (2007): 15–59.

16. McPherson, *Bedside Matters,* 211.

17. Julia Hallam, *Nursing the Image: Media, Culture and Professional Identity* (London: Routledge, 2000), 5.

18. Sheila Mackay Russell, "'The Glass Wall': A New Chapter in the Human Drama in a Hospital," *Chatelaine* (October 1964): 69.

19. Russell, "The Glass Wall," 68.

20. Particularly in the U.S. context, the idea of Black people as socially and biologically inferior has historically been used to justify their subordination. According to Ronald Davis, "This image functioned as the racial bedrock of American popular culture after 1900, especially manifested in minstrel shows, the vaudeville theatre, songs and music, film and radio, and commercial advertising." See, for example, Ronald L. F. Davis, "Popular Art and Racism: Embedding Racial Stereotypes in the American Mindset: Jim Crow and Popular Culture," http://www.jimcrowhistory.org/resources/lessonplans/hs_es_popular_culture.htm (accessed April 2, 2007). On science and racism, see, for example, Stephen J. Gould, *The Mismeasure of Man* (New York: Norton, 1981).

21. Suzanne Lego, "White Nurse Can Help Negro Change Self-Image," *Canadian Nurse* 62 (August 1966): 12.

22. McPherson, *Bedside Matters,* 17.

23. See, for example, Robert Dingwall, Anne Marie Rafferty, and Charles Webster, eds., *An Introduction to the Social History of Nursing* (London: Routledge, 1998).

24. Hallam, *Nursing the Image,* 11.

25. Richard Dyer, "White," *Screen* 29 (Autumn 1988): 44–64.

26. David Roediger, *The Wages of Whiteness: Race and the Making of the American Working Class* (New York: Verso, 1991), 13.

27. "The Atkinson School of Nursing: Toronto Western Hospital Presents: This Was Vaudeville," March 16–17, 1967, *Pulse: The Atkinson School of Nursing Yearbook* (1967): 18–19.

28. "Churches Rapped!!! Grizzle, Moore Speak Out Against Minstrel Shows," *Canadian Negro* 4, no. 1 (March 1956): 1.

29. Hallam, *Nursing the Image,* 25.

30. "Churches Rapped," 1.

31. Ken Alexander and Avis Glaze, *Towards Freedom: The African-Canadian Experience* (Toronto: Umbrella Press: 1996), 150. Viola Desmond's story of being forcibly ejected

from a movie theater in Nova Scotia exemplifies the de facto nature of racial segregation in Canada; see Backhouse, "'Bitterly Disappointed.'"

32. Marlene Watson, interview by author, tape recording, Toronto, Ontario, January 18, 2000.

33. Laura Tynes, interview by author, tape recording, Mississauga, Ontario, December 6, 1999.

34. Virginia Travis, interview by author, tape recording, Windsor, Ontario, June 5, 2001.

35. Travis interview.

36. Ray Greenridge, "Labor, Churches Urged to Back Fight Against Dresden Race Discrimination," *Canadian Negro* 2, no. 1 (February 1954): 1.

37. "The Racial Discrimination Act Adopted in Ontario," http://www.chrcccdp.ca/en/timePortals/milestones/45mile.asp (accessed April 2, 2007).

38. Alexander and Glaze, *Towards Freedom,* 151.

39. See, for example, Ross Lambertson, "'The Dresden Story': Racism, Human Rights and the Jewish Labour Committee of Canada," *Labour/Le Travail* 47 (2001): 1–36; Roger McTair, *Journey to Justice,* National Film Board of Canada, 2000. There is also an earlier version of this film entitled *The Dresden Story,* National Film Board of Canada, 1954.

40. Lambertson, "The Dresden Story," 13.

41. Frieda Steele, interview by author, tape recording, Windsor, Ontario, June 9, 2001.

42. For an excellent discussion of the CCA, which was later renamed the Central Citizens Association for the Advancement of Colored People, see Bristow, "A Duty to the Past, A Promise to the Future."

43. "Prevented Violence at Dresden," *Canadian Negro* 2, no. 3 (February 1954): 3.

44. Darlene Barnes, interview by author, tape recording, Toronto, Ontario, October 22, 1999.

45. Barnes interview.

46. Russell, "The Glass Wall," 66.

47. Tynes interview.

48. Steele interview.

49. Ellesworth interview.

50. See, for example, Flynn, "Race, the State and Caribbean Migrant Nurses"; Shkimba and Flynn, "In England We Did Nursing."

51. "What Is a Student Nurse?" *The Pulse* (1967): 23.

52. Ellesworth interview.

53. Travis interview.

54. Tynes interview.

55. Ellesworth interview.

56. Steele interview.

57. "Girls Nurse Proprietor But Said Not Wanted as Roadhouse Guests," *Windsor Star,* June 14, 1950.

58. Marty Gervais, "My Town—Ugly Incident Didn't Break Spirit or End Friendship," *Windsor Star,* September 18, 2000.

59. Barbara Melosh, *"The Physician's Hand": Work, Culture, and Conflict in American Nursing* (Philadelphia: Temple University Press, 1982), 37.

60. Pat Armstrong and Hugh Armstrong, *Wasting Away: The Undermining of Canadian Health Care* (Toronto: Oxford University Press, 1996), 121.

61. See McPherson, *Bedside Matters.*

62. David Coburn, "Professionalization and Proletarianization: Medicine, Nursing and Chiropractic in Historical Perspective," *Labour/Le Travail* 34 (Fall 1994): 139–62.

63. Ellesworth interview.

64. Travis interview.

65. Steele interview.

66. Russell, "The Glass Wall," 68.

67. Steele interview.

68. Travis interview.

69. Edna Black Searles, interview by author, tape recording, Scarborough, Ontario, September 4, 1999.

70. Hine, *Black Women in White,* xvii.

71. Searles interview.

Alliances of Cooperation: Negotiating New Hampshire Nurse Practitioners' Prescribing Practice

Deborah A. Sampson
University of Michigan School of Nursing

Abstract. Nurse practitioner legislation varies among states, particularly in relation to practice without physician oversight, altering the legal environment within which nurse practitioners can use knowledge and skills to meet patient needs. Using New Hampshire as a case study, this historical analysis of nurse practitioners' negotiations over time for independent practice, defined in state practice acts, illuminates the complex social and economic factors affecting nurses' struggle to gain legal rights over their own professional practice without supervision and intervention from another profession. In New Hampshire, not only did organized medicine oppose nurses' rights to practice, but pharmacists demanded the right to control all aspects of medication management, including who could prescribe and under what circumstances prescribing could occur. Shifting social and political terrain as well as changes in legislative and state professional board leadership affected the environment and negotiations of a small group of nurses who were ultimately successful in obtaining the right to define their own professional practice.

In 1973, the New Hampshire Board of Nursing recognized a new category of nurses called "advanced registered nurse practitioners" when the legislature passed an addendum to the nursing practice act formally recognizing this emerging group of nurses.[1] Following a growing national trend, these nurse practitioners had obtained additional education that enabled them to diagnose disease, order diagnostic tests, and prescribe and dispense medications to patients, activities that had been traditionally designated as only within the realm of medicine. For the next four years, New Hampshire nurse practitioners worked in this expanded role diagnosing disease, dispensing contraceptives and drug samples, and prescribing medications by using physician presigned prescriptions or under physician auspices by telephoning prescriptions to

Nursing History Review 17 (2009): 153–178. A Publication of the American Association for the History of Nursing.
DOI: 10.1891/1062–8061.17.153

community pharmacies under a physician's name. Most often the nurse practitioners were making their own clinical decisions about the drug, prescribing or dispensing without directly consulting doctors. Physicians, who were not always on premises when nurse practitioners examined patients, diagnosed illness, and prescribed or dispensed drugs (and may not even have worked in the same practice as the nurse practitioner), were fully aware and sanctioned this practice.[2] The nurse practitioners reasoned that since the New Hampshire Nurse Practice Act was broadly written and allowed nurses to practice consistent with their education, they were fully within their rights to diagnose and prescribe in the manner that they were doing, even though the practice act did not specifically address diagnosis or prescribing. The nurse practitioners, after all, were educated to perform these functions, and they were bound by state nursing statutes rather than by pharmacy or medical practice acts. The physicians supported these nurse practitioners' actions because, they believed, the Medical Practice Act allowed them to "delegate" with impunity any function they wished to another health care provider, and the physicians with whom the nurse practitioners worked were fully supportive of the practices. Both groups believed they were meeting patient needs without breaking the law.[3]

This practice had been going on for several years without question from any state regulatory office. Community pharmacists, another party to the discussion, occasionally complained to the Commission on Pharmacy, but these rare complaints brought forth no action other than an occasional brief notation in Commission on Pharmacy Board meeting minutes.[4] Both physicians and nurse practitioners were unaware that they were breaking a state pharmacy law that permitted only physicians, dentists, and veterinarians to prescribe and dispense. For almost five years, neither physicians, pharmacists, nor any other professional group seemed interested in ending the nurse practitioners' practices, despite state pharmacy law to the contrary.

But at the end of 1977, the Commission on Pharmacy formally challenged nurse practitioners' diagnosing, prescribing, and dispensing medications. The Commission was under pressure from the New England Regional Drug Enforcement Agency office in Boston and the New Hampshire State Police Drug Investigation Unit to tighten the filling of potentially specious prescriptions for controlled substances through pharmacies in New Hampshire.[5] The Pharmacy Commission, which was charged with inspecting community pharmacies' handling of prescriptions, put pharmacists on notice that prescriptions would be meticulously reviewed at each inspection, a practice that had previously been done in a more random and haphazard way.

During one such inspection in June 1977, a Commission on Pharmacy inspection pharmacist found several prescriptions for controlled substances that, while bearing one physician's name, had markedly different signature styles. Upon visiting the physician's office, the Commission on Pharmacy inspector found that the physician was unavailable. The physician's wife, who worked in the office, claimed to be a nurse practitioner and admitted to signing her husband's name to some prescriptions. She insisted that she had been taught at a prestigious Boston university–based nurse practitioner program that what she was doing was legal. The inspector, in front of the nurse practitioner, called the New England Regional Office of the Federal Drug Enforcement Agency, where an agent informed them both that the nurse was indeed breaking the law, and that she and the physician could be prosecuted under federal statutes.[6]

In July 1977, after discussing the issue at scheduled meetings, the Commission on Pharmacy filed a formal letter of complaint with the New Hampshire Board of Nursing Education and Nursing Registration against the nurse practitioner's practice. The substance of the complaint was that nurse practitioners were prescribing and dispensing drugs, a practice nurses were specifically prohibited to perform by state-mandated Pharmacy Board rules and regulations, and physicians could not abrogate their responsibilities by delegating this task to any person who was not a physician. The Commission moved to pursue a strict interpretation of the law but did not name the nurse practitioner or physician or move to have the nurse practitioner disciplined.[7] Subsequently, New Hampshire nurse practitioners became involved in a lengthy and often contentious legislative process to legally define not only their own practice act rights, but to enlist changes in pharmacy laws.

An examination of the legislative process in a particular state, New Hampshire, can give us information on how nurses cooperate to define their work through legislative negotiations around state practice acts. These negotiations encompass the highly gendered work roles of nursing, medicine, and pharmacy in the health care arena.[8] New Hampshire nurse practitioners' pursuit of prescribing legislation, which began in 1977, demonstrates the power of cooperation that transcends differences in nursing education and experience. Nurses at the New Hampshire state nursing board, most of whom were from academia, provided unqualified support of the nurse practitioners' endeavors. Perhaps most imperative, the cooperative actions of two powerful bureaucrats (Marguerite Hastings, executive director of the New Hampshire Board of Nursing, and Maynard Mires, executive secretary of the New Hampshire Board of Medicine, a leader in the New Hampshire Medical Society and director of New Hampshire Public Health) to support nurse practitioners' prescribing authority demonstrate the power of interprofessional relationships and respect to support change in spite of opposition from state professional organizations and boards.

State Professional Boards and Practice Acts

Professional licensing and oversight by state-mandated boards are an extension of the state's social contract with citizens. The intent of state laws and governing boards is to monitor and regulate professional activity as defined by state regulation. State professional regulation is designed ostensibly to protect the citizens of the state, but also to limit competition so that some groups or organizations are protected.[9] Each state has boards or commissions that oversee regulations for the practice of nursing, medicine, and pharmacy. The names of these boards and their structure, function, power, and laws vary significantly from state to state. Regardless of differences, however, these boards are responsible for administering and enforcing the state practice act. Although many board activities under the act may be mandated, funds may be insufficient to carry out their duties in a comprehensive way, and boards may have to prioritize activities, including oversight of professionals and maintaining boundary infringement by other professionals.

Board members are usually unpaid, overwhelmingly drawn from the professional practitioners the board is charged with overseeing, and often members of the professional organizations involved, a priori, in any legislative activity affecting professional boundaries and practice. A professional group often believes that only those within that profession should have jurisdiction of their practice. Physicians believe that only the medical board and the medical practice act have authority over medical practice. Nurses correspondingly believe that the nursing board and corresponding practice act have sole jurisdiction over nursing. But, in truth, in New Hampshire as elsewhere, the Pharmacy Practice Act also affects all health practitioners' management of drugs requiring a prescription. The boundaries of professional practice are thus not solely defined by one practice act but may extend through those of several professions. Practice acts may delineate the boundaries for each profession, but interpretation of such acts is evidenced by how the laws are clarified through rules and regulations, and board interpretations may conflict with the interests, responsibilities, or rules of other professional boards. In New Hampshire, the Boards of Nursing, Medicine, and Pharmacy all influence legal aspects of medication prescribing and dispensing.

In many states, New Hampshire being no exception, it is common for professional organizations to submit nominations for empty board seats to the governor, and often the nominee is appointed without question. Under this system, the agenda of the professional board may conflict with patient needs. Physician Maynard Mires, director of the New Hampshire Public Health Department and an influential member of both the New Hampshire Medical Society and Board of Medicine in the 1970s and early 1980s, recalled that in New Hampshire in the 1970s,

> members of the Board of Registration and Medicine really came from the Medical Society. So they were together in all of their ideas. I think that the Division of Public Health Services sort of resented time that I would spend with the board or with the Medical Society ... and I almost got into some binds because the Medical Society [and therefore the Board of Medicine membership] would like me to take part in something, which I felt would not be in the best interests of the Division of Public Health.[10]

The ethics of such arrangements, where members of boards charged with protecting the public are intimately involved with promoting the interests of the professions, contains obvious ethical conundrums, but is nonetheless a common occurrence. The actions of regulatory boards, whose formal function is to protect the public, often echo the interests of the profession, particularly when the goals of public safety and protection of the profession conflict.[11] In New Hampshire the practice acts, organizations, configurations, and titles of the boards have changed over time based on legislative mandates. Moreover, state practice acts rarely keep up with "role evolution."[12] Nurse practitioners needed to prescribe before states implemented legal regulations and nurse practitioners found ways to do so.

Cooperation, Coalitions, and Alliances

On July 28, 1977, after receiving the Commission on Pharmacy letter demanding that nurse practitioners no longer prescribe drugs, even under the instructions of a physician, Marguerite Hastings, executive director of the New Hampshire Board of Nursing, sent a letter to the leaders of the New Hampshire Nurse Practitioners Association detailing the Commission on Pharmacy complaint. Hastings informed the leaders that under current statue it was illegal for nurse practitioners to prescribe or dispense medications, practices nurse practitioners had been performing without challenge, sometimes alongside physicians, but also alone in geographically isolated areas or to low-income, underserved patients throughout the state.[13] The nurse practitioner leaders realized that they needed to mobilize their membership quickly to plan a strategy. The law needed not only to be revised but to be crafted and passed in a form that would assure New Hampshire nurse practitioners the legal right to prescribe and dispense under their own names.[14] Nurse practitioner leadership first gathered in October 1977 to discuss the situation.

The New Hampshire nurse practitioner and physician alliance that had worked well, and presumably safely, for both patients and providers was suddenly under threat from the formerly disinterested Commission on Pharmacy, which used state law to halt a practice all stakeholders had tacitly agreed to honor. New Hampshire nurse practitioners found themselves in the middle of a political battle for their livelihood and practice prerogatives. Assumed practice boundaries, within the usual "contested terrain" of medicine and nursing, were suddenly open to interpretation by pharmacists.[15] The nurse practitioners quickly learned not only how to maneuver the difficult, often ambiguous, lengthy, and gritty political process of moving a bill from initial draft into final law, but also how to use intra-, inter-, and extraprofessional networks to negotiate legislation that assured the nurse practitioners prescribing authority without physician oversight. They also had to continue practicing so that patient care would continue without difficulty for patients, physicians, or nurse practitioners.

Hastings was a native of Massachusetts and a 1937 graduate of Newton-Wellesley Hospital School of Nursing. While working as a nursing instructor and nursing administrator in several Massachusetts hospitals and serving as president of the Massachusetts Nurses Association, she earned a Bachelor of Science degree in nursing education from Boston University. After earning a graduate degree in education from Northeastern University in 1966, she moved to New Hampshire to become executive director of the New Hampshire State Board of Nursing, a position she held for 22 years. During her tenure, she also assumed leadership positions in the National Association of Parliamentarians and as chair of the National Council of State Boards of Nursing.[16] Hastings's leadership skills, which she honed through her leadership positions in national and international organizations, earned overwhelming respect and admiration from New Hampshire legislators, the nursing community, and leadership of other state professional boards.[17]

Hastings was never called anything but "Miss Hastings" except by her closest friends and, although she was diminutive, she was known to be intelligent,

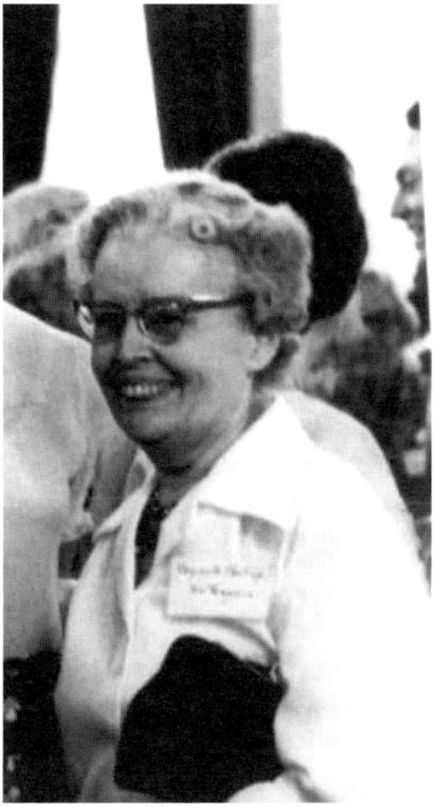

Figure 1. Marguerite Hastings, MS, RN, former Executive Director of the New Hampshire Board of Nursing. Reprinted courtesy of the New Hampshire Historical Society, Tuck Library.

gracious, and poised. Because she frequently visited schools of nursing and hospitals in New Hampshire, meeting with administrators and staff nurses alike, virtually all nurses in the state knew and respected her. The level of respect she engendered translated into significant personal and professional power when negotiating change for New Hampshire nurses. Moreover, Hastings was a shrewd and meticulous planner when developing strategies for change or shaping nursing practice that could cross medical boundaries. She often asked for input from others within and outside the Board of Nursing to assure that she understood all aspects of an issue and had a reputation for always being well-prepared at meetings and when testifying before the legislature.[18] Under Hastings, the Board of Nursing, unlike the Board of Medicine and Commission on Pharmacy, decisively disciplined nurses who violated nurse practice act mandates, particularly those that involved threats to patient safety or nurse substance abuse. Although she was a staunch advocate for nurses, Hastings took seriously the Board of Nursing charge to protect the public. Board of Nursing adjudication often involved license suspensions and revocation, Board actions that rarely happened to physicians or pharmacists.[19]

Hastings worked, often successfully in terms of nurses' position, to negotiate nursing-medical boundaries at fairly regular and amicable Board of Medicine and Board of Nursing joint meetings. For example, in March 1973 the two boards agreed to issue a joint statement that nurses should not be responsible for pronouncing death; that a properly trained nurse was not practicing medicine by inserting a vaginal speculum to perform a pelvic exam; that nurses should not take physician assistants' orders (a practice nurses and the Board of Nursing vehemently opposed); and that nurse midwives were practicing nursing, not medicine, and were exempted from Medical Practice Act, with the Board of Nursing solely responsible for their oversight. The two boards agreed that the issue of a nurse "hanging out a shingle" to give foot care to the elderly should be referred to the Board of Podiatry (nominally under the Board of Medicine), and further that, "If she hangs out a shingle, she could be in trouble."[20] The Board of Medicine often described negotiations with Hastings as "felt meeting was good and were able to discuss and solve problems," and the Board of Nursing, with Hastings's leadership, was able to "win" all the nursing positions.[21]

Hastings undoubtedly had a keen understanding that patients would suffer if nurse practitioners could no longer practice in their full role. She probably also understood that they would no longer have the jobs for which they had recently been educated if they were unable to continue to provide comprehensive care that included prescribing and dispensing. The best interests of the residents of New Hampshire would not be served if these nurses could not continue to dispense and prescribe. Perhaps caught between her roles as state bureaucrat and nursing advocate, Hastings encouraged the nurse practitioners to mobilize to change the nurse practice act to redefine the disputed tasks as sanctioned nurse practitioner practice.

Shortly after meeting with the nurse practitioners, Hastings met with Mires. Their close professional relationship, as noted above, not only facilitated boundary negotiations but also prompted their alliance to promote nurse practitioner practice, even when opposed by pharmacists or the medical society. Mires, appointed director of public health in December 1973, held a position of significant state power. He had an extensive public health background and family ties to New Hampshire, although he was a native of upstate

New York. Before coming to New Hampshire, he had served as a public health physician in the U.S. Navy and subsequently attended Harvard University School of Public Health in the early 1950s. Dr. Alfred Frechette, a former Harvard faculty member and Massachusetts commissioner of public health, encouraged Mires to apply to the New Hampshire Health Department. Undoubtedly Mires's military service influenced his subsequent leadership decisions in New Hampshire. During World War II and after, he worked with military nurses of equal and higher rank who were in leadership positions. Yet he also may have recognized the ambiguities of upholding military regulations while providing health services to individuals and populations.

Mires believed in loyalty to his superiors, in this case the governor, who had administrative oversight of all state boards, but he also believed in "doing his duty" to support unpopular decisions in the best interests of patients, even when this meant defying his colleagues or the governor. Like Hastings, he

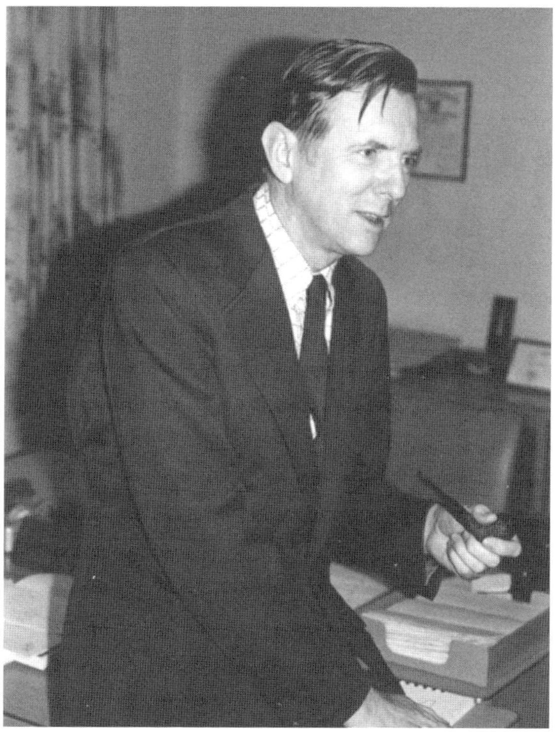

Figure 2. Maynard H. Mires, MD, MPH, former Executive Secretary of the New Hampshire Board of Medicine, leader in the New Hampshire Medical Society, and Director of New Hampshire Public Health. Photograph courtesy of Maynard H. Mires and used with permission.

had the respect of his colleagues, the governor, and legislators. He maintained close personal friendships with politicians, the New Hampshire attorney general, other Board of Medicine members, and the chair of the Commission on Pharmacy, Kenneth Fortier. Mires also had great admiration for Hastings, acknowledging that "Marguerite and I saw eye-to-eye. I worked very closely with her."[22] Whatever the two negotiated jointly, the Board of Nursing and Board of Medicine seemed to approve. Mires affirmed, "The two boards trusted Marguerite and me to the effect they thought, 'You just go ahead and take care of it.' "[23] The Board of Medicine was apparently content to abdicate all nurse practitioner practice issues to Mires and Hastings.

The Hastings/Mires alliance worked well to negotiate, often under the radar, all manner of Board of Medicine and Board of Nursing joint issues. For example, when the Commission on Pharmacy objected to nurse practitioners dispensing contraceptive medications in family planning clinics and private medical offices, Mires and Hastings, with the attorney general's sanction, collaborated to change the Board of Nursing rules and regulations to permit the dispensing.[24] Under the Hastings and Mires alliance, the Board of Nursing led the Joint Practice Committee, comprising the Board of Medicine, Board of Nursing, and New Hampshire Nurses Association, to interpret and implement the amendment to the nurse practice act that defined nurse practitioner status.[25] Mires and Hastings jointly developed protocols for nurse-run immunization clinics, which the Board of Nursing and Board of Medicine approved without fuss. Given that all other Board of Medicine members were practicing physicians with private practices, it is probable that the Joint Health Council medical representation consisted solely of Mires. When Mires, the Board of Medicine, and the New Hampshire Medical Society expressed strong concern that diploma schools of nursing were closing in New Hampshire and community college academic programs were replacing hospital-based training schools, there was little disruption in the cordial relationships between the Board of Nursing and Board of Medicine.[26] Undoubtedly the Mires/Hastings relationship could surmount interboard discord.[27]

When the Commission on Pharmacy complained about nurse practitioner prescribing it also objected to nurse practitioners dispensing medications and contraceptives. Nurse practitioners dispensing medications in public clinics, especially contraceptives at family planning clinics, was critical to meeting patient needs, and physicians would rarely be onsite to oversee the dispensing. Hastings and Mires recognized that patients would suffer needlessly. Therefore, they initiated a process available to state administrative department heads in New Hampshire to facilitate nurse practitioner dispensing of medications without involving the lengthy legislative process or the recalcitrant

Commission on Pharmacy. After consulting with Attorney General David Souter, Hastings and Mires quickly changed administrative rules of the Board of Nursing and the Board of Medicine practice acts to permit nurse practitioners to dispense medications and contraceptives legally under protocols jointly developed with a collaborating physician. The attorney general agreed that physicians could delegate the legal right to dispense, and that defining a process and mechanism to accomplish this only required Boards of Medicine and Nursing agreement about administrative rules.[28] The Commission on Pharmacy, not included in this process, spent the next four years trying to convince the attorney general's office that the rule change should be deemed illegal. The Commission was not successful and New Hampshire nurse practitioners' legal practice boundary was explicitly expanded without the legislative initiative that can often take years in New Hampshire's complex citizen legislature.[29]

What is particularly interesting is that the expansion of nurse practitioner practice was accomplished quickly through the collaboration and cooperation of a physician and a nurse, both state bureaucrats. Mires, a close friend of Attorney General Souter, also believed that the rural center patients needed nurse practitioners to have more freedom in treating and prescribing without physician supervision.[30] Hastings was able to develop a rule that met the needs of clinics and patients as well as legal rulemaking requirements, and was acceptable to Mires. They presented the rule to their respective Boards (incidentally indicating that they had modeled it together), and after approval by Souter it was enacted into law. The Commission on Pharmacy was dismayed and filed a futile formal complaint with the attorney general's office.

The Commission on Pharmacy strongly opposed allowing nonphysician health care professionals, including nurse practitioners, to prescribe or dispense medication.[31] The crux of the opposition was twofold. First, the Commission argued that only physicians had the requisite education for safe medication prescribing. Medications were potentially dangerous, and "patient safety" could be compromised if nonphysicians were allowed to prescribe. Moreover, under current state statutes, prescribing to patients was a legal prerogative limited to physicians and dentists. Any other professional group that prescribed was breaking the law.

Prescribing Medications—Whose Privilege?

The issue of prescriptive privilege for nurse practitioners required a major legislative initiative. Furthermore, New Hampshire Nurse Practitioner Association members had no experience or knowledge about this process. So when Hastings informed the New Hampshire Nurse Practitioner Association leadership that nurse practitioners could no longer prescribe, nurse practitioner leaders Betty Mitchell and Donna White, who worked together at a women's health practice and lived in the same small New Hampshire town, took action. They met with their state representative, George Roberts, Jr., to ask for his guidance for changing the nurse practitioner laws. Roberts, who was not only Donna White's neighbor and high school friend but also speaker of the New Hampshire House of Representatives and former House majority leader, enlisted the help of the legislative attorney to draft a plan for the nurse practitioners to use to change the law.[32] When asked why he bothered to take time to help the nurse practitioners, Roberts said, "My wife was Donna's patient and loved her. I'd have never heard the end of it. I think the local doctors' wives went to her too."[33] Through incredibly valuable community and family networks, these two nurse practitioners were able to enlist the help of a seasoned and powerful legislator and premier legislative attorney to make a solid start in the change process.

In the meantime, the New Hampshire Nurse Practitioner Association leadership continued to hold planning and information meetings for all New Hampshire nurse practitioners and began sending letters to keep them informed and to mobilize political action. The letters urged all nurse practitioners that "this is your chance to participate and whatever happens will affect your nursing practice . . . think about New Hampshire Nurse Practitioner Association's future . . . be prepared to [mobilize] to get through a special [legislative] session" if necessary.[34] This professional network was tapped for practical and financial reasons. Cynthia Cote, former Association treasurer, recalls that members sat around a conference table at the meetings and emptied purses onto the table for postage money to mail the letters. Cote recalls, "I think often a lot of us just paid for the mailings and for any of the supplies and whatever we had to do. We were a very low-budget operation."[35]

The very small group of 20 regular New Hampshire Nurse Practitioner Association meeting attendees had a sparse financial base, but that would not be an obstacle. They had no central office from which to work, so, as women have often done, they met in public spaces such as restaurants and conference rooms in hospitals and clinics, and ran their campaign from their homes, often paying for telephone bills, stationery, and travel out of pocket.[36] The political was indeed both personal and professional, and the boundaries between personal and professional lives were often blurred.

New Hampshire Nurse Practitioner Association leaders immediately formed a Prescription Task Force led by Christine Kuhlman to implement the legislative action plan facilitated by Roberts. Kuhlman and Donna Cassidy, another task force member, worked at the progressive private Concord Clinic with physicians who supported independent prescribing for nurse practitioners. The clinic was often used for strategy meetings; clinic telephones, stationery, copy machines, and other office services were openly used without cost by Task Force leadership with full clinic physician support.[37]

Prescription Task Force members worked hard to organize a successful legislative initiative. They sent frequent information and strategy letters to all New Hampshire nurse practitioners outlining the legislative process, where negotiations and actions stood, names and towns of residence of key state committee legislators, sample letters to send to legislators, and dates of public hearings. The letters stressed that nurse practitioners should let their patients know that their help was needed to assure successful passage of the law. Nurse practitioners also intensively lobbied legislators. Paula Weeman, a member of the Task Force, recalled:

> It seems like, anybody in the legislative process that we needed to talk to . . . well, if we needed to talk in the halls [of the State House], we'd talk in the halls. If we needed to take a senator to lunch, we'd go to lunch; we'd invited the senator to lunch, or a representative. Or we'd go to representatives' breakfasts. We just became much more present, all the while, while we're working, raising families. But we were doing it.[38]

Prescription Task Force members enlisted other tactics as well. They made a presentation to the Commission on Pharmacy, which still actively opposed nurse practitioner prescribing. Hoping to bring the commission into the legislation change support group, the Task Force hoped to increase commission members' understanding about nurse practitioners' practice and the realities of New Hampshire patient care, and convince them that nurse practitioners' education was adequate to assure safe prescribing. Nurse practitioners had been educated to prescribe, and their prescribing practice was safe according to the physicians with whom they worked. Chris Kuhlman recalls "feeling very frustrated because we were taught prescriptive information in school for sure."[39] The Task Force presented details of pharmaceutical education and subsequent practice. Although there were little survey data for nurse practitioner prescribing safety (nor for physicians, for that matter), the Pharmacy Commission may have been mollified. After the presentation, for reasons as yet unclear, the commission neither publicly supported nor actively opposed the legislation during legislative hearings.[40]

The nurse practitioners continued to work with Marguerite Hastings and the Board of Nursing, who in turn continued to work with Maynard Mires and the Board of Medicine. In an interesting contrast to actions in many states, where those groups were opposing camps, in these early years the Board of Medicine and Board of Nursing often presented a united front in support of nurse practitioners against the Commission on Pharmacy. Nurse practitioner leaders used their cooperative networks with patients, physicians, colleagues, and neighbors to coalesce support, develop strategies, and mobilize action, while state leaders Mires and Hastings maintained their support for nurse practitioners' prescribing legislation.

Partial Success

The nurse practitioner practice prescribing legislation passed the House in spring 1979 without difficulty in spite of strong opposition from several powerful and vocal physician and pharmacist representatives from the heavily populated, nurse practitioner-scarce southern tier of the state. But the corresponding Senate bill was defeated on June 6, 1979, delaying hope for legislation until the next legislative session, several years hence.[41] Hamilton Putnam, administrative director of the New Hampshire Medical Society, later took credit for the defeat, insisting that his testimony stressing the need for "safeguards" missing in the bill had influenced the Senate vote.[42] Although Putnam may have had some influence on the outcome, other factors may also have been at play. George Roberts stresses that legislation on new ideas, no matter what the issue, might pass the House but is almost always defeated on the first "go 'round" in the Senate. "In the world of pragmatism [in New Hampshire politics] ... the kill is in the Senate."[43]

Laurie Harding, community health nurse, former lobbyist for the New Hampshire Nurses Association and the New Hampshire Nurse Practitioners Association, and current House representative and member of the Health and Welfare Committee, had insight into why the New Hampshire Senate is traditionally a difficult place to pass a bill.

> The House will study an issue very diligently, because you're only assigned to one committee as opposed to being a Senator and assigned to four committees. They [the Senate] get a hair across their tail end and they make a lot of arbitrary decisions sometimes and they're heavily influenced by outside forces, depending on who is able to influence them at what times, and there have been times when nurses have been able to influence them in a positive way for nursing and for health care. Sometimes it has to do with the numbers, and it's a very individual thing and you really just can't tell sometimes about that Senate. It's highly unpredictable as to what the Senate will do.[44]

The nurse practitioners had been naïve. They had never attempted legislative action and perhaps relied too heavily on the belief that, since what they were trying to do was in the best interests of patients and they were filling a need supported by their collaboration, there would be no question of success. They believed that the backing of Hastings and Mires, representing a medical-nursing alliance, and the support of several legislators who were friends and neighbors, would also guarantee support. They clearly underestimated the possibility of opposition and were unaware of the power of behind-the-scenes political shenanigans that could blindside their attempts. Finally, as nurses often do, they tried to do everything themselves: organizing, testimony, lobbying, strategizing, fund-raising, educating, coalition building, and negotiating in a complex and sometimes covert world, the state legislature, where they had no experience. The term *babes in the woods* comes to mind. They needed more professional assistance than even George Roberts and legislator friends could give, but they did not even know enough on this first go-around to know what they didn't know. They would not be so naïve in the future.

When the bill failed the Senate, the nurse practitioners were discouraged but not defeated. At the next New Hampshire Nurse Practitioner Association meeting, they decided to try again. They discussed what they had learned from the years of strategizing, the lessons in the defeat, and how they could be more successful for their next attempt.[45] They would continue to use cooperation to attempt legislative change to assure their right to cross the medical (and in this case, pharmacy) boundaries for prescribing medications. They would continue to work toward prescribing rights legislation for as long as it took to pass the requisite laws. Unfortunately, they would have to do so without the powerful support of Hastings and Mires.

Hastings was required by state age limitation laws to retire at age 70, effective October 6, 1980. Although she continued to attend Board of Nursing meetings (as can any member of the public), she was no longer in an official leadership position and was unable to participate in a formal way. Mires, who had a close rapport with previous governor Meldrim Thomson, had a less than cordial relationship with Hugh Gallen, elected in 1980. An incident with Gallen changed leadership at the Department of Public Health. Mires evoked the incident, illustrating his own sense of fairness, belief in bipartisan cooperation, and integrity, that led to his leaving New Hampshire:

> The next administration [after Thomson] . . . really caused me to have to leave. I'd never been in a political situation like this before, where Republicans and Democrats really went at it hammer and tongs. I guess I was naïve enough to think they should get along. Anyway, they started saying something that was very untrue about

> the previous administration, that Governor Thomson had approved the dumping of hazardous materials some place. I believe that's what it was about. I knew that was definitely not true. I called Peter Thomson, his son. We met for lunch, and I said, "Peter, they're trying to blacken your father's name, and I don't think it's right." So somehow that word got back to the governor, Hugh Gallen.... I was told that I would have to leave.[46]

When Mires left New Hampshire in early 1981, there was little left of the strong interpersonal linkage and mutual support between the Board of Nursing and Board of Medicine. Stephen Tzianabos, a surgeon in private practice with no personal or professional relationships with nurse practitioners, or physician assistants for that matter, was appointed to the Board of Medicine along with other physicians who were less than friendly to nursing autonomy. Although neither Tzianabos nor other Board physicians were disposed to an alliance with the Commission on Pharmacy, the Board of Medicine became a vocal opponent of nurse practitioner prescribing. Times and leadership in boards and state had changed, and the relationship between the boards would continue to deteriorate.[47] The nurse practitioners needed new strategies.

Perhaps the nurse practitioners did not realize that the Hasting/Mires alliance was a source of power, and that its loss would make the second legislative attempt all the more difficult. Or perhaps they still believed in pursuing the support of the House of Representatives rather than initiating the bill with the more contentious but powerful Senate. Only 2 of the 24 senators attended the Senate Health and Welfare Committee hearings in May; one was Vesta Roy, Senate president. The minimal attendance may have signaled that the Senate decision had already been determined. At the hearing, House health and welfare chair Roma Spaulding unexpectedly introduced an amendment, undoubtedly originating from the New Hampshire Medical Society or Board of Medicine, adding physician assistants to the prescribing bill and requiring both physician assistants and nurse practitioners to be overseen by the Board of Medicine.

The nurse practitioner leaders were blindsided and were not sure how to proceed. If they opposed this arrangement, their hard work could continue to another session. If they agreed, they would possibly be subjected to the supervision of a now-hostile medical board, an abhorrent thought to all. They voted unanimously to oppose any bill that included Board of Medicine supervision of nurse practitioners. This proved to be a moot issue, since on June 12 the prescribing bill was once again "killed in the Senate," when Roy and the Senate Health and Welfare Committee recommended that the bill "ought not pass."[48] Once again, the House had passed the bill only to have it fail in the

Senate. The exact reasons for the Senate defeat are unclear. Perhaps influenced by the Board of Medicine, powerful legislators were content to play politics rather than support the nurse practitioners and the health care needs of the citizens. The nurse practitioners had underestimated the importance of winning over Roy and Spaulding, both powerful women legislators.

Still determined, the nurse practitioners were finally successful on the third try, in the 1984 legislative session. In large part the third attempt was successful because they enlisted initial sponsorship from the dynamic and powerful (and nurse practitioner-friendly) Senator Susan McLane, who was also chair of the Senate Health and Welfare Committee, which would hear the nurse practitioner prescribing bill.[49] Success was undoubtedly also due to the tenacity, cohesiveness, and determination of the nurse practitioners, and their awareness that starting a bill in the Senate, with powerful Senate backing, would be more likely to engender success.

Even though the final bill allowed nurse practitioners to prescribe, the Board of Medicine and Commission on Pharmacy insisted on oversight requirements for ongoing approval of a prescribing formulary. The formulary would define, and therefore limit, the drugs nurse practitioners would be able to prescribe. This was more oversight than the nurse practitioners or the Board of Nursing had hoped, but half a loaf was better than none.[50] Cynthia Cote recalls:

> It was a compromise. I think it was win-win. If you want this, you got to have that. And it was kind of like the safety net.... I think it was some of those back-room kind of deals, and maybe the Board of Pharmacy said as well. "OK, if you say that you, nurse practitioners, are skilled and educated and this is the only way that they really can deliver health care to those that are in need, then we'll go there so long as we have some safeties to protect the citizens from any malpractice on the part of nurse practitioners." And I remember those discussions so heatedly at our meetings, where there were some factions of our group. "We've been through this, didn't make it. Let's come up with a compromise so that we can move." It was a win-win for everybody, and their concerns are being addressed and we can get what we want too, which was to have the ability to write prescriptions legally.[51]

Even though they disagreed in private meetings, the nurse practitioners decided to go along with the compromise and present a united front in public. They had not entirely gained independence over their own practice, but they had made strides toward breaking down medical boundaries over prescribing. The victory they had won would quickly be followed by other major changes, including the legal right to receive direct insurance reimbursement for medical care services in New Hampshire regardless of collaboration with a physician.

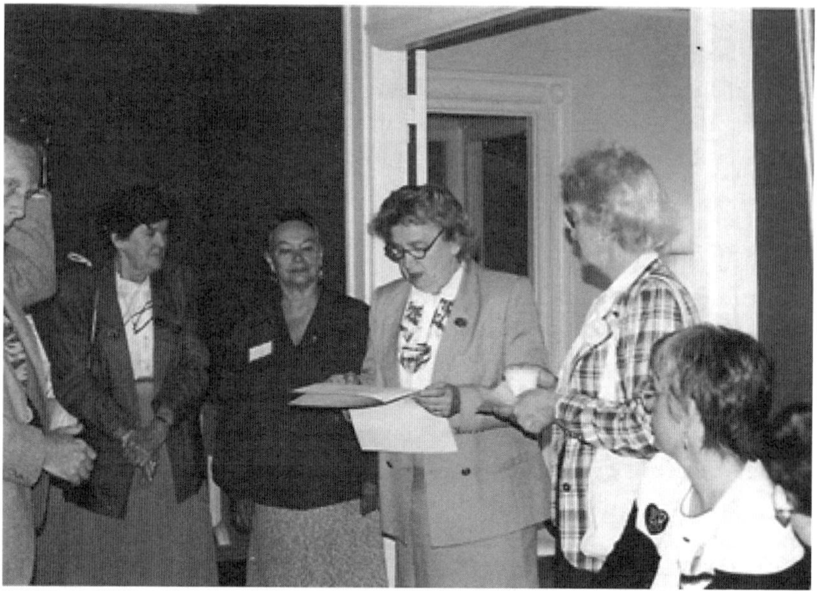

Figure 3. Senator Ruth Griffin, RN, reading recent legislation to nurses and legislators in the New Hampshire State House (approximately 1980). Photograph used with permission of the New Hampshire Historical Society, Tuck Library.

Conclusion

For the most part, specialist nurses, particularly advanced practice nurses, have sought to gain independence from oversight by other health professions. Nurse practitioners seek the legal right to apply *medical* knowledge and practice independent of physician oversight, and have endeavored, state by state, for the right to define their own practice as professionals. The crux of this struggle seems to lie in questions such as what is nursing and what is medicine, who controls the practice of each, how control is implemented, who gets paid, and who gets control of health care access.[52] Nurse practitioners and physicians may not practice in the same physical space, and often do not collaborate to share knowledge. Negotiation was complex and sometimes painful but was a process between intricately related individuals and groups.[53] Although organized medicine has generally sought to maintain control and oversight over nurse practitioners, many other physicians were, and to some degree always have been, supporters of autonomous advanced practice nursing.[54]

New Hampshire nurse practitioners were breaking new ground both politically and in practice. They were pioneering to define new state sanctions for a nursing practice role while negotiating legislative change against some formidable opposition. They were political novices who "really learned a lot through trial and error," becoming more cohesive as a faction and "empowered and assertive and outspoken."[55] A small group, they were determined to have "a big voice," and they "weren't going to go away."[56] Leaders relied on politicians and physicians, other nursing organizations, patients and other community members, state bureaucrats, and each other for political alliances, and these alliances of cooperation shifted and changed over time. Community and professional networks mattered. The nurses formed an identity based on a shared belief about what they, as nurse practitioners, could do to provide care for people in the community, and this care included prescribing medications. Alliances between state bureaucrats of different professional backgrounds, based on respect and common goals, facilitated rules changes supportive of the nurses' goals. The nurse practitioners, with the support of Hastings, Mires, and influential politicians, were ultimately successful in passing the legislation defining new professional responsibilities for nurses.

Nursing history is the history of women (and men) workers in women's sphere in an industry (health care) dominated by powerful traditionally male professionals. It is the story of conflict and cooperation as women negotiate for credibility, economic legitimacy, autonomy, and power in the professional arena, while defining an occupational sphere.[57] It is a tale of women's efforts for professional status in an industry bound in male paradigms of occupational practices, particularly within the parameters of state practice acts. Advanced registered nurse practitioners challenge these male paradigms since they are, first and foremost, nurses, but also have knowledge and skills traditionally identified as reserved for the male physician's sphere.

While nurses have always challenged medical boundaries, the original intent that nurse practitioners could fill medical needs when physicians were not available meant that these nurses would openly diagnose disease and prescribe medications in publicly sanctioned ways. Yet the road to fulfilling their role, particularly around prescribing medications as defined in state practice act law, has been difficult in all states. Advanced registered nurse practitioners have faced opposition by medical and pharmacy organizations and boards, and they have had varying success overcoming this resistance. Current state nurse practice acts vary widely with regard to nurse practitioners prescribing as a nursing activity without state-required physician oversight.[58]

The history of New Hampshire nurse practitioner political activism during a time of significant legislative activity illustrates the concepts of nursing as gendered work, including how women's alliances and cooperation informs negotiations for occupational place in the hierarchy of health professions. This story illustrates the significance of networks and intraprofessional and interprofessional relationships in supporting women's voice and power over their work and stimulating alliances within and across professional lines to influence legislative outcomes.

Deborah A. Sampson, PhD, ARNP
Assistant Professor
University of Michigan School of Nursing
400 North Ingalls
Ann Arbor, MI 48109
734–647–0146
sampsond@umich.edu

Acknowledgments

Funding support for this research was provided by National Institute for Nursing Research/National Institutes for Health predoctoral research training award F31-NR008302–01A1: Doctoral Student Research Award, The American Association for the History of Nursing; Sigma Theta Tau, Xi Chapter.

Signed informed consents and releases of all oral histories are on file in the author's records or at the Tuck Library of the New Hampshire Historical Society.

Notes

1. The New Hampshire 1973 legal designation "advanced registered nurse practitioners" included nurse practitioners, nurse midwives, and psychiatric clinical nurse specialists, adding nurse anesthetists in 1991. Perhaps because there have been few clinical nurse specialists in New Hampshire other than those in psychiatry, they have never been designated advanced practice nurses. For documents related to the 1973 designation, see Box 1–1, folders marked "Legislation 1970," "Charters," "Minutes 1970s," New Hampshire Nurse Practitioners Association (hereafter NHNPA) Papers, archived in the Tuck Library of the New Hampshire Historical Society, Concord, New Hampshire. See also *Registered Nurses and Practical Nurses,* RSA 326-B: 1–22, Laws of the State of New Hampshire (January 1, 1973), Concord, New Hampshire.

2. For documentation of prescribing practices see oral history transcripts of Donna White recorded December 28, 2004 (cited as White), lines 390–408, 445–62; Jeanne

Charest recorded May 15, 2005 (cited as Charest), lines 437–72; Joyce Cappiello recorded August 2, 2005 (cited as Cappiello), lines 229–77; Mary Bidgood-Wilson recorded May 27, 2005 (cited as Bidgood-Wilson), lines 535–45, 574–615; Nancy Dirubbo recorded February 23, 2005 (cited as Dirubbo), lines 240–61; Paula Weeman recorded January 24, 2005 (cited as Weeman), lines 294–381. Transcripts and tapes cited are archived in the Tuck Library of the New Hampshire Historical Society unless otherwise noted.

3. Oral histories from practicing nurse practitioners at this time document the nurse practitioners' prescribing practices and the physician complicity. See, for example, Weeman, Dirubbo, and Charest, also oral history transcript of John Argue, May 3, 2005 (cited as Argue), lines 493–513, 626–49; Maynard Mires recorded April 6, 2005 (cited as Mires), lines 883–944; letter dated July 20, 1977 from Thomas Nadeau, MD, to Commission on Pharmacy, attached to Commission on Pharmacy meeting minutes, July 20, 1977. All Commission on Pharmacy minutes cited are found in the Office of Paul Boisseau, Board of Pharmacy, Concord, New Hampshire. Board of Medicine minutes, December 5, 1977, January 5, 1978. All Board of Medicine minutes cited are found in the conference room, Board of Medicine, Concord.

4. See Commission on Pharmacy minutes, January 17, 1973, December 18, 1974, November 19, 1975.

5. See Commission on Pharmacy minutes, June 10, 1972, all minutes of 1974 and 1975, July 20, 1977, December 13, 1978; Board of Medicine minutes, February 16, 1971, February 19, 1972, December 3, 1973, January 4, 1979; *New Hampshire Medical Society News* 28, no. 4 (October 1977), 1. All *New Hampshire Medical Society Newsletters* cited are found in the Office of the New Hampshire Medical Society, Concord.

6. See a complete discussion of the Pharmacy Commission investigator's report incident in the Commission on Pharmacy minutes, July 22, 1977.

7. An interesting footnote is that the so-called nurse practitioner in question was not licensed in New Hampshire as a registered nurse or nurse practitioner, although she became licensed in both categories. Moreover, the prestigious university she claimed to have attended had no nurse practitioner program at that time. Yet her individual actions, sanctioned by the physician with whom she worked (who also happened to be her husband, a physician well known to the State Drug Investigation Unit), set in motion a lengthy struggle for all New Hampshire nurse practitioners to gain prescriptive authority. It was also at this time that the Board of Nursing was making considerable efforts to address the significant problem of unlicensed nurses working in physicians' offices. According to Board of Nursing minutes, this was a common problem well known to the Board of Medicine. It was not necessarily unusual for an office "nurse practitioner" not to be licensed. See Board of Medicine minutes, May 5, 1977; "Doctor, Is Your Nurse Licensed?" *New Hampshire Medical Society News* 31, no. 1 (February 1979): 2; Board of Nursing minutes, October 1, 1979, May 15, 1980; *Board of Nursing Newsletter* 15, no. 1 (May 1980), 3. All Board of Nursing minutes and newsletters cited are found in the conference room, Board of Nursing office, Concord.

8. For the purposes of this article, the terms *nurse* and *nursing* are used to denote all licensed registered nurses and their practice. Nurse practitioners are one branch of nursing. They are educated to work in capacities that include concepts of nursing care and also provide some components of medical care traditionally performed by physicians, such as diagnosing and treating disease, prescribing medications, and even performing surgery and invasive procedures. While all nurse practitioners are nurses first, not all nurses are nurse

practitioners. Therefore, the concepts and contexts of nursing history are applicable, for the most part, to nurse practitioner history. The converse, however, may not be entirely true.

9. Julie Fairman, "Delegated by Default or Negotiated by Need? Physicians, Nurse Practitioners, and the Process of Critical Thinking," *Medical Humanities Review* 13, no. 1 (1999), 38–58. State regulation is often shared with federal legislation, but states, even in the same geographic region such as New England, can vary widely in their ideology about regulation of citizens.

10. Interview with Maynard Mires, Georgetown, Delaware, April 6, 2005 (cited as Mires 2005), lines 173–82; Ronald L. Akers, "The Professional Association and the Regulation of Practice," *Law & Society Review* 2, no. 3 (1968), 463–482.

11. It is not unusual for professional organizations to form coalitions to combat other competing professional groups, particularly when negotiating mutually amenable legislation. Conversely, professions may introduce or support legislation that is actually detrimental to the public interest. The Commission on Pharmacy introduced legislation in 1975 to prevent outpatient clinics and physicians' offices from dispensing more than a 24-hour supply of medications, including contraceptives from family planning clinics. Patients would be forced to take a prescription to a pharmacy instead. Limiting access to often free or low-cost contraceptives would most certainly be detrimental to patients. Fortunately for many women of New Hampshire, this Commission on Pharmacy initiative failed. Commission on Pharmacy minutes, April 2, 1975, book marked "NH Commission of Pharmacy Minutes January 1975–December 1978."

12. Bobbie Schwaninger Hughes, "Role Evolution vs. Legislation," *Nurse Practitioner* 8, no. 3 (1983), 9, 12.

13. Letter dated July 28, 1977 from Marguerite Hastings, Executive Director of New Hampshire Board of Nursing, to Gloria Klein, President NHNPA, folder "Legislation 1970s."

14. Letter dated November 29, 1977 from Betty H. Mitchell and Donna White to "Dear Fellow Practitioners" sent to all New Hampshire nurse practitioners; letter dated January 24, 1978 from Debbie Clark, RN PNP, Recording Secretary NHNPA, to "Dear Practitioner," folder "Legislation 1970s."

15. For excellent in-depth discussions of nursing and the contested terrain of medical boundaries, see Julie Fairman, "Playing Doctor? Nurse Practitioners, Physicians and the Dilemma of Shared Practice," *Journal of the Massachusetts School of Law* 4, no. 4 (1999); Arlene Keeling, *Nursing and the Privilege of Prescription, 1893–2000* (Columbus: Ohio State University Press, 2007), 27–35.

16. See Obituaries, *Berkshire Eagle* (Pittsfield, Massachusetts), July 7, 1998, Marguerite Hastings, http://oa.newsbank.com.oa-search/we/Archives (accessed December 13, 2005).

17. Hastings was also New Hampshire representative to the National Council of State Boards of Nursing and consulted to the Caribbean Nurses Association. After her retirement from nursing, she was New Hampshire director of the New Hampshire Association of Retired Persons, an active member of the Boston University Alumni Association, and volunteered every winter to help elderly people prepare their federal income taxes. Carolyn Andrews recorded May 16, 2005 (cited as Andrews), lines 480–599.

18. The admiration Hastings engendered is consistently repeated in oral histories collected for this research. For information on Hastings's power, stature, and relationships see, for example, transcripts of Charest, lines 832–937; Andrews, lines 240–309, 971–1020;

Christine Kuhlman recorded November 19, 2004 (cited as Kuhlman), lines 314–32, 882–88; Stanley Plodzik recorded March 4, 2005 (cited as Plodzik), lines 465–529. Also personal communication June 6, 2005 with Doris Nuttelman, former executive director of the New Hampshire Board of Nursing; transcript may be obtained from the author.

19. See, for example, adjudication discussions in minutes of each meeting of Board of Nursing and the Commission on Pharmacy through 1986. Nurses routinely had licenses suspended or revoked for actions including mishandling medications, IRS fraud, or substance abuse. Pharmacists routinely had licenses suspended for similar actions, but often had the majority of the suspension period "stayed" or forgiven. The Board of Medicine, however, rarely suspended or revoked licenses even after Drug Investigation Unit investigations (see Board of Medicine minutes, January 5, 1978). One physician who was found guilty of Medicare and Medicaid fraud had no action (Board of Medicine minutes, December 11, 1978). One who was found guilty of breaking prescription narcotic laws was allowed to "retire with dignity," as were others (Board of Medicine minutes, August 15, 1972, July 7, 1977). Another physician, while spending the night at a patient's hospital bedside, injected himself with massive amounts of Demerol, a potent morphinelike narcotic, while the patient died. Although the physician was subsequently found to exhibit bizarre and unstable behavior and to have a drug and alcohol abuse problem, the Board of Medicine left his license intact for many months (Board of Medicine minutes, July 6, 1978, October 5, 1978, December 11, 1978). These examples are a few of many during the years of study. Mires indicated that there were many "problem" physicians but due to the threat of being sued for an adjudicatory decision, the Board of Medicine was reluctant to take action against physicians (Mires, lines 121–55). Physicians did, however, have licenses revoked if their relicensing fee checks were returned to the Board of Medicine for insufficient funds (Board of Medicine minutes August 7, 1980).

20. Minutes of Special Joint Meeting, Board of Registration in Medicine, Board of Registration in Nursing, Thursday, March 8, 1973, Board of Medicine minutes files, 2.

21. Minutes, March 8, 1973, 3.

22. Hastings died suddenly in 1985, several years after she retired from the Board of Nursing. Although she remained active in the New Hampshire Nursing Association, she spent her time as an H&R Block consultant helping elderly people prepare their federal income tax reports and renovating the house she bought at her retirement (the first she had ever owned). Hastings never married (see Andrews, lines 808–50).

23. Mires was a close personal friend of New Hampshire Attorney General David Souter, who had a hand in backing several rulings supporting nurse practitioners' dispensing in defiance of the Commission on Pharmacy (Mires 2005, lines 18–81, 98–101, 202–25, 380–430, 668–86, 728–840, 1036–40, 1224–29).

24. Letter dated January 9, 1978 from Marguerite Hastings, Executive Director, New Hampshire Board of Nursing, to Deborah F. Clark, RN, PNP, Secretary NHNPA, folder "Legislation 1970s"; letter dated July 5, 1979 from Andrew R. Grainger, New Hampshire Assistant Attorney General, to Maynard Mires, MD, MPH, Executive Secretary, State Board of Registration in Medicine and Miss Marguerite Hastings, Director, Board of Nursing Education and Registration, folder "Joint Regulation Board of Medicine 1979"; letter dated September 13, 1982 from Assistant Attorney General James Townsend to Paul G. Boisseau, Secretary, Commission on Pharmacy, in reply to Subject; "Who Can Dispense," folder "Legislation 1980s." See also *Registered Nurses and Practical Nurses,* RSA 326-B: 4, Powers and Duties of the Board Laws of the State of New Hampshire (January 1,

1974), Concord, New Hampshire, and Commission on Pharmacy minutes, September 19, 1979.

25. See Board of Nursing minutes, January 14, 1974.

26. For comments by Mires and others on the impending closure of the last hospital-based nursing schools, see *New Hampshire Medical Society News* 32, no. 2 (March 1980), 4.

27. See Board of Nursing minutes, February 21, 1974. Selma Deitch, MD, another formidable woman with a national reputation in pediatric health and a significant statewide power base, was director of the New Hampshire Division of Maternal and Child Health services at the New Hampshire Department of Public Health, and reported directly to Mires. Deitch believed strongly in the need for, and abilities of, nurse practitioner care within the public health system, even meeting with Hastings and the Board of Nursing to explore sponsoring a nurse practitioner training program in New Hampshire. Although this idea never reached fruition, Deitch was responsible for facilitating nurse practitioner training for several New Hampshire public health nurses and also for assuring that nurse practitioners held significant positions of power in New Hampshire pediatric programs, public health department administration, and public clinic patient care. It is probable that Mires, when faced with negotiating nurse practitioner practice boundaries on behalf of the Board of Medicine and physicians, was keenly aware that Hastings and Deitch, with whom he had close and often daily working relationships, supported nurses and patients rather than focusing on protecting physician boundaries. Susan McKeown relates how Deitch was responsible for the state supporting education of pediatric nurse practitioners, including Susan herself, to staff federally funded public pediatric clinics in Manchester in the 1970s. McKeown also discusses the remarkable dedication Deitch had to multidisciplinary care for all children in New Hampshire. Transcript of oral history Susan McKeown recorded March 22, 2005 (cited as McKeown), lines 85–626. Kathleen Hoerbinger, former state coordinator and case manager for home care of children with spina bifida, relates that Deitch was "a character. She was dauntless and wouldn't take 'no' for an answer" (personal communication with Hoerbinger, August 22, 2005). Both nurses had great respect and admiration for Deitch.

28. Letter dated January 9, 1978 from Marguerite Hastings, Executive Director, New Hampshire "Legislation 1970s"; see "Joint Regulation of Board of Registration in Medicine & Board of Nursing Education and Nurse Registration relative to definition of professional nursing" discussing the rule for dispensing, attached to letter dated July 5, 1979 from Andrew R. Grainger, New Hampshire Assistant Attorney General to Maynard Mires, MD, MPH, Executive Secretary, State Board of Registration in Medicine, and Miss Marguerite Hastings, Director, Board of Nursing Education and Registration, folder "Joint Regulation Board of Medicine 1979"; letter dated September 13, 1982 from Assistant Attorney General James Townsend to Paul G. Boisseau, Secretary, Commission on Pharmacy, in reply to Subject; "Who Can Dispense," folder "Legislation 1980s." In an interesting coincidence, in June 1978, while Hastings and Mires were negotiating the process to allow nurse practitioners to dispense, the Commission on Pharmacy refused to relicense the State Public Health Department Laboratory (which held pharmaceuticals over which the Commission on Pharmacy had jurisdiction) and required Mires, who oversaw the lab, to close the lab, move the facility, and install expensive and extensive environmental, architectural, and procedural controls prior to reopening. At this same time Mires was also in difficult and contentious negotiations with the Commission on Pharmacy to allow paramedics and

emergency medical technicians to administer medications in emergencies, and the Commission on Pharmacy and Board of Medicine (of which Mires was a member) were disputing Board of Medicine handling of physicians referred for Board adjudication by the Drug Investigation Unit and Commission on Pharmacy, Commission on Pharmacy minutes, April 19, May 10, June 21, July 26, November 8, 1978.

29. Letter dated November 17, 1977 from Attorney General David Souter to Commission on Pharmacy, attached to Commission on Pharmacy minutes, December 14, 1977; Commission on Pharmacy minutes, September 19, 1979, August 13, 1980, May 26, 1982.

30. See Mires 2005, lines 675–91.

31. The Commission on Pharmacy also opposed dispensing, prescribing, or possessing medications by nurses in college health clinics, and by optometrists, chiropractors, paramedics, and emergency medical technicians. Commission on Pharmacy minutes, December 18, 1974, April 19, 1978, July 26, 1978, June 18, 1980, May 7, 1986.

32. See White, lines 909–31; letter dated November 12, 1977 from Betty H. Mitchell and Donna White to "Dear Fellow Practitioners," folder "Legislation 1970s."

33. Personal communication with George Roberts, February 8, 2005. See also transcript of oral history with George Roberts, January 22, 2005 (cited as Roberts), lines 105–50, 415–20, 681–88.

34. Letter dated January 24, 1978 from Debbie Clark, RN PNP, Recording Secretary, NHNPA, to "Dear Practitioner," folder "Legislation 1970s."

35. See transcript of oral history, Cynthia Cote recorded February 11, 2005 (cited as Cote), lines 860–63.

36. Cote, also lines 1353–86.

37. Kuhlman, lines 118–25, 1037–51; Interview with Donna Cassioly, March, 3, 2005, lines 403–24. All NHNPA meetings from January 1977 through September 1983, with the exception of a few dinner meetings at area restaurants, were held after hours or on Saturdays at the Concord Clinic in Concord, where Kuhlman and Cassidy worked with Kuhlman's husband, obstetrician Gerry Hamilton. See NHNPA minutes, January 11, 1977–September 18, 1983. Letters sent to nurse practitioners through January 1980, when NHNPA had its own letterhead printed, were sent on Concord Clinic letterhead.

38. See Weeman, lines 934–41; Cote, lines 617–716; Charest, lines 1060–70, 1500–1580; Dirubbo, lines 440–57, 815–29, 844–80; letter dated January 24, 1978 from Debbie Clark, RN PNP, Recording Secretary, NHNPA, to "Dear Practitioner"; letter dated January 29, 1979 from Kathy Higgins Cahill, President, NHNPA, and Prescription Task Force members Chris Kuhlman, Gloria Klein, and Paula Weeman, to "Dear Nurse Practitioner," folder "Legislation 1970s"; NHNPA minutes May 1, 1979, folder "Minutes 1970–1980."

39. Kuhlman, lines 215–16.

40. See NHNPA minutes September 11, 1978, folder "Legislation 1970s."

41. NHNPA minutes June 5, 1979, folder "Minutes 1970–1980."

42. Reginald W,. Rhein, Jr, "Nurses Colleagues or Competitors," *Medical World News,* 1979, 20–65, 69–71, 73.

43. Roberts 2005, lines 552–54.

44. Interview with Laurie Harding, White River Junction, Vermont, June 14, 2005 (cited as Harding), lines 683–716.

45. NHNPA minutes, January 12, 1980, NHNPA Papers, Box 1–1, folder "Legislation and Minutes 1980."

46. Mires 2005, lines 239–81.

47. Board of Medicine minutes, October 1979, New Hampshire Board of Medicine Minutes, July 6, 1978–December 16, 1979.

48. NHNPA minutes, June 12, 1981, folder "Legislation and Minutes 1981."

49. The June 2, 1981 NHNPA minutes discusses the second legislative attempt and failure. See May 1980 minutes, folder "Minutes 1980s"; minutes, January 1, February 2, September 16, 1983, folder "Minutes & Correspondence 1980–1983."

50. NHNPA minutes June 5, September 11, 1979, folder "Legislation & Minutes 1978 & 1979."

51. Cote, lines 1120–65.

52. Medical-nursing boundaries are further discussed in Fairman, "Delegated by Default or Negotiated by Need?"; Keeling, *Nursing and the Privilege of Prescription.*

53. Julie Fairman, "The Roots of Collaborative Practice: Nurse Practitioner Pioneers' Stories," *Nursing History Review* 10 (2002), 159–194.

54. Susan M. Reverby, "The Sorcerer's Apprentice," in *Prognosis Negative: Crisis in the Health Care System,* ed. David Kotelchuck (New York: Vintage Books, 1976), 170–183. Other scholars disagree with Reverby's analysis in this early work. For example, in more recent scholarly work, Fairman, "Delegated by Default" (1999) has found that nursing academics' dismay at the idea of nurse practitioners was more an aspect of "insecurity" and a "prevailing fear of a middle man between nursing and medicine taking away nurses' power," while physicians were supportive of and encouraged nurses crossing medical boundaries. See also O'Reilly, *Health Care Practitioners: An Ontario Case Study on Policy Making.* (Toronto: University of Toronto Press, 2000).

55. Weeman, lines 1165–74.

56. Cote, lines 1336–86.

57. Nursing history is, of course, more varied and nuanced. For a comprehensive discussion of nurses' work identity intermingled with personal, cultural, and community identity, see Patricia D'Antonio, "Revisiting and Rethinking the Rewriting of Nursing's History," *Bulletin of the History of Medicine* 73 (1999): 268–90, at 270.

58. Nancy Rudner Lugo, Eileen T. O'Grady, Donna R. Hodnicki, and Charlene M. Hanson, "Ranking State NP Regulation: Practice Environment and Consumer Healthcare Choice," *American Journal for Nurse Practitioners* 11, no. 4 (2007), 8–9, 14–18, 23–24.

NOTES AND DOCUMENTS

Pumpkins, Pigs, and People

Amanda Rubenstein
University of Pennsylvania

Fat pigs. Speedy horses. Large pumpkins. If plants and animals could be improved by proper breeding techniques, then why wouldn't the same hold true for humans? In 1927, governor of Kansas Arthur Capper explained to the press, "it is as important for Kansas to grow fine men and women as it is to grow fine cattle and hogs."[1] "Better Baby" and "Fitter Family" Contests that took place at state fairs across early 20th-century America were designed to judge "human stock" to select the most eugenically fit family. While Americans were already exposed to eugenic messages through proeuthanasia films like *The Black Stork,* newspapers, magazines, and biology textbooks, these contests played a pivotal role in popularizing eugenics throughout the 1920s and became increasingly commonplace at international, national, and local fairs.[2] Specifically, eugenics exhibits at the state fairs helped to garner public support for the social reforms such as immigration restriction, marriage restriction, euthanasia, segregation, and compulsory institutionalization and sterilization of those deemed degenerates or defectives.

The Fitter Family Contests actually began as Better Baby Contests that were organized as part of the U.S. Children's Bureau campaign against infant mortality. The Better Baby Contests were originally designed to decrease infant mortality rates, but they changed from this rather benign focus on improving children's health to eugenically oriented Fitter Family competitions with a strong commitment to controlled human breeding.[3] By the mid-1920s, the categorizations used in Better Baby Contests to identify healthy babies and educate mothers about child rearing became a front for the eugenics movement to discourage poor immigrants, Blacks, and the mentally or physically

Nursing History Review 17 (2009): 179–184. A Publication of the American Association for the History of Nursing.
DOI: 10.1891/1062-8061.17.179

disabled from reproducing. When Mary Watts and Florence Sherborn, respectively president and vice-president of the Iowa Baby Betterment Association, joined the American Eugenics Society (AES) Committee on Popular Education,[4] they likely saw themselves as saving infant lives and promoting eugenics as a scientific endeavor to improve the mental and physical quality of the human race.[5] As a result of their partnership with the eugenics movement, the Better Baby Contests eventually became "Fitter Families for Future Firesides" competitions.

The AES used the contests to disseminate practical and scientific information on genetic health, draw attention to eugenics, and promote eugenics research. These contests, along with sermon contests and traveling exhibits, became powerful tools for eugenicists to promote reforms involving the family and reproduction and provided an opportunity to collect detailed family information that could be used for research. At most contests, competitors submitted an "Abridged Record of Family Traits" that was scanned for patterns of presumed inheritance.[6] Favorable capabilities included "[being] generous, self-sacrificing, having strong family ties, and being a successful parent." Negative traits, or "temperamental stigmata" as they were called, included being "selfish, jealous, suspicious, high tempered, and cruel." Also, a team of medical doctors performed time-consuming evaluations of social, educational, occupational, dental, psychological, psychiatric, racial, and medical histories. Each family member was given an overall letter grade of eugenic health, and the family with the highest grade average was awarded a silver trophy. Trophies were typically awarded in three family categories: small (1 child), medium (2–4 children), and large (5 or more children). Childless couples were eligible for prizes in contests held in some states.[7] All contestants with a B+ or better received bronze medals bearing the inscription, "Yea, I have a goodly heritage,"[8] and most winners were White with Western and Northern European heritage.

APS Images of the Eugenics Health Exhibits

The American Philosophical Society (APS) has a collection of scrapbooks maintained by the American Eugenics Society that contains 83 images of the Eugenic Health Exhibits at the 1925 Kansas, Michigan, Texas, and Pennsylvania State Fairs. These images allow one to explore how the fairs visually communicated the hereditary principles on which the Fitter Family Contests were based. They show racial casts and models, pedigree charts, and tables; "Mendel's Theater," where marionettes were used to demonstrate Mendel's principles of genetics; and cages of black and white guinea pigs demonstrating inheritance of dominant and recessive genes and traits. These images also show signs at fairs that compared literacy rates of America's "Native-Born," as the signs screamed, to the "Foreign-Born" and "Negroes."[9] The APS collection provides a window into understanding how such exhibits simultaneously popularized the Fitter Family Contests, promoted the principles of eugenics, and put eugenics in the public eye.

Many visitors found the Flashing Light Exhibit the most compelling (see Figure 1).[10] This exhibit was first displayed at the 1926 Sesqui-Centennial International Exhibition in Philadelphia, an exhibition intended to celebrate the 150th anniversary of American independence. The exhibit received a silver medal as an "advanced educational idea"[11] for its ability to communicate the threat that differential birthrates posed for American society. In fact, it became the prototype for similar exhibits at other state fairs. The exhibit used lights flashing at different intervals to demonstrate that the dangerous and defective were reproducing too quickly, and the normal and advantaged too slowly. At the center in bold letters appeared the words: "Some people are born to be a burden to the rest." At the far left, a light flashed every 16 seconds to indicate, "every 16 seconds a person is born in the United States." At the far right, a light flashed every 7½ minutes to indicate the much lower frequency of the birth of a "high grade person who will have the ability to do creative work and be fit for leadership." Only 4 percent of the American population, according to the AES, fell into this category. Thus, the flashing lights conveyed a sense of urgency and threat by serving as a constant reminder of how quickly the American well-born "stock" was being tainted.

At the top of the poster, a light flashing every 15 seconds marked $100 of taxpayer money spent "for the care of persons with bad heredity such as the feeble-minded, criminals, and other defectives." At a time when social progressives like Jacob Riis were promoting state involvement and welfare

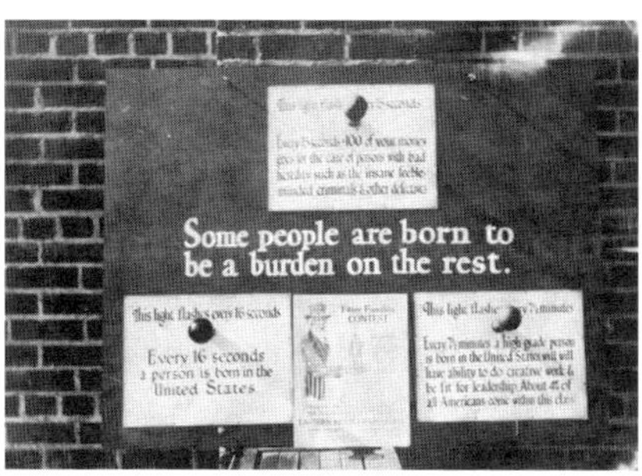

Figure 1. The flashing light sign at the Fitter Families Contest, 1926, Charles B. Davenport papers, Florence B. Sherborn Fitter Families folder, Am3,575.06,49, American Philosophical Society, Philadelphia. Used by permission of the American Philosophical Society.

programs to solve social problems, eugenicists sought to emphasize how much these programs were costing the average American and how selective breeding would reduce the need for them. Eugenicists believed that by intervening in natural selection, these progressives actually promoted "the preservation and care of the feebleminded, the delinquent, the crippled, the insane, and others who varied biologically in the direction of social incompetence."[12]

Flashing Lights Exhibits and Fitter Family Contests sometimes displayed a pocketbook with the flashing light to emphasize how much money was spent on the "unfit." Similar exhibits used lights that flashed every 48 seconds to warn that "every 48 seconds someone is born in America who will never grow up beyond the mental age of 8," that "crime costs America $100,000 every second," and that "very few normal persons go to jail." Many of these had bold letters at the center of the poster that said: "Learn about heredity—You can help to correct these conditions." All these exhibits supported eugenics publications, lectures, and newspaper columns that spoke of a "race suicide" that would result from the reproductive decline of the nation's best "stock." Scientific studies building on Mendel's principles of heredity seemed to validate claims that crime, insanity, mental defects, alcoholism, and indigence were all attributable to bad genes, and that such genes were more prevalent in Blacks and immigrants than in Whites.

The AES wanted Flashing Light Exhibits to make eugenics principles relevant and accessible to a broader American public. Eugenics enthusiasts in the United States were largely middle- to upper-middle-class White, educated Anglo-Saxon Protestants, and the contests presumably attracted a self-selected group very similar to this demographic.

While eugenics was already being taught as a scientific paradigm at elite schools and universities and popularized in the fields of science and medicine, Watts and Sherborn wanted to extend the ideology of "race betterment" to every home. Watts wrote to Charles Davenport, a prominent American eugenicist, "All I dare to hope from our crude plan is the opening of a way for scientific facts to filter into the consciousness of the masses and then the people will save themselves."[13] The exhibits at fairs also seemed like the perfect way to popularize the movement to the "average" American, who did not need to understand science to understand the implications of the flashing lights. The fact that the contests were held at agricultural fairs meant that visitors were mostly from middle-class rural families. Eugenicists wanted the exhibits to appeal to these farmers and their families so that they would recognize themselves as people who had good heredity but bore the burden of those who did not.

Perhaps this need to ensure that farmers would recognize themselves as "good stock" and "high grade" visitors explains why the fairs strategically juxtaposed the idealized White American families who won the contests with freak shows caricaturing criminal and insane grotesques as examples of degenerates.[14] The AES used this contrast as part of its two-pronged approach to popularizing its principles: a *positive* one, which concentrated on exhorting the genetically gifted to reproduce, and a *negative* one, which sought to prevent defectives from breeding. By making native-born White Americans aware of the sacrifices they were making to support the hereditary degenerates and foreign-born, eugenicists wanted fairgoers to leave with an understanding of how hereditary defectives threatened the future racial stock of the country, which would make the American public more willing to support their legislative and social reforms.

Eugenics Is Less Archaic Than We Like to Think

There are still many unanswered questions regarding the impact of Fitter Family Contests and eugenic exhibits. Though contestants did not need to get an A to get a medal, what happened to those who did not get a B+ or higher? Did not receiving a medal greatly affect the way these contestants saw themselves and did it influence whether they decided to have children? How did Blacks and immigrants respond to the exhibits? How often did they participate in the contests and attend the fairs? Were there not psychological implications for people whom the exhibits characterized as "burdens to the rest"?

The rich photographic data available in archives such as the APS collection of AES Records (www.amphilsoc.org/library/mole/a/aes.htm) provide the opportunity to further research these questions and explore the darker side of the Fitter Family Contests. Such data allow us to explore an unanswered question: How did eugenics exhibits transform Better Baby Contests, part of an important health campaign to reduce infant mortality rates, into eugenically oriented Fitter Family Contests? The images also contain clues as to how social mores influenced the interpretation and implications of scientific data.

Amanda Rubenstein, BA
University of Pennsylvania
201 S. 25th Street #209
Philadelphia, PA 19103
949–637–5066
amandar2@sas.upenn.edu

Acknowledgments

I acknowledge the guidance, insight, and support of Julie Fairman, RN, PhD, FAAN, and Patricia D'Antonio, RN, PhD, FAAN.

Notes

1. "Medals Go to 'Fitter Families': Bronze Pins Furnished by Senator Capper," *Topeka Capital,* August 14, 1927.

2. See Martin S. Pernick, *The Black Stork: Eugenics and the Death of "Defective" Babies in American Medicine and Motion Pictures Since 1915* (New York: Oxford University Press, 1996); Steven Selden, "Transforming Better Babies into Fitter Families: Archival Resources and the History of the American Eugenics Movement, 1908–1930," *Proceedings of the American Philosophical Society* 149 (June 2005): 205.

3. Selden, "Transforming Better Babies," 5.

4. "Human Stock at the Kansas Free Fair," *Eugenical News* 7, no. 10 (October 1922): 111.

5. Richard A. Meckel, *Save the Babies: American Public Health Reform and the Prevention of Infant Mortality, 1850–1929* (Baltimore: Johns Hopkins University Press, 1990).

6. "Family History: Nervous and Mental History form" (draft 1920?), "Fitter Families Contests," 1920?, Charles B. Davenport papers, Florence B. Sherborn Fitter Families folder, B: D27 #2, p. 7, American Philosophical Society, Philadelphia.

7. "Fitter Family Contests," 1925, Image Archive on the American Eugenics Movement, Cold Spring Harbor Laboratory, Cold Spring Harbor, N.Y., EugenicsArchive.org.

8. "Family History: Nervous and Mental History form."

9. Publications by the Children's Bureau demonstrate that racial hierarchies were used to classify different traits. See Daniel J. Kevles, *In the Name of Eugenics: Genetics and the Use of Human Heredity* (New York: Knopf, 1985).

10. "Flashing Light Sign Used with Small Exhibits," "Fitter Families Contests," 1926, Charles B. Davenport papers, Florence B. Sherborn Fitter Families folder, Am3,575.06,49, American Philosophical Society, Philadelphia; W. S. Evans (secretary), *Organized Eugenics* (New Haven, Conn.: American Eugenics Society, January 1931).

11. "Flashing Light Sign."

12. Selden, "Transforming Better Babies," 205.

13. Laura L. Lovett, "'Fitter Families for Future Firesides': Florence Sherborn and Popular Eugenics," *Public Historian* 29, no. 3 (Summer 2007): 69–85.

14. Kerry Soper, "Classical Bodies Versus the Criminal Carnival: Eugenics Ideology in 1930s Popular Art," in *Popular Eugenics: National Efficiency and American Mass Culture in the 1930s,* ed. Susan Currell and Christina Cogdell (Athens: Ohio University Press, 2006), 269–307.

IN MEMORIAM

The Path She Tread: Saluting the Lifetime Achievements of Mary Elizabeth Lancaster Carnegie, DPA, RN, FAAN

April 19, 1916–February 20, 2008

Because of the path you tread we are constantly
reminded of the true meaning of being our brother
and sister's keepers. We now know what you have
always known that if we commit to loving each other
as we love ourselves we will succeed. So I thank you
my friend for renewing and rekindling the flames of
unconditional love, faith, hope, charity, and
compassion, which exist in all of us, but too often
are allowed to flicker and die.

Because of the path you tread you fought for us to
be able to participate at the highest levels in
professional nursing when you gave us the tools
to do the important work we were destined to do.
Tools like a legacy filled with information and
instructions to guide and direct us, and tools which
educated and inspired us. So I thank you my friend for
being the ultimate mentor, for your vision, for
your wisdom, for your tenacity, for your
leadership, for your unwavering belief in the
integrity of human beings, but mostly my friend
for cheerfully reminding us that it's not the one who finishes
the fastest, but the one who can endure till the end.
Because of the path you tread you provided opportunities
for us to be able to move from the lowest strata of nursing
education to being able to enter the field with the highest
educational qualifications. So I thank you my friend for
being the perfect role model and sacrificial lamb, showing us
that through perseverance, dedication, leadership, relentless
support, and an undaunted spirit, we too can make the
world of nursing a better place for Blacks.

Nursing History Review 17 (2009): 185–190. A Publication of the American Association for the History of Nursing.
DOI: 10.1891/1062-8061.17.185

Because of the path you tread you unselfishly made
personal and financial sacrifices to give us a
written history. A history which showed us that
"the result of our common striving brings us into closer
relationship and aids us in seeing ourselves as part of
the great whole—the ideal to which we are all striving."
So I thank you my friend for showing the entire nursing
community that Black nurses have contributed much to
our collective profession, to all races in all communities,
throughout the world, past and present, Despite All Odds.
Because of the path you tread, you instilled in me a
burning desire to right the great wrong of race exclusion
in the nursing profession when you gave me stories to
write about. You constantly shared with me stories
of extraordinary Black nurses doing extraordinary things.
Stories that, I promise you, will no longer be lost
to professional nursing history. So I thank you my friend
for writing about our accomplishments thereby
helping me understand the importance of rescuing Black nurses
from historical oblivion and placing them onto the world's stage.

Your life of service to all of mankind was full and
fulfilling, because you truly believed that to whom
much is given, much, much more is expected in
return. God blessed you so you would be able to bless
thousands more. For over seventy years you were that
light which lit our path, and the guardian angel who
guided and protected us. Because you lived we will
face a brighter tomorrow. You are a legend in your
own time, because you cared enough to give us your
very best. Rest in peace my friend, you've earned it.

We remember Mary Elizabeth Lancaster Carnegie, an African American nurse, author, administrator, researcher, philanthropist, pioneer in educational and organizational administration, and a significant leader in struggles to help eliminate discrimination in nursing education, in nursing practice, in society as a whole, and in the national professional nursing organization in this country.

Dr. Carnegie's fight to eliminate exclusionary practices for Blacks in nursing occurred during the time when rigid patterns of segregation and discrimination in nursing education and employment for Blacks existed across this country. Black codes limiting access to institutions of learning and job opportunities, designed to keep Blacks "in their places," were legislated and enforced by laws and customs in the North as well as in the South. Through persistence and dogged determination Dr. Carnegie was steadfast in her efforts to ensure that current and future Black nurses would have the opportunity to become experientially and educationally prepared to assume the highest positions in professional nursing and have the opportunity to do so.

Mary Elizabeth Lancaster Carnegie did not grow up with dreams of becoming a nurse. Her nursing career came about more by chance than by choice; yet, her accomplishments will live long beyond the time she spent here. Throughout her career, she fought injustice and prejudice everywhere she found them, and made a lasting mark on the profession of nursing and the history of Black women and men in it. She has forged a path that many have followed and will continue to follow. The world is a better place because of her determination, strength, and commitment to "fighting the good fight" for what was right and making her voice heard.

Mary Elizabeth was born on April 19, 1916, in Baltimore, Maryland. She was the third child of Adeline Beatrice Swan Lancaster and John Oliver Lancaster. After her parents were divorced, her mother was not physically or financially able to care for her children. All of the children were sent to live with family members. At the age of eight, Mary Elizabeth was taken to Washington, D.C., to her Aunt Rosie who lived on M street in southeast Washington. While at Aunt Rosie's, Mary Elizabeth was determined not to be a burden. To help the family out, at an early age, Mary Elizabeth went to work. She worked at the Allies Inn, a Whites-only cafeteria, after school and on weekends.

After graduating from Dunbar High School in 1933, Mary Elizabeth, growing "tired of working in the cafeteria," went to New York "to find work or further my education." Unable to find work or the opportunity to go to school, she returned to Washington, D.C., and the Allies Inn. But before she returned, however, a cousin suggested she become a nurse. Her cousin encouraged her to apply to Lincoln School for Nurses, a nursing school for Blacks in the Bronx. In July 1934 Mary Elizabeth received a letter from Lincoln informing her that she had been accepted to their nursing school. Unsure if she wanted to be a nurse or even if she would like nursing, she decided she would try it: "Anything would be better than working the steam table at the Allies Inn." At the young age of 17, Lancaster left the security of Aunt Rosie's house and moved to New York City.

During her training at Lincoln, Mary Elizabeth discovered that she genuinely enjoyed her studies at the school of nursing and caring for patients assigned her. It was also during this time that Mary Elizabeth became an activist after learning of the struggle Black nurses were engaged in to gain recognition as full-fledged members of the American Nurses Association (ANA); of major problems Black nurses were having in gaining admission to schools of nursing throughout this country; and the many obstacles Black nurses faced when seeking employment. These and other facts about the Black nurses' dismal plight were revealed to Mary Elizabeth and some of her classmates by Mrs. Mabel Keaton Staupers, Executive Secretary of the National Association of Colored Graduate Nurses (NACGN). The student nurses found out that the NACGN was established in 1908 by Black nurses "to advance the standards and best interest of trained nurses; to break down discrimination in the nursing profession; and to develop leadership within the ranks of Negro nurses." After hearing Mrs. Staupers's lecture, Mary Elizabeth stated, "the information given by Mrs. Staupers was new to us because, even though we had taken a course in the history of nursing, our instructor was White and had made no mention of the contributions of Black nurses to the profession, nor had she mentioned the racial problems that existed." She continued, "shortly after Mrs. Staupers spoke to our class, NACGN held its annual convention in New York . . . and used our school as convention headquarters. Because I was active in student affairs I was selected to serve as one of the hostesses to student delegates, which gave me the opportunity to attend the program sessions and to participate in the social events. The student delegates were from other Black nursing schools in the country. . . . At this NACGN convention, I learned about the problems faced by Black nurses and made a solemn pledge to myself that when I graduated, I would do all within my power to help change the system and break down the barriers that were keeping Black nurses out of the mainstream of professional nursing." And she did!

Always with the love and support of her family and against great odds, Mary Elizabeth courageously pursued her education and career goals. After Lincoln, she attended West Virginia State College full time in return for her work in the school health program. She graduated from West Virginia State College in 1942 with a Bachelor of Arts Degree in Sociology. Using the knowledge about health needs and the care of Black patients acquired during her training at Lincoln, Mary Elizabeth was an unqualified hit with the patients on the Black wing of the Medical College of Virginia. It was on this ward that she worked as clinical instructor for the segregated Saint Philip Hospital School of Nursing. While working at Saint Philip, Mary Elizabeth, despite the fact that she was a professional nurse with a college degree, was not shown the same respect as her White peers. She took offense to the fact that White nurses were addressed as "Miss," "Mrs.," or "Mr.," while she and other Black nurses were referred to as "Nurse" and acknowledged by their first names. Unable and unwilling to tolerate this slight, regardless how small, Mary Elizabeth left Saint Philip.

Always keeping uppermost in her mind the promise she made to herself to "do all within my power to help change the system and break down barriers that were keeping Black nurses out of the mainstream of professional nursing," Mary Elizabeth knew that higher education was crucial. In 1943, Mary Elizabeth initiated the first baccalaureate nursing program in the state of Virginia, at Hampton Institute (Hampton University). She taught less than one year at Hampton when she received the news that she had been awarded a fellowship to continue her education. Carnegie left Hampton to enroll in the School Administration program at the University of Toronto. This opportunity to further her education was provided through the Rockefeller Foundation Fellowship Program. While a student in Canada Mary Elizabeth met and married Eric Carnegie, the brother of a former student. She completed her studies in Canada and received a Certificate in School Nursing Administration in 1944.

Shortly thereafter, Mrs. Carnegie accepted the offer to join the faculty at Florida A&M University (FAMU) in Tallahassee. Mrs. Carnegie initiated the first baccalaureate nursing program in the state of Florida at FAMU. She became the first dean of the newly founded Florida A&M University School of Nursing.

It was while she was at FAMU that Dean Carnegie was pushed onto the world's stage. She became a courtesy member of the Florida State Association's Nursing Board. Courtesy membership was afforded her because she was the elected president of the Florida State Association of the Association of Colored Graduate Nurses; however, courtesy membership came with stipulations. One was expected to pay membership dues but could not vote and was not allowed to speak. According to Carnegie, courtesy membership was "taxation without representation." Again, racism in the nursing profession was raising its ugly head. And again, Carnegie would rebel. Unable and unwilling to tolerate mistreatment from White professional leaders, Dean Carnegie joined forces with the state's Black nurses and fought the injustices being imposed on them. For example, when attending board meetings, Carnegie was not silent like she was directed to be, but was outspoken and outgoing, stating "I don't care about their rules, I spoke up anyway and I also refused to sit in the area designated for Blacks." On many occasions she would tell me, "Before I would sit where they wanted me to sit, I would stand." The following year, Carnegie ran for office and was unanimously elected to the Board of Directors, becoming the first Black State Board member of that or any other state association. While remaining steadfast in her fight for the rights of Black nurses to be included in the mainstream of professional nursing and have the opportunity to do so, Carnegie also continued her education. She earned a Master's Degree in Administration and Higher Education from Syracuse University, New York, in 1952.

In 1953, Carnegie took a leave from academe and applied for a job at the American Journal of Nursing Company in New York City. She was hired, becoming the first Black Assistant Editor of the *American Journal of Nursing*. In 1956, she moved down the hall and joined the editorial staff of *Nursing Outlook* as Associate Editor, and in 1973 she was appointed Chief Editor of *Nursing Research*. Her first editorial in *Nursing Research*, entitled "ANA Directory Identifies Minorities with Doctorates," drew attention to the small number of minority nurses with doctoral degrees. At this time there were no Native Americans, one Hispanic, 12 Asians, and a few Black nurses, most of whom had gone into medicine and were therefore lost to nursing. This prompted the American Nurses Association to write a grant to the National Institute of Mental Health for funding a fellowship program that would increase the quantity and quality of ethnic/racial minority researchers. In 1974, the grant for nearly $1 million was approved and the ANA Ethnic Minority Program was established. In 2008, 34 years after it was initiated, several hundred minority nurses have earned the doctoral degree. After 35 years at the American Journal of Nursing Company, Carnegie retired to begin her second career.

While at the American Journal of Nursing Company, Carnegie noted that there was little to no written data on the contributions of Blacks to the nursing profession. She now knew that all of nursing must know the whole truth about all members of our collective profession; to do less would be a disservice to the entire corps of nursing, past, present, and future. Carnegie also knew that if a complete history, documenting individuals and groups omitted from our history, was to be written, she would have to do it herself. And she did! Dr. Mary Elizabeth Carnegie took thousands of dollars of her own money, and researched, documented, and publicized contributions of Black nurses worldwide in her own book, *The Path We Tread: Blacks in Nursing Worldwide*, and in more than 94 journal articles and editorials, 23 book chapters, 2 other books, 300 speeches, and hundreds of presentations, nationally and internationally.

For her generosity, untiring devotion, and dedicated service to advancing opportunities in professional nursing, Dr. Carnegie was recognized worldwide. She was the recipient of numerous professional and community awards and honors. She also had bestowed upon her eight honorary doctorates. There are 11 distinguished professorships and two endowed chairs named in her honor.

Marie O. Pitts-Mosley, EdD, RN, PNP
Historian, consultant, and retired Associate Professor at Hunter-Bellevue School of Nursing and Howard University School of Nursing
Bowie, MD 20721

MEDIA REVIEWS

Hospital Voices . . . Stories From Nightingale to Now. Held at the Florence Nightingale Museum, London, England, May 12–December 23, 2007. Commissioned by the Florence Nightingale Museum Trustees. Funded by The National Lottery Heritage Fund and Guy's and St. Thomas' Charity. Oral histories collected by Carol McCubbin, Ines Warsop, Kath Start, and volunteers from the Nurses Voices Team Kingston University and St. George's University of London. Carol McCubbin, Project Manager. Designed by DOT. Peter Warren, Designer.

Hospital Voices . . . Stories From Nightingale to Now is an innovative exhibition designed to make the history of nursing and health care more accessible to 21st-century museum attendees. Based on 60 interviews with nurses, patients, and community members related to St. Thomas, Guy's, and Evelina Children's Hospitals and their nursing schools, the exhibit draws on the experiences of people who rarely write histories or memoirs. The typical museum display case is a small part of the exhibit. Rather, seven panels, five interactive kiosks equipped with modified iPods, and 10-minute videos thoughtfully drawing on the oral histories make this an attractive and informative presentation.

The exhibition's focus is the seven well-designed panels, each headed by a quotation from Nightingale and followed by a short discussion of developments since Nightingale. The critical part of these displays includes an index to oral histories that flesh out those developments, excerpts of which can be heard at a nearby interactive kiosk. For example, the first panel, entitled "What makes a nurse?" reminds us of Nightingale's pronouncement: "Nursing is an art. . . . " One excerpt has a nurse remembering the significance of "ward manners," such as having nurses have all nine buttons on each sleeve carefully buttoned and standing erect with their hands behind their backs when the matron or a physician came into the ward. In another excerpt, a nurse describes an early strike, the result of the hospital administration announcing that it would no longer supply the nurses with milk and bread at the end of their shift. The nurses decided to strike; that is, they planned to walk off their posts the next morning at 11 A.M. and report back at 11:30. Medical students agreed to care for patients during the 30-minute strike. When the nurses returned to their

Nursing History Review 17 (2009): 191–200. A Publication of the American Association for the History of Nursing.
DOI: 10.1891/1062–8061.17.191

posts, the matron asked them to visit her that evening, when she quietly asked them what the problem was. After the nurses explained about the milk and bread, the matron served them milk and sandwiches and announced that she agreed milk and bread should be supplied at the end of their shift. And so the food was restored. These and other excerpts demonstrate the strictures under which nurses worked and the methods they used to inform the administration while not sacrificing patient care. The oral histories convey an intimacy, a reality to the history of nursing that is rarely communicated in a printed source. The many ongoing tensions, struggles over what it meant to be a *professional* and everyday frustrations and satisfactions of being a nurse, emerge in the voices of the nurses being interviewed.

The six other panels "Nursing Duties," "Leadership," "Hospitals and Patients," "Infection Control," "Community," and "Progress" similarly connect 21st-century issues and people with the legacy of Nightingale. Interviewees were specifically asked what they saw as her legacy. Interestingly, most saw no direct influence of Nightingale on either their career choice or their career. Yet, the oral histories, with remarks about the Nightingale ward and her stress on cleanliness, make clear many such continuities exist.

The exhibition's insightful presentation adds a crucial dimension to the history of nursing, one that will be appreciated by contemporary nurses and those outside the profession. The kiosks are especially useful. Indeed, we spent much of our time listening to and then discussing the excerpts and their implications for gender, race, class, and professional development. Although this display was not intended for children, evidently children are drawn to it. Since one of us is an educational researcher, the interest among children reminds us that exhibitions may go well beyond their original intentions.

However, as with any such technology, there are glitches. One of the kiosks was not working when we visited. The museum personnel were quick to correct the problem and their commitment to both the museum and the history of nursing was more than a little visible. Also, limited space among the museum's permanent exhibits—this is a very small, compact display—has led to some unfortunate omissions. The excerpts are themselves engaging. Unfortunately, for each excerpt we have only a name and a date and it is not clear whether the date refers to the date of graduation, date of incident being related, or something else. Similarly, because we hear only excerpts, some of which are edited abruptly, we are not clear about the time or place discussed. The histories themselves are available to scholars through the archives at Kingston University, but even a handout listing brief biographies of the various interviewees would have been helpful. However, given the richness of the exhibition, these are minor points.

The exhibition organizers, interviewers, and designers are to be applauded for preserving the lived complexities and intensities of nurses' experiences and their work, ranging from exceptional to menial. Some of the stories present a somewhat romanticized picture of nursing's past; others paint candid views of patient experiences and how they have changed over time. Most important, the exhibition, through its incisive use of oral history, brings alive the experiences of often silent historical actors and immeasurably enhances our historical understanding.

Rima D. Apple, PhD
Vilas Life-Cycle Professor Emerita
University of Wisconsin-Madison
School of Human Ecology and Women's Studies Program
1300 Linden Drive
Madison, WI 53706

Michael W. Apple, EdD
John Bascom Professor of Curriculum and Instruction and
Educational Policy Studies
University of Wisconsin-Madison
Department of Educational Policy Studies
528D Teacher Education
225 N. Mills Street
Madison, WI 53706

Virginia Nursing History. Special Collections and Archives, Tompkins-McCaw Library, Virginia Commonwealth University. Compiled by the Joint History Committee of the Virginia Nurses' Association and the Virginia League of Nursing. Archivist, Jodi Koste; Designer, Andrew Bain, Virginia Commonwealth University (http://www.library.vcu.edu/tml/speccoll/nursing/)

The main purpose of the Web site, *Virginia Nursing History,* is to provide a survey of the history of professional nursing and nursing education in Virginia, including information about nursing organizations, certifications, educational programs, and the accomplishments of selected nursing leaders. The opening page of the Web site orients the visitor to a short description of the site, with information provided about site maintenance, standards, and credits. The site is well organized and divided into seven topical sections, each centering on a particular theme or focus of Virginia nursing history. The first section, *Highlights of Nursing in Virginia,* contains a comprehensive timeline that begins in 1900 and lists important events in the history of Virginia nursing through 2003. Each of the timeline items is accompanied by a short explanation of the event with appropriate embedded links to other sections of the Web site. The *Nursing Schools* section provides maps identifying locations of various nursing programs, both current and defunct, and the years they existed. The educational programs are divided into Doctoral, Master's, Baccalaureate, Associate, Licensed Practical Nurse, and Diploma programs. *Nursing Organizations,* the subject of the third section, identifies 17 Virginia nursing organizations formed over the century beginning with ones organized in 1901. Information on each of the organizations includes summaries on the history of the group, links to past presidents, annual meetings, and if still in existence, a link to the current Web site of the organization. If the organization has merged or is no longer in existence, information is provided concerning that process. The *Virginia Board of Nursing* is the fourth category represented. It presents information concerning the origins of the Board as well as the various names the Board was known by since its establishment in 1903. Named in chronological order of appointment are all the Registered Nurses, Licensed Practical Nurses, and citizen members of the Board. An additional category of this section names the chief officers of the Board from its initial inception. The last three sections of the Web site concentrate on the achievements of individual nurses. The *Fellows of the Academy* lists all Virginia nurses who were named Fellows in the American Academy of Nursing from 1974 to 2001. An *Awards* section lists Virginia winners of national awards in nursing. The final and a most helpful section for the nurse historian is the *Virginia Nursing Hall of Fame.* Fifteen nurses are featured with a short sketch of each along with a portrait, a linked biography, and bibliography for each nurse. The Joint History Committee of the Virginia Nurses Association (VNA) and the Virginia League for Nursing (VLN) developed the selection criteria used for featured nurses and selected the inaugural class of inductees in the spring of 2001.

Created in 2001, the site is overall a very useful research tool that provides a nice perspective on leadership in nursing in Virginia from around 1900 to the near-present. One of the site's major strengths is in its approach to racial inclusiveness. Black and White schools of nursing in the state, outstanding nurses, and organizations that were once segregated are recognized together; blending what were once two separate systems into a whole. The information provided by *Virginia Nursing History* is of interest to historians seeking a snapshot of the development of organized nursing and education in the state, with a focus on major nursing organizations.

The site does contain weaknesses. There are no links to primary documents. Nor does the Web site provide a search function, although it is laid out in an easily navigated format and does include links to outside sites that offer further explanation for entries. Some nursing history pertinent to Virginia is not covered. The years prior to 1900 are omitted from the timeline. This excludes some important early work on visiting nursing in Norfolk. There is little to document the early 20th-century history of state-sponsored public health nursing programs and the important connections that public health nurse leaders forged and the programs they instituted. New educational curricula such as the Clinical Nurse Leader and Doctor of Nursing Practice have not been added to the *Schools* section, and not all *Nursing Organizations*' leaders and meetings are current, though the site is routinely updated. The historical perspective of the site is set by original materials possessed by the VNA/VLN that tend to lean toward organizational history, yet the *Hall of Fame* entries clearly transcend those boundaries.

Despite such limitations, *Virginia Nursing History* remains an important resource.

Many of the more interesting critical events in nursing took place at the state and local levels. Information that focuses on nursing below the national level is sometimes not easily retrieved. Accessible state-level information can lead the researcher to local resources that can reveal unique stories. Numerous state nurses associations across the country are currently celebrating or planning to celebrate 100-year anniversaries as did Virginia in 2001. As they do, disseminating information about the state nursing activities, accomplishments, and issues to a wide audience serves multiple purposes. Web sites such as the *Virginia Nursing History* are welcomed as innovative, readily accessible sources of information on state nursing matters.

Mary E. Gibson, PhD, RN
Assistant Professor
University of Virginia School of Nursing
McLeod Hall
Charlottesville, VA 22908–0782

Influenza, 1918: "The Worst Epidemic the United States Has Ever Known." PBS On-Line, The American Experience. PBS/WGBH. Contributors: Alfred Crosby, PhD, and Jeffrey K. Taubenberger, MD. http://www.pbs.org/wgbh/amex/influenza/

Providing a brief overview of the major events, this Web site chronicles the 1918–1919 influenza pandemic in the United States. A basic introduction to the epidemic, it is designed for use by the general public, with a special emphasis as a source for educators. Particularly impressive is the commentary by Alfred Crosby, author of *America's Forgotten Pandemic,* and Jeffrey Taubenberger, pathologist at the Armed Forces Institute of Pathology, who recently discovered the cause of the devastating illness. The Web site works well, and is accurate in its facts. However, the site provides only a cursory glimpse of the great influenza pandemic, noting contributions of only a few significant physicians, including Surgeon General Rupert Blue and Victor Vaughan, MD. One major omission is the role of nurses and the nursing profession during the epidemic.

The site is easily navigated, but there are some technical difficulties in accessing the audiotaped interviews (at least for this reviewer). Nonetheless, transcripts of these are available. The site contains a "Teacher's Guide" with suggested classroom activities, most useful perhaps, at the high school level. It also contains a map outlining the spread of the disease across the country in various time periods. However, the map moves too quickly and it is difficult to ascertain exactly what is happening and when. What is apparent is that within weeks from its late August onset, the devastating flu covered the entire nation. A bar graph of mortality rates by month is also included on the Web site, as is a timeline of events from March 1918 until January 1919. Again, only very few events are noted—leaving major gaps in the story. One interesting component of the Web site is the detail contained in "City Snapshots," which describes the situation in Boston, Philadelphia, and San Francisco, and includes several photographs of events in these select cities.

The Web site could be expanded considerably. Of particular note, nurses such as Lillian Wald of Henry Street Settlement, Jane Delano of the American Red Cross, and Katherine Tucker of the Philadelphia Visiting Nurses and their work during the pandemic are missing. Also absent is the significant work of the American Red Cross, both at the national and local levels. More important, several major cities, including Washington, D.C., Chicago, and Seattle are not mentioned, nor is there any reference to how small towns across the country were affected.[1] Focusing on White America, the Web site does not discuss the story of Tuba City, Arizona, and the effect of the flu on the Navajo tribes living there.[2] Nor does it pay attention, with the exception of mentioning Brevig Mission, to the stories of devastation in small towns in Alaska, where physicians and nurses from Seattle were sent by ship to treat Alaska Natives.[3]

Links include (1) another PBS site, *The Great War and the Shaping of the 20th Century,* (2) the Centers for Disease Control, and (3) the World Health Organization. While these are all excellent sources for contemporary issues related to influenza, they do not provide historical data. For an historical viewpoint, it would be more helpful to link to such sites as the National Library of Medicine for more on the history of medicine during the pandemic; the Red Cross archives that has a historical timeline of events during the flu; the National Archives and Records Administration, which has a large collection of Red Cross reports from the period (Record Group 75); the Lillian Wald papers at the New York Public Library, which provide an in-depth description of events in New York City; and the Barbara Bates Center for the Study of the History of Nursing, which has a significant collection of Visiting Nurse Association papers about Philadelphia and the flu. Links to historical newspapers of 1918 would also be helpful.

The Web site contains a very short bibliography that could also be expanded to include, among others, such works as John Barry's book: *The Great Influenza,*[4] Carol Byerly's *Fever of War,*[5] Rhonda Keen-Payne's article in *NHR* "We Must Have Nurses,"[6] Gina Kolata's *Flu: The Story of the Great Influenza Pandemic of 1918 and the Search for the Virus That Caused It,*[7] and Rockafellar's "In Gauze We Trust," in the *Pacific Northwest Quarterly.*[8]

The site provides a few original photographs, and one letter sent to a colleague by a physician working in Camp Devens. These primary sources, particularly the letter that describes the author's reaction to caring for hundreds of young, previously healthy soldiers who rapidly succumbed to the illness, add depth and interest to the site's content.

Overall, while accurate in its information, interesting, user-friendly, and easy to navigate, the site does not tell the complete story. It could be made significantly more extensive and would benefit from the inclusion of links to additional primary sources. Nonetheless, it is an excellent starting point for anyone interested in learning more about how the 1918 influenza pandemic affected the United States.

Arlene W. Keeling, PhD, RN
The Centennial Distinguished Professor of Nursing
University of Virginia School of Nursing
McLeod Hall
Charlottesville, VA 22908-0782

Notes

1. See, for examples, R. G. "Experiences During the Influenza Epidemic," *American Journal of Nursing* 19 (March 1919): 203–4; and Beulah Gribble, "Experiences During the Epidemic: Influenza in a Kentucky Coal-Mining Camp," *American Journal of Nursing* 19 (August 1919): 609–11.
2. http:www.pandemicflu.gov/general/greatpandemic3.html, p. 9 (accessed November 5, 2007).
3. See National Red Cross reports, Northwest Division, National Archives and Records Administration, College Park, Maryland, RG, 75.
4. John Barry, *The Great Influenza: The Epic Story of the Deadliest Plague in History* (New York: Viking, 2004).
5. Carol Byerly, *Fever of War: The Influenza Epidemic in the U.S. Army During World War I* (New York: New York University Press, 2005).
6. Rhonda Keen-Payne, "'We Must Have Nurses': Spanish Influenza in America, 1918–1919," *Nursing History Review* 8 (2000): 143–56.
7. Gina Kolata, *Flu: The Story of the Great Influenza Pandemic of 1918 and the Search for the Virus That Caused It* (New York: Simon and Shuster, 1999).
8. Nancy Rockafellar, "'In Gauze We Trust': Public Health and Spanish Influenza on the Home Front, Seattle, 1918–1919," *Pacific Northwest Quarterly* 77, no. 3 (1986): 104–13.

Women and the Holocaust: A Cyberspace of Their Own. Editor, Judy Cohen. Designer, Jeff Freedman. http://www.theverylongview.com/WATH/

The Web site, *Women and the Holocaust: A Cyberspace of Their Own,* is both a source for data and a tribute to women who either survived or were in some way involved or affected by the events of the Holocaust. Its preface, written in 1996 by Joan Ringelheim, lays out the Web site's overall premise: to introduce gender as a category of analysis in the study of the Holocaust, while simultaneously dedicating itself to "women who suffered, fought, died, and triumphed in the Holocaust." All Web site references, therefore, focus on women's experiences, perceptions, and memories through personal reflection, testimony, poetry, film, or other writings.

The Web site, developed in 2001 by Judy Cohen, a Holocaust Witness/Survivor, is separated into 16 sections and maintains its currency. Still, the site is somewhat haphazard in its approach, both by topic area and focus. Some sections are useful and up-to-date, while others lend themselves to redundancy that makes navigating the site somewhat frustrating. For example, the "Women of Valor," "Special Tributes," "Personal Reflections," and "Testimonies" sections overlap significantly even as they aim to provide slightly different foci. One might find the heroines who saved children from the Kindertransport as much a story of "Women of Valor" as they are described as "Special Tributes," or the "Personal Reflections" of survivors of the ghettos and resistance to be "Testimonies" of families torn apart by a brutal regime. While the stories in each section are critical reflections of the female experience during the Holocaust, they might be more easily accessed by reorganizing the Web site's framework.

The book review section, however, though not exhaustive, is an excellent resource for scholars wishing to expand their overall knowledge of the Shoah, particularly as documented by female writers and/or survivors, and about women in the Holocaust more generally. Many of the Web site's listed books have limited market recognition but provide previously unknown information about specific individuals or groups persecuted under Nazi occupation. Simone Liebster's *Facing the Lion: Memoirs of a Young Girl in Nazi Europe,* for example, chronicles the experiences of a young Jehovah's Witness and her family during this period.

In addition to publishing current essays and articles in its "Generation to Generation" section, the site also maintains a fairly up-to-date list of projects and events, highlights conferences related to the topic area, and reviews new books. Though fairly comprehensive, there is also much missing from these sections as well as from the bibliography of secondary sources that might prove useful to nurse historians studying the Holocaust. Nurse historians, for example, will see reference to Roger Ritvo and Diane Plotkin's excellent analysis, *Sisters in Sorrow: Voices of Care* but will not find reference to Bronwyn Rebekah McFarland-Icke's *Nurses in Nazi Germany: Moral Choices in History.* Again, perhaps some of the difficulty finding materials is in the site's organization. Johanna Kruse's new book, *Twice Persecuted,* for example, is described in the "Projects and Events" section where it would best be placed under the book review section. The "Bibliography" section, updated annually, could be married with the book review section as well, so that Web site users could more easily locate materials that might be missed upon initial search.

On the whole, the Web site attempts to bring together unusual and diverse materials that would be scattered and difficult to access otherwise. Students and scholars across various disciplines—history, literature, women's studies, to name a few—will find the site a useful resource for their research as will those who simply have an interest in women and their experiences during the Holocaust. Many sections need to be updated but, by and large, the site is well maintained and provides ongoing new materials. An addition to the Web site might be in guiding interested parties to archives for more primary sources.

The Web site's strength is in its ambition to pull together vast materials from a variety of sources and venues to help create a broad analysis of the female experience during the Holocaust; its weakness is in the site's overall organizing framework for these significant sources of data.

Barbara L. Brush, PhD, RN, FAAN
Associate Professor
University of Michigan School of Nursing
400 N. Ingalls Building
Ann Arbor, MI 48109

BOOK REVIEWS

Eighteenth Century British Midwifery, Part I, Vols. 1–4

Edited by Pam Lieske

(London: Pickering & Chatto, 2007) (1,600 pages; $595.00 for vols. 1–4 cloth)

Eighteenth Century British Midwifery is a four-volume collection that is the first of a planned three-part, 12-volume set concerning British midwifery and childbirth between 1650 and 1800. The remaining volumes are due to be published during the next two years. Editor Pam Lieske, Director of Women's Studies and an associate professor of English at Ohio's Kent State University, merged her interests in women's studies and history to embark on this ambitious project. The books are primarily composed of high-quality facsimiles of primary texts on midwifery and childbirth, which Lieske arranged thematically and chronologically. The materials are of an impressive and fascinating variety and include lectures; pamphlets; treatises; works concerning the establishment of lying-in hospitals and midwifery training; and works from popular culture such as midwifery service advertisements, medicinal cures, monstrous births, and midwifery satire. The first volume consists of three categories of works: "Popular Culture and Medicine"; "Midwifery and the Law"; and "The Maternal Imagination: The Daniel Turner-James Blondel Controversy." The second volume chronicles "The Mary Toft Affair." The third volume considers "Continental Midwives in Transition." And the fourth consists of "Midwifery Texts for Women."

Far from being simply a catalog of republished midwifery texts, though, these volumes are rich with analysis and historiographic context. Lieske's general introduction at the beginning of the series introduces many concepts that are important in placing the primary sources in the proper framework. Included are a brief review of Egyptian, Roman, Greek, German, and French antecedents of British midwifery; an introduction to the gendered discussion of male versus female midwifery; a discussion of some of the licensing and marketplace concerns of midwifery; an introduction to statistical methods used in the 18th century to determine maternal and infant mortality rates; and a discussion of 1700s state-of-the-science including infections, procedures, equipment, and knowledge of anatomy and physiology. It is tempting to skip ahead directly to the facsimile texts, but readers of these volumes are well served to carefully and thoroughly read this general introduction.

Although these midwifery texts are separated in time from today by hundreds of years, Lieske demonstrates their relevance. She links these works to contemporary care of pregnant and birthing women through a hope that the volumes will help today's care providers to remember that women should be at the center of their practice. The author ends her general introduction by stating: "When reviewing the following collection of texts, my hope is that readers will continue to keep in mind the real-life experiences of pregnant

Nursing History Review 17 (2009): 201–244. A Publication of the American Association for the History of Nursing.
DOI: 10.1891/1062–8061.17.201

and labouring women so that they gain deeper empathy for, and understanding of, their experiences" (p. xxvi).

Although the volumes are very comprehensive, Lieske notes that it was a difficult task to narrow her choices of primary texts for inclusion in the books. She explains her reasoning for the selection of various texts and her inclusion of rare and seminal works along with those not previously republished in the modern era. The many works that Lieske believes to be important but had to exclude due to space constraints will be listed in a volume-12 bibliography.

Due to the cost, these volumes may be more suitable for purchase by libraries as references than by individuals. Nonetheless, the books will be interesting and instructive to a wide audience that includes historical scholars interested in the history of women, nursing, midwifery, obstetrics, the 17th and 18th centuries, and culture. The primary sources contained in these volumes will be a valuable resource to many, and Lieske's thoughtful indexing and analysis make the sources accessible for use in related studies. Indeed, Lieske states that her intent with the volumes is "to provide scholars with a readily accessible source for further study of particular themes and topics of interest, as well as prompting a deeper, more nuanced understanding of the history of British midwifery, and encouraging new avenues of investigation and new ways of thinking about midwives, midwifery students, pregnant and labouring women, and the experience of childbirth" (p. xiii).

Anne Z. Cockerham, CNM, MSN
PhD Candidate
University of Virginia School of Nursing
Charlottesville, VA 22911

The Great Stink of Paris and the Nineteenth-Century Struggle Against Filth and Germs

By David S. Barnes

(Baltimore: Johns Hopkins University Press, 2006) (314 pages; $35.00 cloth)

During a research trip to Paris, I made sure to visit the sewers, a tourist destination since the 19th century. For years, I displayed on my office door a postcard from the Paris sewers museum depicting men and women going underground to visit the famed tunnels and to view the fascinating equipment contained therein. David S. Barnes's *The Great Stink of Paris and the Nineteenth-Century Struggle Against Filth and Germs* brought back memories of that excursion and the memento I purchased. His book is an intriguing exploration of a time when *merde* and manure, sewers and stink, were the main actors in political, medical, and cultural transformations affecting 19th-century France. The text not only provides the reader with a history of the medical, political, and cultural issues related to dirt and disgust, but also offers a fascinating analysis of etiology. Finally, the book is timely in terms of its discussion of the longevity of what Barnes characterizes as the "sanitary-bacteriological synthesis (SBS)" (p. 3).

Barnes employs the Great Stink of Paris of 1880 to explore the medical, political, and cultural changes affecting France and its people in the late 19th century. In 1880, a stench pervaded Paris and disgusted and terrified the city's residents, who feared for their health and their lives. The most important figures in science and medicine, including Louis Pasteur, weighed in with their advice and opinions. What emerged from the discussions and debates was the sanitary-bacteriological synthesis, or "a new way of understanding, explaining, and combating disease in society by integrating the old concerns of the sanitary movement (filth and contamination, cleanliness and morality) with a new germ-centered focus" (p. 3). Not content to deal with the crisis alone, citizens demanded assistance from the government. Authorities agreed that it was their duty to protect the lives of French citizens. They realized that science and medicine might assist them in the fight against disease *and* in the struggle to establish a healthy, secularized, and republican France. Thus, political leaders throughout France depended on public health experts and epidemic doctors to bring "civilization," including new cultural standards of cleanliness, to the country's residents.

In addition to his interesting explanation of the sanitary-bacteriological synthesis, Barnes deftly analyzes etiology. In showing how germ theory arose, Barnes describes the etiologies that can be deployed to understand disease. He notes four "levels of causal explanation": academic, which stresses "current research agendas" (p. 108) of a given historical period; individual, which "explain the origins of single cases within a framework dictated by the life circumstances of the individual patient" (p. 108); folk, which "reinforce behavioral and cultural strictures or … rationalize regional and seasonal health disparities" (p. 109); and local, which "reveal scientific knowledge … in tension and dialogue with social transformations, political agendas, and cultural norms" (p. 109). What is significant about Barnes's analysis is the notion that scholars must understand the medical truths of a given period and people, and resist applying modern medical standards to the past.

Barnes's book resonates with present-day concerns about drug-resistant strains of disease and about infections, like MRSA, that are plaguing hospitals and that are shutting down schools. Nineteenth-century sanitarian techniques like disinfection and isolation are alive and well in modern America. In medical centers across the United States, hand-sanitizing lotion dispensers are mounted everywhere. Health care workers and visitors don gowns, gloves, and masks simply to enter the room of an infected person. The book's relevance to modern-day medical concerns will make it appealing to nurses, public health experts, and medical professionals in general. Finally, historians of medicine and scholars who specialize in French historical studies will find an intriguing investigation into the medical, political, and cultural affairs of late 19th-century France.

Karol K. Weaver, PhD
Assistant Professor
Susquehanna University
Selinsgrove, PA 17870

Race and Medicine in Nineteenth- and Early-Twentieth Century America

By Todd L. Savitt

(Kent, Ohio: The Kent State University Press, 2007) (453 pages; $49.00 cloth)

In *Race and Medicine in Nineteenth- and Early-Twentieth Century America,* Todd L. Savitt presents a reorganized, revised, and updated collection of his seminal papers on the intersections of race, racism, health care, and the experiences of different health care practitioners in the American South. Savitt is best known for his seminal *Medicine and Slavery: The Diseases and Health Care of Blacks in Virginia,*[1] his important edited collection (with Harvey Young) on *Disease and Distinctiveness in the American South,*[2] and his career-long attention to ways in which region and place shape historical practices.

Race and Medicine, however, highlights less well-appreciated aspects of his scholarship: a commitment to translating the implications of historical research to clinical and regional as well as academic audiences; and an equally compelling commitment to understanding the significance of the failures as well as successes that dot the historical landscape. This collection replaces the dog-eared copies of articles that many of us use in our own research. It adds new ones found in places we may never have thought to look—in other historians' edited collections and in journals ranging from *Civil War History* to the *Journal of the American Medical Association* and the *Journal of the National Medical Association.* As important, it provides a model of how a research trajectory develops over a career, and a different way to understand and perhaps even rethink the meaning of *failure* in nursing as well as in African American health care history.

Part One, "Diseases and Disorders of African Americans," presents Savitt's earlier works on the smothering of Virginia slave children, filariasis (or elephantiasis), and sickle cell anemia. These chapters are interesting in their own right. But they also provide exemplars of that which Savitt does particularly well. They show how to weave historical evidence with current clinical research and explanatory paradigms (in many cases updated for this collection) in nuanced yet informative ways.

Part Two, "Health and Health Care During Slavery and Reconstruction," begins with Savitt's widely reprinted article on the health and health care of African Americans on slave plantations. He then brings in other articles based on data that either did not make it into *Medicine and Slavery* or that extended his research focus into Reconstruction. "Medical Experimentation and Demonstration on Blacks in the Old South," for example, contains the (in)famous case of J. Marion Simms, but it also contains less well-known examples that point to the strength with which entrenched racism could override inherent contradictions. To quote Savitt: "despite the political rhetoric then in the Old South about a separate medicine for blacks and whites, the research and teaching, in fact, reflected the opposite. Blacks did not seem to differ enough from whites to exclude them from extensive use in Southern medical schools and in research activities" (page 77). This section also contains Savitt's less well-known work on slave life insurance, and the political and social entanglements that compromised the promise of the Georgia Freedman's Bureau's attempts to deliver health care to African Americans during Reconstruction.

Parts Three and Four, "African American Medical Schools" and "The Black Medical Profession," contain both Savitt's earliest and most recent publications. These sections represent both a reemergence of his initial interest in African American medical education and his current effort to understand how, as the failed promise of Reconstruction gave way to the hardening of the racial color line in the "New South," African Americans—and particularly African American medical practitioners—negotiated entry into a private and ruthlessly competitive health care system that had previously and, in now many cases even more vigorously, excluded them. Savitt builds these two sections largely around case studies of small, regional, largely ignored, and, in most cases, ultimately unsuccessful medical schools, hospitals, and African American medical publications. On the one hand, each of these case studies tells its own particular story. In Savitt's assessment, some medical schools run by and for African Americans—schools such as Hannibal Medical College in Memphis, Tennessee—deserved to fail: they were mismanaged and offered poor quality instruction. But others, such as the Leonard Medical School of Shaw University in Raleigh, North Carolina, failed even though its graduates were performing well both on licensing exams and in the communities in which they practiced.

Insufficient finances are a large part of Savitt's stories of failure. The *Medical and Surgical Observer,* the first African American medical journal in the United States, failed when it could not maintain its subscription and advertisement base. Medical schools founded by Northern religious groups floundered when denominational interests shifted in the late 19th and early 20th centuries to the plight of eastern and southern European immigrants. But money is not the entire story. Racism looms large. But this racism was not just centered on White physicians' refusal to assist their African American colleagues. Many potential African American patients, raised within slavery, were often suspicious about the quality of care provided by African American physicians.

Some African American medical schools, Savitt argues, could have and should have succeeded—if offered not just money, but, more important, the time to continue their clear movement into the categories of Class A medical schools—that ranking needed for the accreditation required for state licensing exams. But time was the one commodity not provided. The AMA's Council of Medical Education (CME), as active as Abraham Flexner in the reform of American medical education and, in many ways, even more aggressive than Flexner, refused to compromise; and several very promising medical schools had to close their doors. By 1919, only Howard and Meharry's medical schools remained. And one is left wondering if, in the end, what has been frequently characterized as nursing's failure to ensure the same tight control over its education as that of the CME over medical education might not have worked to nursing's advantage: our history might be that of (whether we wanted to or not) allowing promising but still struggling schools the time to develop their financial, institutional, and educational infrastructures needed for professional practice.

Patricia D'Antonio, RN, PhD, FAAN
Associate Professor of Nursing and
Associate Director
Barbara Bates Center for the Study of the History of Nursing
Claire M. Fagin Hall
University of Pennsylvania School of Nursing
Philadelphia, PA 19104

Notes

1. Todd Savitt, *Medicine and Slavery: The Diseases and Health Care of Blacks in Virginia* (Urbana: University of Illinois Press, 1978).

2. Todd Savitt and Harvey Young, eds., *Disease and Distinctiveness in the American South* (Knoxville: University of Tennessee Press, 1991).

Covenant of Care: Newark Beth Israel and the Jewish Hospital in America

By Alan M. Kraut and Deborah A. Kraut
(New Brunswick, N.J.: Rutgers University Press, 2007)
(304 pages; $37.95 cloth)

Alan and Deborah Kraut have set forth a detailed and fascinating account of how the Beth Israel Hospital of Newark, New Jersey, was established by the Jewish community as an exemplary medical facility that has played, and continues to play, a vital role in the lives of the people of that city and state. The story of the hospital, from its earliest beginnings in 1902, spans the entire 20th century. The authors highlight how it grew and developed into a first-rate modem institution, equipped to move into and to meet the new and daunting challenges of the 21st century's complex health care delivery system.

The authors start with a brief description of the origin of Jewish hospitals, and they aptly assert that Jewish hospitals in the United States, existing "at the intersection of immigration history, Jewish history, and the history of the voluntary hospital," make up "a critical chapter in the larger history of U.S. medicine" (p. 2). By the mid-19th century, anxiety was growing within the Jewish population over the issue of discrimination against Jewish patients in other religiously based hospitals. Soon, members of Jewish communities in several major cities began to establish their own hospitals in order to meet their needs. This movement gained momentum with the rising tide of Jewish immigrants who flocked to the major cities of the United States during that era. By the 1920s, Jewish hospitals existed in cities throughout America, including New York, Philadelphia, Chicago, Los Angeles, and many others.

In Newark's Jewish community, the health and social welfare needs had mushroomed with the great influx of immigrants from Eastern Europe. Measures to meet these needs were very often sparked by the efforts of the Jewish women in the community. Thus, Jewish philanthropists and physicians were spurred on by women in organizations such as the Daughters of Israel to join forces and to create a community hospital. The early days were not conflict-free as various groups jockeyed for supremacy, but, soon, leadership emerged to unite them and to lay the groundwork for the Beth Israel Hospital. One of its distinguishing features was that, like Jewish hospitals in general, its doors were open, without discrimination, to patients of every religion, ethnicity, and race.

From the outset, it was understood that the Beth Israel Hospital would provide a welcome setting for Jewish physicians to practice medicine. The American medical profession, throughout a large part of the 20th century, had placed barriers to admitting Jews into its ranks by setting restrictions on admissions to medical schools and appointments to hospital staffs. The ranking physicians at the newly established Beth Israel Hospital were determined to establish and maintain a first-rate medical staff and medical education program. Despite numerous difficulties and frustrations, their efforts were successful. Thus, the authors point out that the hospital appeared on the following lists: (l) the 1906 AMA *American Medical Directory* of hospitals and sanatoria, (2) the 1921 AMA Council on Medical Education hospitals approved for internships, and (3) American Council of Surgeons (ACS) first year accredited 1919 (Appendix Table 1).

Nursing education and the nursing program at the Beth Israel Hospital also come under the authors' scrutiny. The early presence of nursing is described as follows:

> Daily operation of Beth Israel was the responsibility of Caroline Feitzinger, the nursing superintendent. The title was a misnomer: Feitzinger, a trained nurse, served as hospital manager, chief operating-room nurse, and founder and chief instructor of the new nursing school.... Feitzinger was a formidable presence. (p. 26)

In May 1906, commencement exercises were held for the first graduating class of three nursing students. But there were still many challenges and obstacles on the road to the development of the nursing school. Nursing directors were recruited to make improvements. Often, however, the reforms that they recommended were not approved, their jefforts were stymied, and they would soon leave. For example, in response to the *Goldmark Report,* the hospital hired an experienced nursing director whose proposals were received with praise. However, the hospital Administrative Committee did not support her efforts, and she resigned after two years. The authors point to some later successes, such as the1943 approval of the school by the U.S. Public Health Service for the U.S. Cadet Nurse Corps, and the exceedingly good performance by the graduates on the January 1943, state board examinations. The school continued to function until 1968, when it became clear that professional nursing education for the future would be moving into academia. Two minor errors in the text are noted: Josephine Goldmark was not a nurse, as cited on page 108; the correct designation is American Nurses Association and not American Nursing Association, as cited at the top of page 147.

In 1996, the Beth Israel Medical Center was sold to the Saint Barnabas Healthcare System, but the original name and the Star of David would remain on the premises. The authors have presented a lively and informative narrative about this vibrant institution whose "service to the people of Newark was a gift of the city's Jewish community" (p. 9). It still stands as a tribute to the pioneer spirit of its founders.

Evelyn Rose Benson, RN, MPH
1 Longfellow Pl. #418
Boston, MA 02114

Colonial Pathologies: American Tropical Medicine and Race Hygiene in the Philippines

By Warwick Anderson

(Durham, N.C.: Duke University Press, 2006) (355 pages; $84.95 cloth; $23.95 paper)

With *Colonial Pathologies,* Warwick Anderson examines early 20th-century American notions of race and health confronted by the colonial realities of a postwar Philippines. From the medical-surgical fronts of the Philippine-American War (1898–1900) to the trenches, rivers, and streams of malarial control, Anderson presents a measured, intelligent account of the changing racial and medical perceptions of Philippine-based American colonizers. The book is organized topically, consisting of eight chapters with a short introduction and conclusion.

The first two chapters detail the experiences of American military medicine, as it struggled to orient itself among an unfamiliar tropical environment. Anderson presents the ecologic perceptions of several military medical officials, along with the deleterious effects upon health these officers attributed to the environment. Anderson argues that these perceptions of American military medicine, along with its consequent reactions, positioned it as a precedent-defining force in future Filipino public hygiene initiatives.

The middle chapters reflect the various public health activities undertaken during the colony's gradual demilitarization. Accompanying this change is a shift, with public health officials turning to racial rather than ecologic preconceptions of health and illness. Here, much of the story revolves around Victor G. Heiser, director of health in the Philippines from 1905–1915. The focus of the colony's biomedical research, fixed upon the ramifications of the tropics and the local population upon the White man's health, is the focus of Chapter 3. In Chapter 4, Anderson explores the scatological obsessions of colonial public health officials. Convinced of the deleterious effects of the locals' disregard of Western standards of sanitation, public health officials developed a series of sanitary interventions, introducing the "sanitary pail," an annual Carnival with increasingly propagandist overtones, and national Clean-Up Week (p. 119). Chapter 5 details the psychological struggles and reactions of the White colonizers, convinced of the superiority of their hygienic interventions yet presented with both an unfavorable ecologic reality and uneven colonial sanitary reform. The oft-fascinating account of the Culion leper colony is presented in Chapter 6. Upon this small island in the south, Heiser attempted to "sanitize" the local patients, to make them both less ill and less Filipino. According to Anderson, it was Heiser's hope that they would then serve as a model for the health all Filipinos could achieve with Western medicine and sanitation. The final two chapters detail the Rockefeller Foundation's hookworm and malaria programs in the Philippines. Here Anderson presents the "disintegration, repair, and persistence" of White American ideas regarding Filipino capability and culpability (p. 10).

Throughout *Colonial Pathologies,* Anderson contextualizes his writing, often providing relevant contemporary parallels from the continental United States. Though much of this work describes the paternalistic, pejorative, and often condescending actions of the colonial public health officials, Anderson avoids polemics. Instead, he infuses the book with quotes, photographs, and subtle humor, leaving much of the emotional interpretation to the reader. While some readers may enjoy this, others may find themselves questioning Anderson's even-handed delivery of contentious material. Also, with few exceptions, Anderson delivers his accounts squarely from the perceptions of the White colonizers. Perhaps his sources did not speak to their story, but there is a noticeable dearth in the accounts and perceptions of the Filipino people.

Overall, Anderson delivers an impressive account of the evolving nature of early 20th-century American colonial medical and public health thought as its authors observed, interpreted, and interacted with an unfamiliar people and place. As such, this book will be of great interest to any historian interested in the social construction of health and illness, as well as to those interested in tropical and/or colonial American medicine. Though intended for an academic audience, it is clearly written and quite suitable for a more general audience, especially those with an interest in military, colonial, or medical history.

Keith C. Mages, MSN, MLS, RN
Doctoral Candidate
Barbara Bates Center for the Study of the History of Nursing
University of Pennsylvania School of Nursing
Philadelphia, PA 19104

Lucy Osborn, a Lady Displaced: Florence Nightingale's Envoy to Australia

By Judith Godden
(Sydney, Australia: Sydney University Press, 2006) (373 pages; $34.94 paper)

This book is a detailed biography of the first St. Thomas nurse that Florence Nightingale sent to a British colony in the 19th century. Arriving in Australia in March 1868, nurse Lucy Osborn eventually fell out of favor with Nightingale, and, as the foreword correctly states, the book "has all the ingredients of Victorian melodrama" (p. ix). Judith Godden, a historian of Australian women and nursing, has written a chronological narrative that includes the successes and failures of early Nightingale nursing with all its class, gender, and religious overtones. Godden effectively weaves together the stories of Osborn and Nightingale throughout her analysis. For this reason, the book is perhaps mistitled. Should it be *Lucy Osborn and Florence Nightingale: Reforming Nursing in Australia in the Nineteenth Century?*

The two women are intricately linked in the book, and indeed, the sources consist mainly of hundreds of long letters to Nightingale from Osborn during her 17 years there. This is admittedly biased evidence, in part because no letters back to Osborn from Nightingale survive. And Osborn's letters gave a false impression because they were almost always litanies of her political and interpersonal problems, rather than discussions of her successes with improved patient care, for example. Godden also makes use of official photographs of Lady Superintendent Osborn, in order to show her High Church, "popish" religious beliefs as exemplified in the large cross around her neck and her upper-class dress. Such High Church belief was not acceptable in the colony and this was a constant issue for Osborn.

Having never nursed much herself as a new graduate, Osborn's experience was rather harrowing because she had arrived in the colony to reform nursing, specifically by establishing a training school in the Sydney Infirmary under the same rules and frameworks as St. Thomas's Hospital School. Such a huge task was complicated by the specter of the iconic Nightingale and by the five nurses she led to Australia at the request of the Colonial secretary, Henry Parkes. Four of these nurses "were more experienced … than Osborn," Godden notes, but she was a "lady" who claimed her right to authority "over issues that women would best understand" (p. 3).

As an upper-middle-class, educated, pious woman, Osborn was automatically the leader of the other five, who were working-class women. These "sisters" would later cause Osborn much trouble because they all "sank into a squabbling mass of scandal and pettiness" after the training school admitted its first probationers and the nurses began to work with the colony's poor (p. 82). The newspapers of the day pilloried Osborn and her nurses for the scandals (e.g., one nurse got pregnant) and for allegedly bad nursing care. But Osborn's main opponent was Dr. Albert Roberts, an "honorary" or consultant surgeon who, according to Osborn, had made the Infirmary his "hobby." He wanted control over the nurses and did not understand nor accept the Nightingale model of the female hierarchy. Osborn's personality was feisty and "boyish"; she was blunt about her opinions and in her criticism of those who opposed her, namely, Roberts. She was forced to endure a large-scale parliamentary inquiry into her management of the Infirmary nursing in 1870, and although she was vindicated, the stress affected her health. Nightingale had effectively cut her off by 1870, because the bad publicity reflected negatively on the Nightingale model of nursing.

Godden's purpose is never stated, but it appears to be a corrective to the previous heroic, but partial, tales of Osborn's life. Godden sees her as "a forerunner of the professional women who emerged in the 1880s and 1890s" (p. 2), and she writes with empathy and affection for her subject, calling her "a highly attractive woman" (p. 7). Perhaps this is a bias. Godden's historiographic framework is feminist and the thesis of the book, as noted in the conclusion, is that Osborn created a new professional space for laywomen to practice nursing in Australia.

My criticisms are that the book is too long and detailed, and perhaps it needed strong editing to keep the story clear. No context is provided with regard to other countries, including Britain where medicine, nursing, and politicians clashed. Nonetheless, it is an important book for Nightingale scholars and for colonial nursing history.

Meryn Stuart, PhD, RN
Associate Professor
Director, Associated Medical Services Nursing History Research Unit
University of Ottawa
School of Nursing
Ottawa, ON K1N 6N5
Canada

Saving Sickly Children: The Tuberculosis Preventorium in American Life, 1909–1970

By Cynthia A. Connolly
(New Brunswick, N.J.: Rutgers University Press, 2008)
(176 pages; 10 illustrations; $39.95 cloth)

In December 2007, Aisha Malone of Oakland, California, surrendered custody of her six-year-old son to the state's child and family services. Malone was charged with child abuse because she allowed her son to reach 140 pounds. She had also failed to keep appointments with nurses and nutritionists to develop a diet plan for her son.[1]

At first glance, this case would appear to have nothing to do with caring for tubercular children in the early 20th-century United States. *Saving Sickly Children* persuasively argues that contemporary interventions for "the best interest of the child" are very similar to those in the early 20th century. Connolly's main thesis is that while tuberculosis has largely disappeared as a public health problem among the nation's children, "the set of issues that led to the inception of the preventorium continues to pervade American society" (p. 8).

Connecting the past and present in this manner allows Connolly to provide a nuanced view of early 20th-century efforts to rescue children from the "certain doom" of tuberculosis. According to the "standard of care" of the era, institutionalizing children judged "at risk" was commonplace. Connolly acknowledges that Progressive reformers were motivated by a desire to shape the lives of the poor by educating indigent children in White, middle-class, Protestant values of health and hygiene. Yet she also demonstrates the limitations of applying a social control model to early 20th-century child saving. Connolly persuasively argues many reformers recognized the broader social factors that made it difficult for poor families to provide adequate care for their children, and saw the preventorium as an imperfect solution to health disparities among the American population.

The book is organized chronologically, tracing the preventorium's origins in the evolving science of tuberculosis prevention and treatment in the early 20th century, the development of a nationwide network of these institutions, and the decline of this preventive strategy in the late 1930s. Connolly draws upon a rich variety of published and archival primary sources to illustrate her major points. As a historian of childhood and youth, I was especially impressed by her ability to capture the perspective of the young patients.

Connolly explores how scientists in the early 1900s challenged the prevailing assumption that childhood was a "golden age" of immunity from tuberculosis. The development of the tuberculin skin test in 1907 greatly aided in the effort to identify "pretubercular" children, that is, those who tested positive for TB antibodies but had no symptoms of active disease. Unlike most other histories of tuberculosis care, she shows the key role public health nurses played in the preventorium movement. Not only did nurses provide intensive care to the young patients, they also served as cultural ambassadors between institution and home. Consequently, these public health nurses enjoyed a high degree of autonomy and job satisfaction that was rare in the nursing profession at this time. Nurses recognized that their legal authority to remove a child from home was limited, so some degree of cultural sensitivity was needed to convince parents to send their children away from home. Yet, like other reformers and professionals at this time, public health nurses believed they had a duty to ensure clients fully adopted "modern" American hygienic practices before they would return the child to the home. The preventorium declined not because this attitude toward child saving disappeared, but because other diseases—most notably polio—replaced tuberculosis as the most feared public health threat to the nation's children.

Connolly concludes her brilliant study by asking about how the preventorium should be remembered. Her answer avoids the standard whiggish notion that the preventorium was a "bad" public health strategy that belongs in the dustbin of U.S. history. She argues that, above all, the founders of the preventorium were motivated by the same humanitarian impulse that inspired movements against child labor and family violence. Then, as now, the United States provides an inadequate safety net for the nation's most vulnerable citizens. Although many practitioners recognize that health problems of the nation's young are shaped by a combination of genetic, social, and environmental factors, their ability to "do something" about problems like childhood obesity are limited by our government's tendency to frame public health problems in terms of personal responsibility. Connolly's book provides a valuable service to modern nurses by showing the ways in which their present-day choices are shaped by political constraints developed over a century ago.

Heather Munro Prescott, PhD
Professor of History
Coordinator, Women, Gender, and Sexuality Studies
Central Connecticut State University
1615 Stanley Street
New Britain, CT 06050–4010

Note

1. Lyanne Melendez, "Should a Parent Lose Custody of an Obese Child?" KGO-TV, December 5, 2007, http://abclocal.go.com/kgo/story?section=news/assignment_7&id=5817191&pt=print (accessed February 22, 2008).

Nursing and the Privilege of Prescription, 1893–2000

By Arlene W. Keeling
(Columbus: Ohio State University Press, 2007)
(218 pages; $42.95 cloth; $9.95 CD)

Late 20th- and early 21st-century professional nurses are all too familiar with the many contentious battles fought to secure legal prescriptive privileges for advanced practice nurses. It was, in fact, a 2000 legislative fight waged by Virginia nurse practitioners to obtain expanded prescriptive authority that inspired author Arlene Keeling to examine nurses' work with medications. The result of that research, *Nursing and the Privilege of Prescription, 1893–2000,* is a fascinating look at the long-time involvement with and struggles over nurses' work related to medical therapeutics.

Keeling's purpose in writing this book is straightforward, focusing on "the formal and informal roles nurses played over the course of the century in dispensing, furnishing, and prescribing medications" (p. xvi). As such, this book is not an exhaustive analysis of 20th-century prescriptive authority, something Keeling notes could have become quite complicated, lengthy, and tedious. Rather, Keeling skillfully uses a series of case studies to chronicle the work of six groups of nurses who practiced in expanded roles at different points in time throughout the United States, examining how those nurses incorporated medication dispensing, furnishing, and prescribing into their practices. This approach works. Keeling uncovers the often invisible yet central role medications and activities surrounding them had for nurses. She highlights the ways in which previous generations of nurses worked or at times fought with physicians to ensure that their patients had full access to appropriate treatment, including drugs and medications.

The case studies, which are presented in a loose chronological order, center on nurses who practiced in independent situations from the turn of the century to current times. The first groups of nurses featured shared several similarities in terms of populations treated and the ways in which nurses approached the provision of medications. For example, the Henry Street Settlement nurses, the Frontier Nursing Service nurses, and the nurses employed by the Bureau of Indian Affairs all worked with indigent populations who were either financially or geographically remote from conventional sources of health care. Although nurses realized medications were critical components of their patients' care regimens, the relative isolation of the patients served made access to medications difficult, if not impossible. So nurses learned to carry a supply of commonly used drugs in their bags, or saddlebags as the case might be, thus becoming diagnosticians, prescribers, and dispensers of medications. As Keeling astutely notes, it was at this point that nurses crossed the "fluid boundary lines" between medicine and nursing. Nurses, respecting physicians' professional sensibilities, solicited cooperation from physician groups, collaborated with them, and developed and adhered to protocols involving standing order regimens. Keeling notes that collegial relationships, careful attention to the legal confines of practice acts, a high level of trust between nurses and physicians, and the relative isolation and impoverishment of the populations served enabled nurses to practice relatively freely.

Yet, problems did occur. Physicians sometimes viewed nurses as interlopers and potential threats to their economic well-being. Even nurse anesthetists, the topic of Chapter 2, seemingly safe from challenges by practicing within hospitals under the direct supervision of surgeons, were subject to lawsuits alleging they were practicing medicine without a license. Despite such occurrences, the boundaries between medical and nursing practice were fluid enough to move back and forth, depending on the type of patient, health care setting, and time. For the most part, particularly in areas where nurses were the sole health care practitioners or when the position of the nurse enabled the work of physicians to proceed more smoothly, nurses prevailed.

The second half of the book covers the work of cardiac care nurses and advanced nurse practitioners. By the mid-20th century, innovations in medical treatment resulted in the ability to administer life-saving drugs. When physicians delegated to nurses, who were the health care practitioners always present at the bedside, the administration of drugs such as quinidine, lidocaine, and nitroglycerin via standing orders and protocols, patients received immediate treatment in dire situations, thus enjoying better outcomes. The success in using hospital nurses in expanded roles easily transferred to community settings where the modern-day nurse practitioner was introduced. Several factors led to the rise and acceptance of nurses in these positions, not the least of which was the proximity and accessibility of nurses to patients. As access to care rose to prominence as a major health care issue, it was to nurses that the public turned for primary health care services.

The growth of the nurse practitioner movement intensified debate over prescriptive authority. Nurse practitioners, who directly diagnose and prescribe treatments, require legal prescriptive authority to carry out their work. Increased utilization of nurse practitioners highlighted the need to resolve long-standing problems with medical therapeutics. However, achieving prescriptive authority proved to be an onerous task, complicated by the state, the nature of nurse and medical practice acts, physicians' fears about encroachments on their practices, and a myriad of other issues. Although successful at gaining prescriptive rights in many states, the battles have not been easy and remain ongoing.

Keeling has effectively mined an impressive amount of evidence to support her major thesis that nurses' freedom in dispensing, furnishing, and prescribing medicines is dependent on "the particular setting in which they practiced, on individual practice negotiations between physicians and nurses at the grassroots level, and on the level of trust that developed between them" (p. xviii). Within the narrative, a number of themes, such as the promotion of access to care, responsibility for care, the importance of advanced knowledge for safe practice, economic determinants of care, and interdisciplinary cooperation, collaboration, and conflict are expertly weaved throughout each case study. In particular, Keeling emphasizes the importance education had for nurses as a means of validating their competence to prescribe medications. Keeling notes that all of the nurses qualified for their positions through some type of advanced training, such as taking public health courses in the case of the early 20th-century nurses, or the late 20th-century convention of obtaining a master's degree for advanced nursing practice. This additional preparation ensured that nurses practiced in a proficient manner and encouraged physicians to trust nurses as they carried out more advanced responsibilities. And, it was the trust established between nurses and physicians that provided the environment in which nurses were free to prescribe medications.

This book should appeal to a wide audience. Obviously, nurse practitioners and those who study that movement will be interested. The detail with which Keeling approaches the case studies results in a book that is more than a history of nurses' involvement with medications. The everyday practices of nurses are meticulously described, providing the reader with an excellent sense of how earlier generations of nurses worked, the problems they encountered, and how challenges to effective practice were approached. This serves as an outstanding source for those interested in the working lives of nurses and the conditions under which they were employed. As well, for those interested in health care policy, the book advances understanding of earlier health care access problems in its depiction of the plight of patients with minimal access to health care services. Keeling's work illuminates how populations left without ready access to conventional health care services managed. They turned to nurses.

My only disappointment with the book was the absence of any mention of how the majority of early working nurses handled medication issues. In the late 19th and early 20th centuries, most nurses worked independently in patients' homes as private duty nurses. Some attention to how these nurses worked with or around medication issues would have strengthened this story. Most likely, the case study approach used prevented their examination.

Despite this omission, this is a strong work, which was highly enjoyable to read and provided an excellent analysis of a significant piece of nursing history. As the first and at this point only full-length examination of prescriptive authority, *Nursing and the Privilege of Prescription, 1893–2000,* which received the prestigious 2007 American Association for the History of Nursing's Lavinia L. Dock Award, is a winning contribution to a growing body of historical scholarship investigating the history of advanced practice nursing.

Jean C. Whelan, PhD, RN
Assistant Adjunct Professor
University of Pennsylvania School of Nursing
Philadelphia, PA 19104–6096

Black Physicians in the Jim Crow South

By Thomas J. Ward, Jr.
(Fayetteville: University of Arkansas Press, 2003) (368 pages; $34.95 cloth)

Thomas J. Ward has produced a useful and fascinating history of individuals who shared a profession and lived in a unique period of American history. He tells the story of the men and women who pioneered as African American physicians during the repressive years of segregation in the South from the 1890s to the 1960s. This book grew from doctoral research at the University of Southern Mississippi and reflects the writer's interest in the region, the period, medical history, and the lived experience of African Americans in the study period.

The book is divided into three major parts: "Education," "Professional Life," and "Community Life." Each unit surveys the topic throughout the study period. The first unit profiles the development, tribulations, and achievements of historical Black medical schools, the entrance of minority students into traditionally White programs, and the issues faced by doctors seeking postgraduate education and fellowships. Each chapter is illustrated and personalized with details from the students, physicians, and educators. The role of philanthropy, changing professional standards, and balancing demands and resources are given faces with personal sagas. This practice continues throughout the work.

The second part highlights how these physicians established their practices, struggled to make a living, and developed either their own hospitals or related to the few segregated facilities in the region. The stories in this section graphically demonstrate how many historically Black institutions were established and how the physicians gradually gained a foothold in what had been a totally White world. What is striking about this part of the book is how much discrimination these doctors faced from both races. The degradation of people for their skin color was truly illustrated by the fact that the Black patients would put up with discrimination and backroom segregated facilities in order to see a White doctor because there was a belief that they were better than any Black doctor in the community. In addition, the few White patients wanting the attention of Black practitioners had to come to the office after dark to avoid public scrutiny for their care-seeking behaviors.

In this second section on medical practice and hospital development, there are many strong glimpses of nursing and the environment in which nursing evolved with medicine for Blacks in this period. The nurses are well placed in the saga of the system that functions in spite of discrimination and the limitations of segregation. One can view the early hospitals as both centers for medical practice and environments for early nursing education. The author also covers early public health efforts in the Mississippi Delta and nursing activities that were needed in those programs.

The closing section of the book highlights the roles and status of these pioneer physicians as elite members of the leadership in their communities. In spite of the struggles in their professional lives, they did generally enjoy a better socioeconomic status than their peers locked into the sharecropping system of the South. They also played a significant role in the development of public health efforts and were generally recognized leaders in their segregated communities. The evolution of this group of professional/civic leaders led some into the Civil Rights arena as doctors sought integration of medical facilities and opportunities in the last years of the study period.

If there is a limitation in this study, it is one common to most regional studies for this period: they are forced to rely on urban sources. In the Preface (p. xiv), the author notes that most of his doctors and data came from the cities and large towns in the region. There are so few surviving resources on the lived experiences of rural people in this period that it is difficult to profile them in this type of study. This reader has had similar difficulties in studies of nursing activities in the region.

Black Physicians in the Jim Crow South is a valuable resource for any nurse historian focusing on the South in the late 19th and early 20th centuries because Ward has set his doctors, hospitals, and disease experiences in their time and society. The reader can view the demands, structure, and challenges of a human service profession set in the segregated South where every aspect of daily life was affected by skin color. What pleased this reviewer were the graphic descriptions of the poverty, social isolation, and disease demands on this generation of professionals and how they coped with and overcame the problems of ignorance and fear. The findings support those of earlier studies that looked at nursing and hospital development.

Ward has provided the nursing profession with a valuable background work that is richly documented from an extensive study of the resources in the region and can give direction to any researcher wishing more answers about the lived experience of health care providers in the South during the era of Jim Crow.

Linda E. Sabin, RNC, PhD
Professor of Nursing
University of Louisiana at Monroe
Monroe, LA 71209

Japanese American Midwives: Culture, Community, and Health Politics, 1880–1950

By Susan Smith
(Urbana: University of Illinois Press, 2005) (280 pages; $25.00 paper)

In *Japanese American Midwives,* Susan Smith weaves a fascinating tale of the professionalization of midwifery in Japan (1880–1920) and its ultimate demise in the United States (1930–1950). Smith skillfully uses race, gender, and transnationalism as interpretive frames to render a conceptually complex yet personal reconstruction of the challenges that certain Japanese immigrant midwives faced, their negotiations with American health officials and their communities, and the shifting meaning of midwifery in the American West and Hawai'i'. Although Smith does not speak Japanese, with the help of translators, she used a wide array of sources, including interviews, diaries, government records, and archival material. As a result, she renders a deeply contextualized portrayal of how and why these midwives worked within a marginalized subculture not just as public health workers but as cultural brokers. As such, they helped to build ethnic communities and maintain Japanese cultural traditions while serving as professional role models for Nisei women (second-generation Japanese Americans) and encouraging them to adopt new birthing traditions in accordance with American norms.

In the first chapter of the book, Smith begins with a careful analysis of the emergence of the *sanba,* or the state-certified midwife in Japan during the Meiji Period (1868–1912). In keeping with the Japanese quest for empire and modernity, the *sanba,* or modern, well-educated midwife, was created to replace the traditional and "untrained" midwife, or *toriagebaba.* In this case, the impact of the state on midwifery in Japan benefited some midwives; primarily younger, urban-dwelling *sanba* at the detriment of older, rural *toriagebaba.* Smith argues that *sanba* played an active role in midwifery reform, with their legitimacy and cultural authority stemming not just from Western medicine, but also from the birthing women who appreciated the class distinctions made between the traditional birth attendants and the modern midwife. The chapter thus sets the stage for understanding the centrality of midwifery in Japanese birthing culture, transitions brought about by midwifery reform and the commitment of Issei *sanba,* first-generation Japanese immigrant midwives, to serve their communities in the United States (p. 30).

The next three chapters explore the intersection of Japanese immigration and race, gender, and health politics and how these shaped the lives and practices of Issei *sanba.* Embedding the *sanba* experience within the regional and multicultural history of midwifery in the United States, Smith persuasively argues that the American *sanba* were both constrained by and benefited from the racial and health politics of the day. For example, although anti-Japanese sentiment was growing in the early 20th century and exclusion policies were enacted with the 1924 immigration act; many Americans did not view Japanese Americans as being a "health menace." The author contends that they did not pose a threat to White physicians who typically did not serve Japanese American communities. *Sanba* were well trained and educated midwives imbued with the values of Western science. As such, they were not targeted by middle-class American reformers who were more concerned with medicalizing birth than professionalizing midwives. In Smith's words, "western dissatisfaction with or indifference to midwifery was a sign of admiration and racism" (p. 58).

Smith's characterization of the mainland *sanba* experience is greatly enhanced by her use of the 56-year diary of *sanba* Toku Shimomura. She uses this and other firsthand accounts to build a vivid picture of the mainland *sanba,* at least the ones that she studied as being ruggedly independent and decidedly entrepreneurial. At times they eschewed traditional gender roles and helped to build ethnic communities, evoke cultural change, and expand employment opportunities for women. Yet, their history is not monolithic and their experiences varied significantly across geography and class lines. Those who lived in rural impoverished areas were geographically isolated from other midwives, typically attended births on a part-time basis, and infrequently received remuneration for their work. By contrast, their urban counterparts were well organized, autonomous, and availed themselves of the economic opportunities afforded to them both in their own and multicultural communities.

Less well developed, but nevertheless fascinating, is her portrayal of the Hawaiian *sanba* experience. Smith addresses some of the differences in the contexts confronting Hawaiian versus mainland *sanba,* including differences in population racial composition and balance, the early involvement of the state in controlling midwifery practice, and the expansion of Sheppard-Towner funds to Hawaiians in 1925. Yet, she does not fully explicate the impact of the sociopolitical upheaval brought about by the overthrow of the indigenous monarchy and subsequent colonization of Hawai'i' during this era. This critique notwithstanding, she provides insight into the social, cultural, and political conditions that they encountered. Although Hawaiian *sanba* certainly faced difficulties not encountered by mainland *sanba,* they successfully negotiated with public health officials to shape state regulations and supervision of their practice by assuring that the midwife supervisor was at least as qualified as they (p. 141).

In the final chapter, the author investigates the role of World War II in the demise of Japanese American midwifery. While the impact of mainland internment and martial law in Hawai'i' certainly "marked the beginning of the end" of the *sanba* (p. 143), Smith contends that it affected the pace of the end, but not the direction (p. 183). She points to other forces from within and outside the Japanese American community that set the stage for the cultural shift in birthing practices. As non-Whites, Japanese Americans were clear targets of the early 20th-century Americanization campaigns; and by 1945, the dangers of not adopting mainstream American cultural birthing norms, namely giving birth in hospitals, were very real (p. 181). Lastly, Smith argues that the *sanba* encouraged the abandonment of midwife-attended home births in favor of the modern medicalized birth for Nisei women. It was, after all, in keeping with the dynamic modern scientific tradition that they were trained in.

In closing, Susan Smith has once again made a significant contribution to the history of midwifery in the United States. The book is meticulously researched and adds to the limited scholarship on Issei women as well as to a greater understanding of the multi- and transnational nature of American midwifery. The book is unique in that it weaves the voices of Issei and Nisei women into the history of international, racial, and health care politics. The beautifully written narrative and smart analysis is relevant to multiple fields of historical study and would be of interest to Asian Americanists as well as historians of nursing, medicine, health care politics, and race relations.

Joy Buck, PhD, RN
Associate Professor, West Virginia School of Nursing &
Robert C. Byrd Health Sciences Center, Eastern Division
2500 Foundation Way
Martinsburg, WV 25401

Healing Henan: Canadian Nurses at the North China Mission, 1888–1947

By Sonya Grypma
(Vancouver: University of British Columbia Press, 2007)
(288 pages; $85.00 cloth; $32.95 paper)

Between 1888 and 1947, 30 Canadian nurses went to China, most of them single women sent out by the Women's Missionary Society (WMS) to work as missionaries and nurses at the North China Mission (NCM) in Henan. Some were married to NCM missionaries but continued to use their nursing skills within the missionary families.

In *Healing Henan: Canadian Nurses at the North China Mission, 1888–1947,* Sonya Grypma argues that though the closure of the NCM in 1947 was fatal to missionary nursing there, the Canadian nurses in Henan contributed to the development of modern nursing in China through their work in hospitals, establishment of nursing training schools, and organization of professional nurses. Grypma also argues that the history of Canadian nursing in China has remained untold due to the missionaries' fear of harming their Chinese friends under the Communist regime and the shift in attitude in Canada toward Christian mission work from a heroic task of promoting Western and Christian values and culture in China to cultural imperialism. Under this premise, Grypma constructs a historical account of Canadian nurses' work in China while exploring the interplay of professional nursing with issues such as religion, gender, culture, health, and nation.

The book is organized into seven chapters, and Grypma uses both primary and secondary sources as well as one interview in order to "highlight ways in which the missionary nursing movement influenced the development of nursing in one region of China" (p. 3). In the first two chapters, Grypma examines the establishment of the NCM medical mission in Henan. The first nurse was sent out not for her nursing skills but because the NCM realized the need for female missionaries. Grypma shows that the number of nurses in China was dependent on the doctors' attitudes toward having nurses, the interest for missionary nursing in Canada, and the view of the mission board on the role of missionary nurses. Grympa identifies a difference in focus between the mission board in Canada, which saw the goal of medical care to be a part of the evangelistic strategy by gaining the trust of prospective converts, and the doctors and nurses in Henan whose focus became treating physical ailments. When the doctors specifically asked for nurses for medical care, this was considered a nonreligious purpose by the board and the grant was not accepted.

In the 1920s, the obstacles on the road toward modern nursing in Henan disappeared as three hospitals were founded in North Henan. This development was made possible by funding and moral support by supporters in Canada, the recognition of the need for nursing in China based on scientific evidence delivered by the Chinese Medical Missionary Association (CMMA), and the Nurses Association of China (NAC) and the International Council of Nurses provision of a national and international professional network.

During the late 1920s and early 1930s, nursing within the NCM in North Henan peaked due to increasing Chinese independence of foreign missionary leadership, especially in the Nurses Association of China, and with the promotion of health and education of nurses becoming a priority to the Chinese authorities. The Canadian nurses in China also began to identify more with nurses in the homeland, which becomes evident through their communication to colleagues not only through church journals but also through the *Canadian Nurse.* They also began using furloughs in Canada to speak at nursing alumnae events and not solely at church gatherings.

From 1937 until the end of the missionary period of the NCM, China was at war. The Sino-Japanese War, Japanese occupation, and the Communist Revolution made the nurses' and doctors' work increasingly difficult. New obstacles arose as the missionaries under the Communist Revolution were seen as opposing Chinese independence. The missionaries experienced great disappointment when Chinese brothers and sisters in Christ chose to leave the mission and to allow nationality to rule over religion. At the same time, Grypma notes, the support from Canada began to crumble as the economic crises of the 1930s made supporters focus on problems closer to themselves. The military attack of the Communists on the compounds in Weihui and Anyang in 1947 was the final stroke to a mission that had been weakened for years.

In her epilogue, Grypma brings the remains of Canadian missionary nursing in Henan up to date. During a visit to Henan, she learned that the local Chinese authorities are hoping to reopen the Weihui Hospital as a tourist site to depict—not mission history—but an example of older Chinese hospitals.

Grypma makes a strong case for her argument through excellent documentation and evidence. *Healing Henan* is well written and exciting reading, and it sheds new light on the significance of the efforts by nurses and doctors in a Chinese province. The book also provides the reader with a close view of the ambitions, struggles, and accomplishments of Canadian nurses in Henan, and it will appeal to anyone interested in the history of religious nursing.

Anne Marie Overgaard, MA
Curator
Museum Soenderjylland Kulturhistorie Toender
Kongevej 51
DK-6270 Toender
Denmark

Suffering in the Land of Sunshine: A Los Angeles Illness Narrative

By Emily K. Abel
(New Brunswick, N.J.: Rutgers University Press, 2006)
(176 pages; $ 24.95 paper)

Illness narratives, reports of disability or sickness from the perspective of the sufferer or close family member, provide a unique dimension through which historians can analyze changing conceptualizations of disease and the way in which variables such as culture or gender, for example, shape meaning for particular individuals. Emily Abel has uncovered the story of Charles Dwight Willard (1860–1914), a prominent California newspaperman and author who traveled to the state as a "health seeker," seeking relief from tuberculosis

(TB). Abel discovered Willard's letters, housed at California's Huntington Library, while gathering data for a broader study of the social history of TB in Los Angeles. Surprised that his public boosterism of California differed substantively from the way in which he reported his own experiences to close family members, Abel grew intrigued. In Abel's deft hands, his weekly letters to family members, written between 1886 and 1914, are interpreted through the lens of social history. They provide a rich context through which we can not only appreciate Willard's private world, but also that of a chronically ill individual living in the late 19th and early 20th centuries whose condition was undergoing a major shift in cultural representation and societal meaning.

Suffering in the Land of Sunshine, the title drawn from a journal founded by Willard extolling California's health properties ("Land of Sunshine"), is organized chronologically, beginning with Willard's arrival in southern California in 1886 soon after being diagnosed with consumption, as most people still called TB in that era. Upon his arrival, Willard began a pattern of slow improvement accompanied by optimism, followed by despair and a sense of powerlessness and frustration, as his symptoms always returned. Despite his disease, however, he was able to obtain paid work, first as a tutor and then as a journalist and writer. He also married and became a father, all the while struggling to prevent TB from controlling his life.

Through Abel's analysis of Willard's letters, the reader gains insight into the way in which the gendered norms for his era compelled White men such as Willard to embrace the Rooseveltian ideal of robust health, even in the face of manifest illness. Abel argues that because he accepted the notion that illness and failure were intertwined, Willard's only recourse was to rail against his disease and redouble his efforts to maintain a positive attitude and get well. His support for the era's reform movement, Progressivism, and its optimistic ethos only strengthened his conviction that this approach made sense as the many passages from his letters that Abel pieces into the larger narrative reveal. Although Willard's personal story remains in the foreground, his life and times are well chronicled in the context of major political, economic, cultural, and social events of his era. For example, Willard's experiences are interpreted within the history of California, Progressivism, and changing ideas concerning the etiology of TB as well as its treatment, including the work of TB nurses.

Abel also draws attention to Willard's many contradictions. He disdained, for example, the indigent tubercular and others whose illness or infirmity made them dependent on others. But had his class status not meant that he possessed a social network of friends who offered assistance, adversity in the form of financial problems and a house fire might have meant that he and his family would have descended into poverty themselves. Further, he accepted the germ theory but still felt a need to convince himself that he was not constitutionally disordered because he suffered from TB. He believed in his superiority as a White, Protestant male, even as Japanese servants, his wife, and other caregivers made it possible for him to maintain his lifestyle and profession.

Lucidly written in an accessible style, this superb book should have wide appeal to historians, medical anthropologists, sociologists, those interested in disability studies, and anyone interested in the lived experience of disease. For clinicians, this book is especially thought-provoking. Not only does this study remind us of the enduring U.S. practice of "blaming the victim" for his or her plight when recovery fails to materialize, it reveals how easy it is to internalize that and other cultural messages, as well as the sometimes surprising places from which they arise.

Cynthia A. Connolly, PhD, RN
Associate Professor
Yale University School of Nursing
Assistant Professor
Yale University School of Medicine
PO Box 9740
100 Church Street South
Yale University School of Nursing
New Haven, CT 06536–0740

Promise on Parnassus: The First Century of the UCSF School of Nursing

By Marilyn E. Flood
(San Francisco: UCSF Nursing Press, 2007) (191 pages; $35.00 cloth)

Promise on Parnassus examines the development of the University of California, San Francisco (UCSF) School of Nursing from its founding amidst the rubble of the 1906 earthquake to its present-day status as one of the leading academic nursing programs in the United States. Written in anticipation of the school's 100th anniversary, author Marilyn Flood combines UCSF's archival resources with accounts from faculty and rich photographic documentation into a balanced combination of heritage and history. The chronological progression of the narrative unfolds as an organizational history interspersed with explanations of how various statewide and national events either curtailed or accelerated the school's development.

Like many school histories whose origins emanated from training schools, issues surrounding its mission—whether to educate nurses or provide labor for hospitals—provided the necessary ingredients for much of the story. A fair portion of the book chronicles faculty attempts to gain professorial status and shed the training school image and expectations. The school, in some capacity, had to continually strategize and update the curriculum in order to answer potential critics as well as defer attacks on its emerging growth. Whether it was the denial of the undergraduate curriculum as being equal to a typical University of California (UC) bachelor degree, unwillingness of UC Regents to promote nursing faculty past the rank of associate professor, or numerous other politically motivated attempts to keep the School of Nursing from gaining full academic status, the faculty had to face many challenges to their credibility as scholars if they were to become full-fledged members of the university community. Flood aptly argues that this purposeful blockade spurred the development of faculty and eventually made their participation on the Faculty Senate, not only desirable, but also inevitable.

Equally convincing is Flood's account of the school's long-standing clinical focus. Dean Margretta Madden Styles pushed during the early 1970s for the school to have essential clinical connections. Building on existing collaborations with the hospital, Styles expanded clinical liaisons through hiring new faculty and collaborating with the School of Medicine and other health care agencies in opening a diabetic clinic, an independent pediatric practice, and an adult clinic in a low-income area of San Francisco. These clinical activities drew on a wide range of faculty expertise and speak to the school's present-day ability to attract students.

Throughout the introduction and conclusion, Flood asserts two key points about the general construction of the narrative. The first, that this is a survey history that largely reports the events of interest to the school's development; and second, that upon her own admission to the faculty at UCSF, she halts her historical examination in the early 1970s and essentially switches to wrapping up the narrative with more of a heritage slant than critical historiography. She pertinently identifies that at the conclusion of this historical survey there are more questions than answers.

However, this is perhaps the more interesting contribution of the book to nursing history. While Flood accomplishes what she set out to do with clean writing and attention to quick and interesting progression of the story, she also leaves us with fodder for future work. For example, the reader is left wanting to understand more about the significance of the interdisciplinary nature of the school's faculty and the influence this might have had on the development of the school as a whole. Additionally, Flood mentions the influence of California's political geography on the school's development: events like the emergence of the two-year associate degree programs, programs that at present day outnumber baccalaureate degree programs 4 to 1 in the state, and, in general, the progressive nature of California's health care policy initiatives, likely produced an altogether different set of circumstances for the development of the school. Moreover, there were intimations about the region's early and sustained diversity that seemed to differ from schools in other areas of the United States. All of these issues, while touched on by Flood in some capacity, were left largely unexplored.

For those readers who take interest in the development of nursing education and women's inclusion onto university campuses, Flood's work is well worth the read. And for those readers eager to explore political and cultural issues, Flood puts forward some interesting information and jumping off points for future works. All in all, *Promise on Parnassus* makes for a substantive addition to histories of academic nursing.

Jennifer Lynn Hobbs, RN, MSN
Doctoral Candidate
Barbara Bates Center for the Study of the History of Nursing
University of Pennsylvania School of Nursing
Philadelphia, PA 19104
VA Pre-Doctoral Nurse Fellow
VA San Diego Healthcare System
3350 La Jolla Village Drive, Bldg. 13, 111N-1
San Diego, CA 92109

Passing the Legacy: A History of the Last Fifty Years of the School of Nursing of the Hospital of the University of Pennsylvania

By Eleanor Crowder Bjoring

(Philadelphia: Alumni Association of the School of Nursing of the Hospital of the University of Pennsylvania, 2006) (205 pages; $25, cloth)

Eleanor Crowder Bjoring writes a history about the well-respected School of Nursing of the Hospital of the University of Pennsylvania (HUP Training School). Focusing on this one school's last 50 years, Dr. Bjoring captures the essence of the transformation of nursing education in the United States. The history of this school highlights the apprenticeship nature of nursing education that existed in this country well into the 20th century. It also illustrates how this method of education was more congruent with the needs of the hospital rather than with the educational philosophy of the university. Using this local history, the author shows the dilemma nursing leaders faced when confronted with a seemingly outdated but traditional apprenticeship method of education, strong alumni, and changing social values about nursing education and nursing roles.

Bjoring does an excellent job of framing the history of the school within the context of the history of nursing education during the 20th century. She provides the reader with the background of nursing education, including the move by newly formed nursing organizations at the beginning of the 20th century to standardize nursing education and practice as well as the mid-century studies that advocated baccalaureate education in nursing.

The book focuses on the last 50 years of the HUP Training School beginning with 1928 and ending in 1978 when the school closed. Bjoring's story overlaps a previous history that covered the school's earlier years. She renders a vivid account of how life within this three-year diploma program tried to accommodate to a rapidly changing modern world. During this period, the school had to contend with coexistence with other schools of nursing within the same HUP system and, in particular, one where nurses were prepared at the baccalaureate level, and education rather than service was the goal. Maintaining the status quo created tension among those who advocated the continuation of HUP Training School and those who sought a more progressive route in higher education.

The school's leaders sought support from the accrediting body as they continued to inculcate students with the importance of service to the institution. They were successful in their efforts as they were recognized and valued for many years by the hospital they serviced, the nursing students they recruited, and the community they served. By 1978, however, they closed their doors succumbing to the efforts in nursing at both the national and local level to educate nurses at the baccalaureate level. It became more difficult for HUP Training School to meet the demands of an increasingly complex health care delivery system and a university system that could no longer support the ideals of diploma education.

Bjoring captures this remarkable history with depth and breadth as well as with the wisdom of someone who experienced part of that history. She chronologically organizes the history according to decades starting with the 1930s, titling this chapter, "A Period of Introspection." The titles of each subsequent chapter, including the 1940s "War and Its Aftermath," the 1950s "Challenges of a New Decade," the 1960s "Nursing Education in a

New Light," and then ending with the 1970s "A Painful Passing of the Legacy," inform the reader of the issues related to that particular period in history.

The research is well supported by the many primary and secondary sources that Bjoring uses, including minutes of various constituent groups, annual reports, published articles, mid-century nursing studies, alumni letters and reports. Her own voice can also be heard throughout the narrative, which further enriches the story. For example, she makes an excellent point describing how too few hospitals distinguished between the educational levels of nurses when hiring. Supported in the literature by nursing leaders such as Martha Rogers, Bjoring's own voice rings out in the following excerpt:

> Nurses, constrained by hospital rules, were restricted in their ability to implement creative solutions to nursing problems. For graduate nurses to do so might have set a bad example for students and, God forbid, administration did not want three hundred or so nursing students running about being "creative." (p. 143)

HUP Training School maintained its 100-year tradition of educating nursing professionals until they could no longer serve their constituency. *Passing the Legacy* tells an excellent story about this school, including the nostalgia surrounding its history. Yet, Bjoring wants us to remember that this school must be "credited with laying the foundation of nurses education at the University of Pennsylvania" (p. xiii), and this clearly resonates in her excellent historical account. Scholars interested in the history of nursing education and leadership during the 20th century in the United States will find this book an important one to read and consider.

Sandra B. Lewenson, EdD, RN, FAAN
Professor of Nursing
Lienhard School of Nursing
Pace University
New York, NY 10038

Marriage of Convenience: Rockefeller International Health and Revolutionary Mexico

By Anne-Emanuelle Birn
(Rochester, N.Y.: University of Rochester Press, 2006) (434 pages; $95.00 cloth)

A "marriage of convenience," described by Anne-Emanuelle Birn as "contracted for practical reasons" (p. 2), describes the relationship between Mexico and the Rockefeller Foundation that was formed to improve public health and modernize the nation. Although not always agreeing on issues and maintaining outside relationships, like a marriage, they worked together and ultimately influenced and shaped each other during their work together that lasted from 1921 to 1951. The Rockefeller Foundation, incorporated in 1913, has interested readers from its beginning, including newspaper articles; professional journal articles written by foundation staff; and books written by historians analyzing the work, politics, leadership, and science of this philanthropic organization. *Marriage of Convenience* uses Mexico as a case study to examine the work of the international division of the Rockefeller Foundation as an interchange, presenting evidence that it was not a one-sided authoritarian approach but a relationship to improve the delivery of public health. It is a story of the grab for power and influence by both the Mexican leaders and the Rockefeller staff, each seeking to place public health under their authority to implement their programs using their personnel.

The book presents a look at the development of state-supported public health in Mexico and brings into the analysis the smaller players that affected program planning and implementation. It starts with the large, governmental *Departamento de Salubridad Pública* (Department of Public Health) and includes nurses, midwives, alternative healers, medical elites, and politicians. The light coverage of public health nursing includes an analysis of the "bridging" role held by Mexican nurses as they connected citizens to physicians and aided the importation of modern public health practices determined by the Rockefeller Foundation and absorbed by the Mexican physicians and State.

By the 1920s, the U.S. government and business interests developed an interest in Mexico because of the threat of the spread of disease across the border and the threat of disease to workers needed for U.S. production in the area. Mexico, however, was very suspicious of U.S. involvement in the country after years of land seizures and business manipulations that took money and resources out of Mexico without benefiting the country. The goal of the Rockefeller Foundation was to break through this deep-seated resentment and suspicion to bring public health campaigns to Mexico. As the author points out, the interactions shaped both the philanthropy and the Mexican state institutions.

Although their campaigns against yellow fever, hookworm, and the push for development of local health units were accepted by Mexican medical elites, the Rockefeller Foundation came up against the refusal of the Mexican people to adhere to their regulations and recommendations. This refusal was, in part, due to the lack of knowledge of the potential benefits, but many times it was in defiance of U.S. involvement. The people believed the campaigns were a "prelude to U.S. invasion" of their country (p. 58).

The international division of the Rockefeller Foundation became a source of information for leading Mexican physicians hoping to use the transplanted knowledge, power, and resources to establish themselves as the authorities in public health. The Rockefeller Foundation work did help to break down the ill feelings toward the United States held by Mexicans and created a relatively cooperative atmosphere for further interaction through the years.

Birn's book is an analysis of the Rockefeller Foundation's quest to spread international health cooperation through its goals and principles; the national doctors, nurses, dentists, and other health care workers then translated the information and applied it according to Mexico's needs. The value of this book is in the analysis and explanation of how cooperative international health developed during the 20th century, as the author puts it, "not bound by colonial strictures, proselytizing mandates, or military objectives" but along "strictly official terms" (p. 267). By offering insight into the effects of foreign influence, this book is valuable for those interested in international public health work, especially in light of the increased interest by schools of nursing and public health to offer global experiences for their students as well as those heading for work in the international setting of a nongovernmental agency.

Jeannine Uribe, PhD, RN
Barbara Bates Center for the Study of the History of Nursing
University of Pennsylvania School of Nursing
Philadelphia, PA 19104

American Babies: Their Life and Times in the 20th Century

By Elizabeth A. Reedy
(Westport, Conn.: Praeger, 2007) (216 pages; $39.95 cloth)

Elizabeth Reedy has accomplished a remarkable feat. She has taken her pediatric clinical nurse expertise and her historical scholarship on the hospitalized care of premature infants[1] and melded them into a comprehensive book on infancy/babyhood in the United States. *American Babies* opens in 1906 when the birth of a baby, with the aid of kin, midwife, or a physician, occurred in the home. It was usually a time of family joy, but often sorrow lurked in the background because babies could, and did, develop life-threatening problems within the first year of their lives, problems that physicians lacked the skills and knowledge to remedy. A few pediatricians had begun to devote their skills and talents to the exclusive care and understanding of the health of children, but they were few and existed only in metropolitan areas. This factor plus numerous others accounted for the high infant mortality and morbidity statistics of the era.

Using a social and medical history format Reedy explores, throughout the century, a wide range of factors that she deems essential to the well-being and development of babies, including changing parental and societal attitudes toward babies, availability of health information and medical expertise to treat babies, the economics of infancy, racism, population numbers, immigration in both the early 20th century and in the current era, and more contemporary issues such as infertility, adoption, foster care, and obesity.

The strongest chapters of the book are those that focus on the dramatic increase in the capability of public health and medical leaders to address the health needs of infants. Advances in public health and medical science led to clean water and food supplies for babies. The discovery of vitamins, immunizations against lethal infectious diseases such as diphtheria and polio, and the creation of the modern hospital with its surgical and medical sophistication aided physicians and nurses in successfully treating infants' congenital anomalies and prematurity. In addition, governmental initiatives, beginning with the establishment of the U.S. Children's Bureau in 1912 and the creation of various states' health department's maternal and child bureaus in the 1920s, brought needed health care and information directly to families. All of these initiatives and the passage of the Federal Social Security Act in 1935 that provided financial Aid to Families with Dependent Children increased the survival and quality of lives of infants and children.

Reedy clearly substantiates the claim of many that the 20th century significantly improved the survival and lives of children. In 1915, out of 1,000 White live births, 100 of them would not survive to reach the age of one. For Black births the ratio was 200 infant deaths for every 1,000 births. In 1998 the mortality statistic had changed to 6 deaths per 1,000 White births, and slightly more than 14 deaths per 1,000 Black births. This dramatic improvement in the survival of infants reflects the success of our efforts to improve the lives of the country's babies, but it also demonstrates that there is still a glaring inequity in the availability of quality care and society's interest to the needs of babies of different races and classes.

Reedy is to be commended for her ability to create a book that introduces recent historical scholarship on the health care of children to a larger general audience than historians and social scientists. She has captured the dramatic growth of the nation in the 20th century and its changing views of how its youngest citizens and their families should be valued and treated. In closing, she outlines the challenges facing the country as it continues to meet the special needs of babies, while at the same time, moving a tremendous amount of its resources into the care of its exploding aging population of citizens. Rather than feeling overwhelmed by the task, one leaves the book believing that the experience of our past should aid us in meeting the needs of both generations of Americans.

Barbara Brodie, PhD, RN, FAAN
Madge M. Jones Professor Emerita
University of Virginia
Associate Director
Center for Nursing Historical Inquiry
Charlottesville, VA 22903

Note

1. Elizabeth Reedy, "Ripe Too Early: The Expansion of Hospital Based Premature Infant Care in the United States, 1922–1950" (PhD diss., University of Pennsylvania, 2000).

Psychiatric Cultures Compared: Psychiatry and Mental Health Care in the Twentieth Century

Edited by Marijke Gijswijt-Hofstra, Harry Oosterhuis, Joost Vijselaar, and Hugh Freeman (Amsterdam: Amsterdam University Press, 2005) (456 pages; $50.00 paper)

Psychiatric Cultures Compared is based on a series of papers first presented at an international workshop entitled, "Cultures of Psychiatry and Mental Health Care in the Twentieth Century: Comparisons and Approaches," held at the University of Amsterdam in 2003. Offering a wide range of sophisticated analyses by leading scholars in the field, the book's specific focus on the history of mental health care in the 20th century makes it a valuable addition to the literature. This time period is still an underexplored terrain in psychiatric history. The collection contextualizes important transformations of 20th-century psychiatry, using a comparative approach to topics such as institutional and outpatient care, funding, legislation and welfare politics, patient rights, the role of professional groups, antipsychiatry and deinstitutionalization, and the broader social, political, and cultural context of care. It provides historical overviews of psychiatric care in the Netherlands, Britain, the United States, Germany, and France, as well as focused studies on patient experiences in the Netherlands, Japan, and Italy and—of particular interest to the audience of *Nursing History Review*—two analyses of psychiatric nursing in Sweden and in the Netherlands, as well as a chapter on the history of psychotropic drugs. The book concludes with two reflective chapters, which synthesize the main themes and discuss various methodological issues in comparative historical research. According to the editors, "this collection of essays offers one of the first attempts in the history of psychiatry towards a more systematic comparison of national developments in a number of major Western countries during the twentieth century" (p. 12). As such, it is an innovative work that explores some new ground in historical research.

The first section of the book examines changes in institutional and out-patient care and the role of the state in mental health care in various national contexts. Dutch scholars Marijke Gijswijt-Hofstra and Harry Oosterhuis provide an analysis of institutional and out-patient psychiatry in the Netherlands, describing how psychiatric institutions gradually opened up during the course of the 20th century, eventually differentiating into a range of community and specialized services. Gemma Blok's chapter on the antipsychiatric movement in the Netherlands is a fascinating critique of this underexamined trend and offers much opportunity for comparison. Hugh Freeman looks at the relationship between the state and care of the mentally ill in Britain, especially following the establishment of the National Health Service in 1948. Gerald Grob gives an in-depth analysis of deinstitutionalization policy in the United States, arguing that *trans-institutionalization* is perhaps a better term to describe the shifting patterns in postwar residential mental health care.

Three chapters in this section are devoted to German psychiatric history. Volker Roelcke examines the role of institutions, Greg Eghigian analyzes East German psychiatry during the Communist era, and Franz-Werner Kersting studies asylum psychiatry in West Germany from 1940 to 1975, from the Nazi euthanasia program to reform in the postwar era. Jean-Christophe Coffin describes trends in the organization of French psychiatry in the 20th century. The emphasis on national psychiatric cultures and changing dynamics between professionals, patients, families, and institutions in these chapters, especially as of the 1950s, constitutes a compelling overview. The analyses clearly demonstrate that general trends and transformations must be understood in their local and regional context.

In the second thematic section, new studies by Joost Vijselaar, Akihito Suzuki, and Patricia Guarnieri on patient records and asylum admission patterns confirm the recent insight in psychiatric historiography that the family remained of central importance in negotiating care and admission. Asylum admission was but one strategy families used in a range of options. Gender and welfare policy have a particular emphasis in these studies. Vijselaar also includes an interesting discussion of the value of qualitative database research tools for analysis of patient records.

An exciting part of this section is the new research on psychiatric nursing history. Cecile aan de Stegge analyzes trends and transformations in the use of restraints in 20th-century Dutch psychiatry. In the postwar era, nurses took on innovative new roles in patient care, reconceptualizing the meaning of *nursing* care and patient responsibility in dealing with difficult patient behavior. Gunnel Svedberg describes trends in the professionalization of psychiatric nursing in Sweden, which was heavily influenced by ideals about femininity from the Nightingale legacy. As a result, female nurses obtained leading positions in asylums whereas male nurses remained in the role of attendants. During the 1960s more gender-neutral terminology emerged to refer to trained nurses, and career opportunities for male nurses increased.

In the final section, the reflective chapters by Frank Huisman, Ido de Haan, and James Kennedy provide a critical discussion of assumptions about progress and the complexity of making cultural comparisons in the historical analysis of mental health care. This book is a "must read," especially for scholars interested in a critical analysis of the deinstitutionalization era, which recently has received new interest in North American psychiatric historiography. However, considering the broad, international scope of the book and the inclusion of discussions of methodological and conceptual issues in comparative historical research, the book also is a rich resource for all scholars and clinicians interested in new developments and trends in the historiography of international health care.

Geertje Boschma, RN, PhD
Associate Professor
School of Nursing
University of British Columbia
T201–2211 Wesbrook Mall
Vancouver, BC V6T 2B5
Canada

Polio: An American Story

By David M. Oshinsky
(New York: Oxford University Press, 2005) (342 pages; $16.95 paper)

Salk, Sabin, FDR—famous faces that arise when one hears the word *polio.* Many reading this can recall the panicked headlines and restrictive municipal measures taken to prevent polio's spread and devastation during the 20th century. Jonas Salk and Albert Sabin are the victorious faces of successful polio vaccines. David M. Oshinsky's engrossing 2006 Pulitzer Prize–winning book, *Polio: An American Story,* provides a comprehensive timeline and examines, in depth, the national approach taken by the United States to mobilize social, medical, and scientific resources directed at solving the polio epidemics that created public health crises in the 1930s, 1940s, and 1950s. These epidemics resulted in near-panic and hysteria in the populations where they occurred.

Prominent and famous scientific names and their efforts are examined as they sought to find the answer to combating polio: Abraham Flexner, who until his death steadfastly believed only one polio virus strain existed; and Sister Elizabeth Kenny, the Australian nurse whose methods of polio treatment and personal manner alienated the majority of the medical community. Less well-known names and their efforts within the polio race are presented: David Koprowski, whose unsuccessful vaccine trials in Belfast, Ireland, made him a pariah within the polio research community; Isabel Morgan, whose personal decisions led to her retiring from the scientific arena; Basil O'Connor, the charismatic fund-raiser for polio research; David Weaver, the National Foundation director whose grants funded medical research; and others whose scientific and publicity efforts kept the momentum going to seek a successful vaccine for polio.

The most famous face of polio, Franklin Delano Roosevelt (FDR), and his popularity spearheaded national efforts to fund and underwrite the research for a polio vaccine, ultimately gained by Salk and Sabin. The March of Dimes with the Marching Mothers and poster children raised public awareness and galvanized national fund-raising activity across all segments of society to contribute dimes to fund vaccine research, which ultimately led to the development of national funding for scientific research. Oshinsky thoroughly explores the rival team efforts headed by Salk and Sabin and the tensions between them as to who was the better scientist. Oshinsky does not shield Salk from the unsparing criticism arising from his failure to acknowledge his successful vaccine was a team effort and not the single effort as was perceived.

Efforts to have the first viable vaccine exposed some questionable ethical concerns about vaccine testing. Salk, after inoculating his family, did early testing of his three-injection killed-virus vaccine on institutionalized children. Sabin's efforts to mass test his vaccine found fertile ground in the Soviet Union where he was invited to test his attenuated oral vaccine. The rush to bring the approved vaccine to the public led to the Cutter Laboratory fiasco where contamination of several lots of the Salk vaccine led to outbreaks of polio among those vaccinated for prevention of the disease. Ultimately, the debate over which vaccine was the more effective, oral-attenuated (Sabin) or killed-virus injection series (Salk) led to a change in polio vaccination protocols in the United States. The Sabin oral vaccine, as the preferred protocol until the 1990s, has now been supplanted by the Salk injection vaccine as research demonstrated its better effectiveness in eradicating polio.

Polio: An American Story is a comprehensive and succinct detailing of a disease that caused public panic and a national mobilization of all arenas to research and find a solution to this menace. In placing polio and the efforts to seek a viable vaccine against the social history context of the United States, Oshinsky has elegantly crafted a compelling story with riveting elements and also with sufficient science for the reader to comprehend the depth, passion, excitement, failures, roadblocks, dead ends, and major and minor successes that characterize vaccine research. Exploring the scientific, political, and social personages who utilized their energies and intelligence to find a solution to a public health problem, *Polio: An American Story* serves as a blueprint for confronting future public health challenges and a reminder of the success that can be achieved when all efforts are mobilized to work toward a solution for a problem affecting a nation's population.

Teresa M. O'Neill, RNC, PhD
Associate Professor
Our Lady of Holy Cross College
New Orleans, LA 70131

Vom "Liebesdienst" zum modernen Frauenberuf: Die Reform der Krankenpflege nach 1945 [From "Labor of Love" to a Modern Female Profession: Nursing Reform After 1945]

By Susanne Kreutzer
(Frankfurt/New York: Campus Verlag, 2005)
(306 pages; 34.90 Euro; 54.70 USD paper)

Susanne Kreutzer examines the transformation of nursing in West Germany after 1945. Offering an analysis of German nursing history during the 1950s and 1960s, a period of profound change, the book explores how a new generation of women took up nursing in different ways, moving away from the long-standing traditions of religious and charitable nursing bound by a motherhouse structure. Once dominated by a work ethic grounded in principles of religious calling, charitable service, and self-sacrifice, nursing began to be reconceptualized and reworked into a modern female profession with an image more appealing and acceptable to a new generation of women as well as men during this time.

Because of the powerful influence of the motherhouses, nurses had a unique position in the German health care system. Motherhouses followed a centuries-old model in which single women devoted their lives to charitable service and received board and lodging in return, while being assured of lifelong care by the sisterhood. They negotiated their own contracts with hospitals, since they were not a part of the regular labor and social security regulations negotiated by trade unions that had become the regulatory structure for most laborers and employees in state or municipal service. As health care and social welfare expanded during the 1960s, this system, grounded in the idea of self-sacrifice, was increasingly perceived as outdated, if not exploitive. The quest for more individual independence, less rigid living and working conditions, and better education grew—a process of modernization closely linked to broader social changes taking place in women's work. The formation of the welfare state, the profound shortages of adequately trained health care personnel, the growing number of married women entering the workforce, and the new educational demands generated by an increasingly medical and technological hospital environment created strains on traditional constructions of nursing work.

Focusing on these transformations in German nursing, the book provides new and compelling perspectives on a period in nursing history that has largely been unexplored. The focus of the study places the book at the crossroads of health care, women's history, and labor history, providing an important historical context to a question that has not lost its relevance: how care of the sick and elderly can maintain its appeal as an attractive occupation in the face of current pressures on the workforce.

To explore these changes, Kreutzer conducts a case study of one organized nursing group that reflected the changes typical of the time. She examines a nursing league [*Schwesterschaft*], established as a grassroots organization shortly after the end of the Second World War and incorporated into a larger union by the late 1940s, the League of Free Sisters in the Trade Union for Public Service and Transport [*Bund freier Schwestern in der Gewerkschaft Oeffentliche Dienste, Transport und Verkehr*]. Kreutzer analyzes how nurses' work arrangements changed in response to new demands, and were renegotiated by the nurses who took up leadership positions in this trade union, as well as by the largely male union leadership. Significantly, at the time this League was established in 1946, the German word for "sister" [*Schwester*] was still the common term to refer to a female nurse. It had a more general meaning than the literal English translation suggests. At that time, *sister* meant nurse, which could be either religious or secular, and it was not until the 1960s and 1970s that the more general term *Krankenpfleger* or *Krankenpflegerin,* which also means nurse (male or female, respectively) emerged. This term became more commonly used, in part reflecting the transformation Kreutzer is studying. Rather uniquely, nurses were organized as a separate section within this larger trade union, seeking to reconcile the traditional ideals and goals of an organized sisterhood with the new interests and demands of a modern professional group. In 1968 the League was opened up to male membership.

The book has three main chapters. Following an introduction sketching the main focus of the book, Chapter 1 outlines how the traditional image of nursing was transformed into a modern professional one. Chapters 2 and 3 form the main body of the book. Chapter 2 examines how the League of Free Sisters obtained its organizational structure and was embedded in the larger union structure, initially supported by union politics that were favorable to women. This helped nurses to negotiate better working conditions and highlighted their important role in people's health and well-being, in a sense still drawing on traditional images. Although the working conditions were gradually transformed and renegotiated, the fact that the League never fully broke with traditional values might explain why the initial innovative efforts came to a halt during the 1960s, and why the nurses, in many ways, lost their unique position in the union. Nurses' ideals, objectives, and bargaining strategies were more closely aligned with those of other union members. This chapter includes a detailed reconstruction of the work and leadership of nurses within the union.

The act of carefully balancing nursing ideals and union demands created dilemmas of its own, as Kreutzer points out in the third chapter. The demand for reasonable hours, salaries, and working conditions went hand in hand with pointing out the need for more nursing education, but the focus was more on the length of the training than on envisioning changes in the conceptualization of the content of nursing. Chapter 3 analyzes in more detail the profound legal, social, and cultural implications of turning a charitable field into a profession. Giving numerous examples, Kreutzer examines how the League's leaders and members renegotiated the regulation of nurses' working conditions. Eventually the laws regulating nursing and nursing education changed. Yet, the changes also generated concern over the loss of nurses' traditional emphasis on "total patient care" in light of a health care system that was increasingly dominated by pressures of bureaucracy and efficient organization, as well as leveling and division of labor within the nursing profession itself.

Although the League was an innovative alternative for women who no longer were attracted to the traditional motherhouses during the 1950s, a decade later it had a hard time keeping up with the rapid changes in health care, and it seemed to have lost its momentum. Some improvements had been achieved, such as instigating a 48-hour work week, treating nursing as a "normal" occupation. But when push came to shove, the League was not prepared to entirely give up on some of the long-standing values of service, and it still held on to traditional expectations: nurses, for example, should not "watch the clock" when it came to patient needs. How to materially value work that always had seemed to be a natural ability of women was not a simple matter, and hence not easily translated into negotiable demands. The nursing shortage rather than proactive labor negotiations was the decisive influence on the abandonment of many of the strict rules.

With regard to nursing education, the League often perceived practical experience to be of higher value than theoretical knowledge, despite the changing demands of increased medical and technological care. Often the League remained firmly attached to ideals of "total care" nurses once provided, and it lacked a vision, for example, of how an increased division of labor within nursing and introduction of nurse assistants could serve the profession or should be negotiated in labor contracts. Rather, a differentiation between basic and specialized technical care became the basis for a quest for professionalization and enhanced education, with basic care considered to be of lower complexity and lower responsibility. Hence, basic care was almost naturally left to less educated and less well-paid women. Within the union itself, nurses remained something of an anomaly, neither in full alignment with the interests of other female workers in cleaning or secretarial jobs, nor gaining the full respect and support of their male counterparts when it came to sharing power and influence. Moreover, as a conceptual vacuum arose over the content of nursing, nurses had difficulty gaining full autonomy over substantial domains of nursing care.

Kreutzer concludes that the modern image was not without its new dilemmas. The transition from a "labor of love" to a modern female profession was a highly complex process in which there were gains for women, for sure, but also undeniable losses for nurses as well as for patients, leaving a void as to how to conceptualize and claim authority over (good) care in the current health care system (as opposed to good medical treatment alone). This well-written and well-documented book will be of interest to a wide range of academic and professional audiences in nursing, social science, and health care history, and it provides a compelling analysis of relatively recent changes in nursing and health care. It is a critical and valuable contribution to the history of nursing, substantially augmenting the international nursing history scholarship.

Geertje Boschma, RN, PhD
Associate Professor
School of Nursing
University of British Columbia
T201–2211 Wesbrook Mall
Vancouver, BC V6T 2B5
Canada

Making Room in the Clinic: Nurse Practitioners and the Evolution of Modern Health Care

By Julie A. Fairman
(New Brunswick, N.J.: Rutgers University Press, 2008)
(255 pages; $45.95 cloth)

Making Room in the Clinic examines the emergence of the nurse practitioner movement in the 1960s and 1970s. The author uses this phenomenon as a lens to examine the negotiated boundaries of professions, in this case nursing and medicine, and the connection between microlevel, local decisions about which provider thinks about and does what for patients and macrolevel factors such as the context of social movements, national professional organization interests, politics, and economic factors. Ultimately, this is a study of the dynamics of change in the cultural institution of health care.

This spontaneous movement in nursing and medicine bubbled up in many places, taking several forms in the early 1960s. Initially these were local, often dyadic arrangements between one physician, who wanted to be able to serve more patients and/or concentrate his practice on things he found more challenging, and an experienced, imaginative nurse who wanted more tools, both in clinical reasoning and in technical skills, to provide broader or better care to patients, even though this involved practice at the borderlands of nursing and medicine. Patients, both as individuals in innumerable clinics and doctors' offices, and as "the public" in governmental, regulatory, and funding mechanisms, weighed in on the side of adjusted boundaries.

The author has sculpted this comprehensive account from a mass of source material, giving shape to the story and prompting intriguing historical questions. This analysis includes the intersecting circumstances of both medicine and nursing, inasmuch as the movement had roots equally in both. The narrative traces development from the earliest, localized arrangements to coalescence into a movement, which in turn led to gradual establishment and standardization as training programs developed, funding sources emerged, and practice arrangements became codified.

The introductory chapter lays out the perspective, parameters, questions, and arguments of the study. Chapters 1 and 2 describe the atmosphere in health care and clinical practice in which the many local negotiations and arrangements began. They explore the circumstances of larger collectives such as professional organizations and academic institutions that had a stake in this new phenomenon. Chapter 3 focuses on academic health centers as sites of innovation using University of Florida and University of Rochester as exemplars to look at the importance of individual relationships and local organizational politics. Chapter 4 examines the evolution of physician assistant training programs, with a focus on the first one at Duke University, noting this as another response to the same forces encouraging nurse practitioner (NP) development and referencing the initial conceptual fuzziness about the characteristics of the two roles. Chapter 5 shifts the focus to the national professional organizations, the AMA and the ANA, and the circumstances that gave rise to nursing specialty organizations. Chapter 6 describes the work of the National Joint Practice Commission from 1972–1981, which gave advice on revision of state practice legislation. Chapter 7 is a case study of the initially triangulated but gradually changing relationships of the National Association of Pediatric Nurse Associates and Practitioners (NAPNAP) with ANA and the American Academy of Pediatrics. Certification was the need that drove NAPNAP toward initial close alliance with the Academy. Chapter 8 touches on trends since the 1970s that have supported demand for NPs and capacity to prepare them. It underscores and illustrates with recent examples the thesis that local practice negotiations are still the engine of change for the borders of practice.

Other elements are of interest in themselves, beyond their contribution to the overall argument. These include:

- While fully acknowledging the broad social, economic, and political factors involved in the rise of the movement, this account highlights the difference that individual persons and local combinations of persons made in the course of events.

- The author explicates the centrality of the diagnostic reasoning process to the identity of physicians and medicine, and within that understanding describes the significance of beginning to teach this to nurses.
- This is not a story of gendered conflict between medicine and nursing, by and large. Rather, it is one of constructive creativity around meeting patient needs at the point of care.
- The federal funding policy decision to focus on cost containment and competition rather than on access to health care shifted the forces surrounding the NP role, creating substantial changes in its clinical practice and in relationships with physicians in the 1980s and beyond.

I am hard pressed to think of a *Nursing History Review* reader who would not value this volume. Consumers of nursing history will enjoy the engaging narrative. Historians of health care, medicine, and nursing will appreciate the framework, analysis, evidence, and substantive endnotes this work provides.

Marilyn E. Flood, RN, PhD
Emeritus Associate Dean
School of Nursing
University of California San Francisco
2 Koret Way
San Francisco, CA 94143–0604

Mental Health Policy in the United States Since 1950: Better but Not Well

By Richard G. Frank and Sherry Glied
(Baltimore: Johns Hopkins University Press, 2006)
(183 pages; $39.95 cloth; $21.95 paper)

Mental Health Policy in the United States Since 1950 is a data-driven assessment of mental health care in America since 1950. It examines the changes in the lives of people with mental illness and the factors that have affected their lives. The book approaches the history of mental illness in America from a different perspective, drawing heavily on economic theories in explaining changes in the mental health field over time.

The chapters discuss economic policies that, in turn, affected mental health policy in the United States. Chapter 1 provides an overview of the factors that affected people with mental illness. Chapter 2 describes people in America with mental illness, and Chapter 3 discusses explanations for change over time in the lives of people with mental illness. Chapter 4 covers the financing of mental health services, and Chapters 5 and 6 describe the changes in providers of mental health care since 1950 and the consequences of changes in financing of mental health services, respectively. Chapter 7 considers treatment and living conditions of people with mental illness since 1950, with the concluding chapter taking a look into the future.

Overall, the book is written on a positive note, clearly stating that people with mental illness are better off than they were 50 years ago. It also has recommendations for the future that may further enhance the lives of people with mental illness.

The strongest feature of the book is its use of data to guide the discussion of the complex topic of mental health in America. Within the economic framework, a very clear and concise picture of the changes in mental health policy and in the lives of Americans with mental illness over 50 years emerges as one reads the book. Efficacy of treatments for mental illness, federal insurance programs, changes in mental health care workers, distribution and coordination of mental health services, and mental health policy are well presented. The focus of each of these topics is how it affected the lives of Americans with mental illness.

Mental Health Policy in the United States Since 1950 is a well-written and important work that provides a definitive look at the past and a glimpse into the future of mental health policy in America. Anyone interested in people with mental illness in this country will find the book useful, including those who participate in the care of people with mental illness and those who are involved in health care policy. In addition, people interested in the historical aspects of the lives of persons in America with mental illness will enjoy reading it.

Kathleen Brown, RN, MSN, PhD
Practice Assistant Professor
University of Pennsylvania School of Nursing
418 Curie Blvd.
Philadelphia, PA 19104

Daring to Care: American Nursing and Second-Wave Feminism

By Susan Gelfand Malka
(Urbana and Chicago: University of Illinois Press, 2007)
(219 pages; $25.00 paper)

Traditional wisdom holds that nursing and feminism are naturally antithetical to each other. Yet in this work, based on her doctoral dissertation, Susan Gelfand Malka argues that the relationship between nursing and feminism was in part mutually beneficial. As the strident feminist movement of the 1960s evolved into the softer feminism of the 1980s, nurses were empowered. They "Dared to Care."

Daring to Care addresses the impact of the women's movement of the 1960s to the 1980s, feminism's "second wave," on nursing education and practice. (The women's movement of the 19th and early 20th centuries is known as the "first wave.") From historical and feminist perspectives, Malka describes how nurses evolved during these years from submissive handmaidens to scientific professionals, partially in response to second-wave feminism. Acknowledging this link between feminism and nursing will inform the current debate surrounding issues such as the escalating visibility of nurse practitioners, the shortage of bedside nurses, and the proposed professional doctorate in nursing.

Daring to Care opens by introducing the reader to Nightingale's founding of modern nursing, constrained as it was by gender and class. For women trained in the Nightingale model, moral superiority was paramount. Technical nursing expertise was of secondary value. Nursing was thus grounded as women's work with the angelic attributes of sacrifice, obedience, and discipline. This quasireligious aura attracted impressionable young women while impeding nursing's professional growth and autonomy. Malka then explains how nurses remained true to their founding mother over the succeeding decades. In the post–World War II period of the 1950s and 1960s, nurses were predominantly female, White, and subordinate by gender, class, and division of labor within the hospital hierarchies. Malka points out the inherent contradiction for these postwar nurses. While other women were expected to abandon their wartime jobs to resume their "rightful" work in the home, nurses were needed in civilian nursing—although they worked without the relative autonomy of wartime nursing practice. Thus nurses were expected to be workers in a society that devalued working women and failed to recognize the monetary worth of caring.

Along with the upheaval of the Civil Rights movement and the unrest surrounding the war in Vietnam, second-wave feminism shook the tradition-based world of nursing. Malka describes two sequential manifestations of second-wave feminism. The first, from the early 1960s to the 1980s, pursued total gender equality. Feminists, many of whom perceived nursing as the epitome of gender inequality, viewed nurses with disdain—and the feeling was mutual. However, by the third decade of the feminist movement, in the 1980s, feminism had evolved into a gentler, more caring movement, which accepted a plurality of female ideals. Malka contends that this new face of second-wave feminism significantly contributed to the growth in nursing autonomy and increased professional status. Many nurses, whether or not they identified themselves as feminists, could identify with feminism's softened image and the new value placed on caring. Nurses were emboldened to value their work of caring and extend that work beyond nursing's long-held boundaries. Nurses developed new roles in the community; they started to embrace technology and scientific knowledge; they ventured into the management of health care; and they increasingly trained as advanced practice nurses. Further, as second-wave feminism impacted nurse educators, new nurses graduated with career aspirations that would have been foreign to many of their predecessors.

This book, supported by a range of sources, convincingly defends its central argument that second-wave feminism impacted the growth and maturation of nursing over the second half of the 20th century. As a historian who used to practice nursing, Malka infuses her historical scholarship with an awareness of what she describes as nursing's "group identity." This identity, born of nursing's traditions, surfaces as another element, perhaps impediment, in nursing's tenuous hold on parity with other health care workers.

Through *Daring to Care,* Malka addresses an area of women's and feminist history—nursing and second-wave feminism—that has called for further analysis. For nurse historians, her work contributes to an understanding of nursing's search for its professional identity. Malka's analysis will also provide guidance for nurse leaders as nursing struggles with issues of education and practice, specifically those related to autonomy such as advanced practice nursing and the doctorate of nursing practice. This book should have broad appeal to social historians, particularly those researchers and students engaged in the fields of women's studies, labor, and nursing history. As a text for students, it invites discussion and reappraisal of the traditional view of nursing and the women's movement.

Brigid Lusk, PhD, RN
Professor and Chair
School of Nursing and Health Studies
Northern Illinois University
DeKalb, IL 60115

Capturing Nursing History: A Guide to Historical Methods

Edited by Sandra B. Lewenson and Eleanor Krohn Herrmann
(New York: Springer, 2008) (236 pages; $45.00 paper)

The editors of *Capturing Nursing History,* Sandra Lewenson and Eleanor Herrmann, are both accomplished researchers of nursing history. Through this book we learn of their personal journeys in nursing history and what led them to become researchers in the field. That journey is what forms their perspectives on why the nursing profession needs to do historical research. Additionally, embedded in their enthusiasm for historical research is their hope that researchers of nursing history will not only inform novices of the profession but will capture their imaginations about their professions and perhaps create a researcher or two.

The editors' intent in creating this text was to present the collected wisdom of experienced researchers regarding how to do historical research in nursing. Someone interested in doing this kind of research could be mentored by works collected in this text. The editors assembled 18 leading scholars in the history of nursing, including themselves, to create this valuable resource. Each chapter is devoted to different aspects of the enterprise of nursing history. The authors present their conception of historical research within the context of their own research, describing the process and methodology used. In essence, each chapter is a case study. The authors demystify doing historical research. The material presented can be read in any order, and "each chapter can be read as a stand-alone" essay (p. xiii). However, my sense of the book is that each chapter builds on the previous one creating a coherence I was not expecting.

Even though each chapter could stand alone, I find a division between the conceptual and methodological issues, then a potpourri of other pieces that surround the history of nursing research. In Chapter 2, Patricia D'Antonio sets the stage for the succeeding six chapters that go into greater depth about methodological issues. She presents five key conceptual issues and three methodological ones. With each, she uses examples from existing nursing history research to explicate her arguments.

For most of the researchers who present in Chapters 3 through 8, the self-reflection embedded in their research continues as if they jumped into a gem-polishing canister with their ideas, and they continue to be shaped by the process that enlightens and energizes their research as well as making it more interesting. These chapters begin examining the process of doing historical research by starting with Lewenson's description of moving from the beginning to the end of her work in nursing education. Joy Buck, through her work on the history of hospice, presents social and political frameworks. Sonya Grypma takes us through the process of using the biographical method, which is closely related to the following chapter on the use of oral history research presented by Geertje Boschma, Margaret Scaia, Nerissa Bonifacio, and Erica Roberts. Each of these four authors tackles oral history from a different point of view. The reflective process needed by a researcher of history is fleshed out in greater detail by Boschma, Grypma, and Florence Melchior. Researchers always need to be aware of the subjectivity they bring to the research. Herrmann, in Chapter 8, examines conducting historical research in developing countries.

Chapters 9 through 14 discuss resources available to the researcher. We find information about working with primary sources (Keith Mages and Julie Fairman), working with archival materials (Christine Hallett), artifacts (Herrmann), ethical guidelines and standards (Nettie Birnbach), the use of those guidelines and standards (Lewenson and Herrmann), and funding for historical research (Jean Whelan and Cynthia Connolly).

Finally, three appendices will help researchers find resources to aid them in research. In Appendix 1, there is a list of additional artifact resources. Appendix 2 cites sources for nursing history centers, museums, and archives. Appendix 3 references nursing history Internet sites, including the American Association for the History of Nursing Web site (www.aahn.org).

Sandra Lewenson's disarming comment in Chapter 1 about how too many nurses remember nursing history as being boring or they do not remember learning anything at all about it touched an important cord for me in terms of my own journey in embracing the history of nursing and then engaging in historical research. There is nothing boring about *Capturing Nursing History.* It is a significant, valuable, and thought-provoking look at the myriad issues facing those undertaking nursing historical research. I recommend it for undergraduate and graduate students as well as those already conducting historical research. I expect that it will be a volume that will become well worn from use as a resource for researchers.

Carla Schissel, PhD, RN
Adult Nurse Practitioner, retired
Grady Health System
Atlanta, Georgia

New Directions in the History of Nursing: International Perspectives

Edited by Barbara Mortimer and Susan McGann
(London/New York: Routledge, 2005) (224 pages; $150.00 cloth)

In the past, several books have claimed to provide new directions in the history of nursing, but none have done it with as much clarity and foresight as this one edited by two British seasoned researchers, Barbara Mortimer and Susan McGann. *New Directions in the History of Nursing* opens and closes with sophisticated and nuanced analyses of the history and current state of the field of nursing history written in English. Mortimer begins this task by examining nursing's most iconic and mystical figure, Florence Nightingale. Mortimer states that because earlier historians of Nightingale valorized her for her efforts to improve the health of patients, this theme of valorizing has permeated the body of nursing scholarship.

In 1980, Celia Davies helped move nursing history into the mainstream of historical and social scientists' analytic work, and in so doing, she provided new opportunities for nurse historians to study subjects such as asylum nursing and traditional women healers rather than great leaders. Davies challenged nurse historians to follow the work of mainstream historians and produce work that was analytic, intellectually rigorous, balanced, and utilized the scholarship of other colleagues in the historical academy. Evidence that today's nurse historians have followed this path is illuminated in Mortimer's examination of historical studies done in the last decade or so. She found such powerful factors as gender, professionalization, race, ethnicity in the global world of nursing, plus the history of caring, carefully scrutinized and analyzed in their work.

On the other side of the Atlantic, American dean of modern nursing history, Joan Lynaugh, offers a complementary and cogent essay on what she views as the "common working ground" that historians can build upon to create an international community of nursing scholars. Drawing on her own extensive historical experiences, while acknowledging the valid differences in worldviews held by other historians, Lynaugh proposes a series subjects for study that could dramatically enhance the level of communication among scholars.

The first of the proposed subjects is the universal relationship between *nursing and the state.* Using the example of the legal and social networks of countries, she demonstrates how these networks have shaped the profession and forged nursing's interdependence on the government. *Religious influences, economics and nursing, social welfare,* and *gender* are also discussed as subjects that will enrich the shared common ground of historians. Lynaugh also introduces two new subjects that she believes are common to nursing. The first is the impact of *changes in* medicine, beginning with the scientific advancements that created and now sustain the modern hospital. The rapidness of scientific change today, however, is increasing the level of stress on hospitals, the insurers who pay for services, the patients who reside in them, and the health professionals who struggle to provide quality care to patients within them. The second subject is the elusive subject known as *nursing knowledge,* which nurses claim as their common heritage and which serves to bind and guide nurses in their decisions and activities.

Between these two essays is a collection of 17 original studies that represent the growing sophistication and analytic power of nurse historians to explore diverse subjects in different parts of the globe. There are interesting and insightful contributions from Norway, Japan, South Africa, Europe, New Zealand, and North America that cover nursing events from the 19th and 20th centuries. Readers are able to learn much about how nurses of other lands function in their culture while at the same time appreciate the activities all nurses' share.

This insightful book will appeal to the seasoned historiographer and those who simply enjoy learning more about the history of nursing in other countries. I believe it would serve as a wonderful text for nursing history doctoral students to read and debate. The book challenges readers to rethink what they believe, and it offers new insights and modes of thinking about why events occurred, and how they shaped or didn't shape the world of nursing. Unfortunately, this book, because it costs $150, will not be read by many or found on personal and library bookshelves. Before too much criticism is heaped on the publisher for making the book so costly, it is important to remember that the falling value of the U.S. dollar plays a large part in making the book so expensive for American readers.

Barbara Brodie, PhD, RN, FAAN
Madge M. Jones Professor of Nursing Emerita
Associate Director, Center for Nursing Historical Inquiry
University of Virginia
Charlottesville, VA 22908–0782

El Género en la Socialización Profesional de las Enfermeras [Gender and the Professional Socialization of Mexican Nurses]

By Maribel Rios Everardo
(Cuernavaca, Morelos: Universidad Nacional Autónoma de Mexico, Centro Regional de Investigaciones Multidisciplinarias, 2001)
(224 pages; Spanish-language version only; $12.50 + shipping, paper)

Through an elegant blend of historical and contemporary analysis, Rios Everardo, a cultural anthropologist, explores how issues of gender in Mexico influenced the professional socialization of nurses in that country. The purpose of her study is to describe and analyze the socialization processes of Mexican nurses in relation to their sociocultural experiences of gender as men and women in Mexico. The research and subsequent book emerged in conjunction with the implementation of the North American Free Trade Agreement (NAFTA), concerns about the overall quality of nursing care provided by nurses working in the state-funded health system, and formal acknowledgment by the Mexican State that the country had a huge professional nursing shortage. New investment by the State in developing professional infrastructure and nursing human resources helped address these issues, but also increased the potential for Mexican nurses to migrate abroad to work and send home remittances—a critical part of the Mexican economy.

Given the context and timing of the work, the main strength of Rios Everardo's work is how she systematically pieces together key historical moments in Mexican nursing's history with the social advancement of women in Mexico. Through a critical interpretive feminist approach in the analysis and substantive examples, Rios Everardo delves into Mexican nursing history in critical detail to explore the roots of Mexican nursing and explain some of the present challenges the country faces in developing nursing human resources. She successfully argues that there is a strong link between nursing socialization processes in Mexico and the overall status of women—something tacitly acknowledged in the literature but not often overtly stated.

A key point of the analysis is that, in many ways, Mexican women who choose nursing become the embodiment of the Great Mother figure, an image found both in indigenous and Catholic religions in the country. The Great Mother brings care and well-being to others even as she sacrifices her own needs. To show the contemporary consequences of this sacrificial image, she blends the historical findings with data from 15 interviews with nursing faculty residing in Mexico City. Her interviewees describes their professional challenges as rooted in a conceptual war between professional development and vocational sacrifice. Rios Everardo's analysis suggestively hints that the struggle to blend the female-gendered

Great Mother image with the more male-gendered structures of a profession is the root of Mexican nursing's development dynamics.

Of the flaws in the work, class in relation to gender receives less attention than it should. Mexico has a highly class-stratified society, and Rios Everardo only cursorily examines this factor in relation to gender. Class becomes important because of issues related to educational access for women of all classes in Mexico and its influence on who became a nurse at different points in Mexican history. She also interviewed only one male nurse, so that limits the generalizability of the findings to the male nursing experience in Mexico. Finally, readers unaccustomed to the presentation of Latin American scholarly work may find the book's organization unusual, but it fits with the academic tradition of the region.

Nonetheless, by blending historical and contemporary data, Rios Everardo illustrates the consequences of the deeply rooted cultural tendencies about gender socialization on modern Mexican nursing. An important finding from Rios Everardo's work is that without factoring in the historical and contemporary status of Mexican women in society and the social acceptability of males working in nursing, policymakers miss a critical component in planning for the development of nursing human resources.

Researchers from any discipline have produced few studies about Mexican nursing and its development. Historical research about Mexican nurses trends toward the chronological, with only significant dates reported and little critical analysis of the related context. Of the few historical analyses about Mexican nurses, this is one of the best. Even though the work is only available in Spanish at this time, nurse historians with even basic Spanish-language abilities will find the work a valuable read and contribution to their knowledge base. Nursing human resources policymakers will receive additional insight into the social challenges involved in producing nurses, a problem that, as Rios Everardo's work demonstrates, is not simply a matter of a lack of physical infrastructure and capital.

Allison Squires, PhD, RN
University of Pennsylvania
Center for Health Outcomes & Policy Research
418 Curie Blvd., Floor 3R–338
Philadelphia, PA 19104

Final Exam: A Surgeon's Reflections on Mortality

By Pauline W. Chen
(New York: Alfred A. Knopf, 2007) (268 pages; $23.95 cloth)

Final Exam is one of several new medical narratives that hold growing market allure. Divided into three sections and nine chapters that guide the reader through the author's process of professional development and identity, it is both the story of Dr. Chen's own experiences as a medical student and liver transplant surgeon and a personal essay about a physician's discovery of humanity. Section One, "Principles," discusses Chen's medical student years and her experiences with cadaver dissection and many "firsts" such as her first resuscitation and first death pronouncement. Weaving her tale with literary mastery, she shares the sights, sounds, and smells imprinted on her memory as vividly as she does the depth of her emotional growth in facing mortality. Those of us who have ever dissected animals in anatomy and physiology, for example, can certainly relate to the description of formaldehyde as "the olfactory version of a high-pitched shriek" (p. 9) or the heart as "a ball of muscle barely the size of a fist squatted like a bulldog guarding a house" (p. 27).

The early lessons learned in medical school are in sharp contrast to the "Practice" that Chen encounters as an intern and surgical resident. It is here that Chen's narrative about her struggles with mortality is the most poignant and serves as the book's central thesis. She illustrates the paradox between medicine's focus on cure and the reality of death and dying and how unprepared she and her colleagues were in dealing with terminally ill patients. Describing medicine as "a discipline of action" and surgery as a "doer's paradise" (p. 147), she underscores the need for a "Reappraisal" of how physicians prepare for and approach end-of-life care and how the system supports "hope driven treatment" (p. 157) in the face of conflicting evidence.

Narratives expose one's failures and expectations to public scrutiny and these are Chen's most compelling passages. It is through her shortcomings and errors that she provides the most insight and self-reflection. We feel her relief and confusion when she avoids uncomfortable situations such as the death of a friend and former neighbor or telling a family about the death of a loved one. We also share her surprise in discovering that patients are "whole beings" rather than the body parts or diagnoses (p. 137) and how positive role modeling from a physician colleague changed her approach to end-of-life care (he actually sat and talked to the patient's family after a death).

Indeed, as a nurse whose preparation and practice focuses on family and individual *care* giving, I was amazed at times by the divide that still exists between caring and curing in physician training and practice. As Chen discussed her own process in learning to *care* for dying patients instead of focusing on curing and saving, I could not help but formulate my own narrative experiences with dying patients and how considerably divergent they were from hers. This is the power of narrative to transform and inform, not only the writer but the reader. Personal essays provide an insider view to understanding how practice and policy play out in practical terms and what emotions they evoke. They provide windows to daily experiences and intimate thoughts that are typically missing in scientific writing. Chen opens a window into her own mind and soul and allows the reader to self-reflect in parallel time.

Final Exam is a well-written book that portrays the complex and often paradoxical reality of physician training and practice, particularly as it relates to caring for dying patients. It is also an excellent example of a genre of writing that needs further expression and participation by others whose stories can inform and transform. *Final Exam* may help medical and nursing students and others confront their own perceptions about dying and humanity in the care of terminally ill patients and provide a model for critical self-reflection. While not historiography, the personal essay can highlight values and ideas around subject matter that is typically unrecognized or insufficiently understood. Its autobiographical nature, while meant for public consumption, is critical and reflective, and can serve the historian as a contextual springboard.

Barbara L. Brush, PhD, APRN, BC, FAAN
Associate Professor
University of Michigan School of Nursing
400 N. Ingalls
Ann Arbor, MI 48108

NEW DISSERTATIONS

Compiled for the *Nursing History Review* by Jonathon Erlen, PhD, History of Medicine Librarian, Health Science Library System, and Assistant Professor, Graduate School of Public Health at the University of Pittsburgh, Pittsburgh, PA. These dissertations can be obtained through Proquest Dissertations.

James Patrick Ronan, "Nursing, society, and health promotion—healing practices: A constructionist historical discourse analysis," 2006 PhD dissertation, The University of Arizona (Publication Number: AAT 3237461).

Nicole Bernadette Hansen, "Motherhood in the mother of the world: Continuity and change of reproductive concepts and practices in Egypt from ancient to modern times," 2006 PhD dissertation, The University of Chicago (Publication Number: AAT 3240093).

Joseph Michael Gabriel, "Gods and monsters: Drugs, addiction, and the origins of narcotic control in the nineteenth-century urban North," 2006 PhD dissertation, Rutgers The State University of New Jersey–New Brunswick (Publication Number: AAT 3240213).

Derek S. Oden, "Harvest of hazards: The farm safety movement, 1940–1975," 2006 PhD dissertation, Iowa State University (Publication Number: AAT 3243574).

Courtney Q. Shah, "'This loathsome subject': Sex education in Progressive-Era America," 2006 PhD dissertation, The University of Houston (Publication Number: AAT 3242261).

Takakazu Yamagishi, "World War Two and the health of the state: The development of health insurance in Japan and the United States, 1931–1952," 2007 PhD dissertation, The Johns Hopkins University (Publication Number: AAT 3240815).

Laurel Lee Lewey, "Nothing to fear but fear: Social work in Cold War Canada, 1945–1960," 2006 PhD dissertation, The University of Calgary (Canada) (Publication Number: AAT NR19582).

Ruth E. Simpson, "The germ culture: Metaphor, modernity, and epidemic disease," 2006 PhD dissertation, The State University of New Jersey–New Brunswick (Publication Number: AAT 3240278).

Judith Ann Fruiterman, "The lived experiences of nurses who cared for victims of the World Trade Center attack, September 11, 2001," 2006 PhD dissertation, George Mason University (Publication Number: AAT 3240144).

Nursing History Review 17 (2009): 245–253. A Publication of the American Association for the History of Nursing.
DOI: 10.1891/1062–8061.17.245

Jan-Louise Leonard, "The role of professional nursing in the origin of the Newborns' and Mothers' Health Protection Act of 1996 from a feminist perspective, 1981–1996," 2006 PhD dissertation, The University of Massachusetts at Amherst (Publication Number: AAT 3242345).

Nikki Levy Miller, "The American Civil War and other 19th century influences on the development of nursing," 2006 PhD dissertation, The University of Arizona (Publication Number: AAT 3243878).

Ombasie Sedlacek, "A comparison of HIV knowledge, HIV beliefs and risk behaviors among low income African American and Hispanic women in 1997 and 2005," 2006 PhD dissertation, Touro University International (Publication Number: AAT 3243224).

Christy Bryceland, "From 'gunslingers' to 'policed professionals': The historical and institutional development of professional psychology in Alberta," 2006 PhD dissertation, The University Calgary (Canada) (Publication Number: AAT NR19148).

Marc H. Zelenka, "Prescription for a profession: The educational philosophy of Abraham Flexner and cogency in medical education," 2006 PhD dissertation, Indiana University (Publication Number: AAT 3238508).

Michael Robert Blackie, "Rest cures: The narrative life of a medical practice," 2006 PhD dissertation, University of Southern California (Publication Number: AAT 3236481).

Lesley Ann McBain, "Providing care in divided space: Nursing in Northern Saskatchewan, 1944–1957 and beyond," 2006 PhD dissertation, The University of Saskatchewan (Canada) (Publication Number: AAT NR18151).

Anna K. Kuxhausen, "Raising the nation: Medicine, morality, and vospitanie in eighteenth-century Russia," 2006 PhD dissertation, The University of Michigan (Publication Number: AAT 3238005).

David G. Schuster, "Neurasthenic nation: The medicalization of modernity in the United States, 1869–1920," 2006 PhD dissertation, The University of California, Santa Barbara (Publication Number: AAT 3238802).

Alexandra Cornelius Diallo, " 'More approximate to the animal': Africana resistance and the scientific war against black humanity in mid-nineteenth century America," 2006 PhD dissertation, Washington University in St. Louis (Publication Number: AAT 3238641).

Sharon L. Hadenfeldt, "A historical study of nurse anesthesia education in Nebraska," 2006 PhD dissertation, The University of Nebraska–Lincoln (Publication Number: AAT 3237556).

Anne Meredith Stiles, "Neurological fictions: Brain science and literary history, 1865–1905," 2006 PhD dissertation, The University of California, Los Angeles (Publication Number: AAT 3234346).

Ellen Griffith Spears, “Toxic knowledge: A social history of environmental health in the New South’s model city, Anniston, Alabama, 1872–present,” 2006 PhD dissertation, Emory University (Publication Number: AAT 3234046).

Nicole Rousseau, “A historical materialist analysis of the commodification of Black women’s biological reproduction in the United States,” 2006 PhD dissertation, Howard University (Publication Number: AAT 3235562).

Alice Schoonbroodt, “Baby busts and baby booms: The fertility response to economic shocks,” 2006 PhD dissertation, The University of Minnesota (Publication Number: AAT 3235425).

Alexander R. Bay, “The politics of disease: Beriberi, barley, and medicine in modern Japan (1700–1939),” 2006 PhD dissertation, Stanford University (Publication Number: AAT 3235179).

Robert P. Stolz, “‘Yanakagaku’: Pollution and environmental protest in modern Japan,” 2006 PhD dissertation, The University of Chicago (Publication Number: AAT 3231466).

Monica Ann Black, “The meaning of death and the making of three Berlins: A history, 1933–1961,” 2006 PhD dissertation, The University of Virginia (Publication Number: AAT 3235103).

Rachel Faircloth Green, “‘There will not be orphans among us’: Soviet orphanages, foster care, and adoption, 1941–1956,” 2006 PhD dissertation, The University of Chicago (Publication Number: AAT 3231399).

Melissa Eden Gormley, “Motherhood as national service: Race, class and public health policy in Brazil, 1930–1945,” 2006 PhD dissertation, The University of California, Davis (Publication Number: AAT 3235998).

Shae Davidson, “Eating democracy: School lunches and the social vision of the New Deal,” 2006 PhD dissertation, Ohio University (Publication Number: AAT 3234224).

Marni Davis, “‘On the side of liquor’: American Jews and the politics of alcohol, 1870–1936,” 2006 PhD dissertation, Emory University (Publication Number: AAT 3234014).

Joanna Leslie Dyl, “Urban disaster: An environmental history of San Francisco after the 1906 earthquake,” 2006 PhD dissertation, Princeton University (Publication Number: AAT 3236174).

Erika Lorraine Milam, “Looking for a few good males: Female choice in evolutionary biology, 1915–1975,” 2006 PhD dissertation, The University of Wisconsin–Madison (Publication Number: AAT 3234794).

Heather Green Wooten, “The polio years in Harris and Galveston counties, 1930–1962,” 2006 PhD dissertation, The University of Texas Medical Branch Graduate School of Biomedical Sciences (Publication Number: AAT 3234208).

Ellie Christine Schemenauer, "Gender, identity, and the security state: The politics of international drug trafficking," 2006 PhD dissertation, Florida International University (Publication Number: AAT 3235616).

Lorna M. Ronald, "Empowered to consume: Direct-to-consumer advertising and pharmaceutical governance," 2006 PhD dissertation, Rensselaer Polytechnic Institute (Publication Number: AAT 3232622).

Dejun Su, "Old-age mortality in a life course perspective: Union Army veterans, 1805–1946," 2006 PhD dissertation, The University of Chicago (Publication Number: AAT 3231467).

James Owen Ross, "The impact of the nineteenth-century public health movement upon American architecture: Theories of disease, ventilation, and sunlight, 1840–1944," 2006 PhD dissertation, Brown University (Publication Number: AAT 3227923).

Tywanna Marie Whorley, "The Tuskegee Syphilis Study: Access and control over controversial records," 2006 PhD dissertation, University of Pittsburgh (Publication Number: AAT 3232820).

Marika A. Seigel, "Reproductive technologies: Pregnancy manuals as technical communication," 2006 PhD dissertation, The Pennsylvania State University (Publication Number: AAT 3229336).

Asha Nadkarni, "Reproductive nationalism: Eugenic feminist literature in the United States and India," 2006 PhD dissertation, Brown University (Publication Number: AAT 3227901).

Kameelah L. Martin, "Conjuring moments and other such hoodoo: African American women and spirit work," 2006 PhD dissertation, The Florida State University (Publication Number: AAT 3232419).

Charlotte Anne Biltekoff, "Hidden hunger: Eating and citizenship from domestic science to the fat epidemic," 2006 PhD dissertation, Brown University (Publication Number: AAT 3227800).

Roberto Abadie, "A guinea pig's wage: Risk and commoditization in pharmaceutical research in America," 2006 PhD dissertation, City University of New York (Publication Number: AAT 3231981).

Christin Lee Hancock, "Sovereign bodies: Women, health care, and federal Indian policy, 1890–1986," 2006 PhD dissertation, Brown University (Publication Number: AAT 3227840).

Amanda Hope Littauer, "Unsanctioned encounters: Women, girls, and non-marital sexuality in the United States, 1941–1963," 2006 PhD dissertation, University of California, Berkeley (Publication Number: AAT 3228403).

Don Alan Romesburg, "Arrested development: Homosexuality, gender, and American adolescence, 1890–1930," 2006 PhD dissertation, University of California, Berkeley (Publication Number: AAT 3228476).

Susan Marie Groppi, "The science of mind: Exploring the influence of the academic environment on the development of research psychology in America, 1880–1910," 2006 PhD dissertation, University of California, Berkeley (Publication Number: AAT 3228344).

Karen Deane Ross, "Making medicine scientific: Simon Flexner and experimental medicine at the Rockefeller Institute for Medical Research, 1901–1945," 2006 PhD dissertation, The University of Minnesota (Publication Number: AAT 3230247).

Matthew Thomas Whittaker, "Lights, camera, bureaucratic action! Politics, demographics, and two decades of Superfund operations," 2006 PhD dissertation, The University of Iowa (Publication Number: AAT 3229711).

Joanna Z. Mishta, "Contradictions of democratization: The politics of reproductive rights and policies in postsocialist Poland," 2006 PhD dissertation, The University of Colorado at Boulder (Publication Number: AAT 3239386).

Joshua A. Dolezal, "The re-imagination of the scientific physician in American literature, 1850–1930," 2006 PhD dissertation, The University of Nebraska–Lincoln (Publication Number: AAT 3176774).

Elisa Munoz Franco, "Women's education, first sex, and family formation in Mexico: 30 years of stability . . . and change," 2006 PhD dissertation, Brown University (Publication Number: AAT 3227897).

Wyatt John Bonikowski, "Traces of war: Shell shock, death drive, and narrative after the First World War (Rebecca West, Ford Madox Ford, Virginia Woolf)," 2006 PhD dissertation, Cornell University (Publication Number: ATT 3228126).

Lisa Hope Harris, "Challenging conception: A clinical and cultural history of in vitro fertilization in the United States," 2006 PhD dissertation, University of Michigan (Publication Number: ATT 3224897).

Stephanie A. Limoncelli, "The politics of humanitarianism: States, reformers, and the international movement to combat the traffic in women, 1875–1960," 2006 PhD dissertation, The University of California, Los Angeles (Publication Number: ATT 3224339).

Michele Elaine Morales, "Persistent pathologies: The odd coupling of alcoholism and homosexuality in the discourses of twentieth century science," 2006 PhD dissertation, University of Michigan (Publication Number: ATT 3224705).

Jennifer Lynn Muller, "Trauma as a biological consequence of inequality: A biocultural analysis of the skeletal remains of Washington, D.C.'s African American poor," 2006 PhD dissertation, The State University of New York at Buffalo (Publication Number: ATT 3226897).

Katherine H. Nelson, "The temperance physicians: Developing concepts of addiction (Benjamin Rush, William Clark, Thomas Sewall, Reuben Mussey, Charles Jewett)," 2006 PhD dissertation, The American University (Publication Number: ATT 3227753).

Deborah Ann Sampson, "Determinants and determination: Negotiating nurse practitioner prescribing legislation in New Hampshire, 1973–1985," 2006 PhD dissertation, The University of Pennsylvania (Publication Number: ATT 3225536).

Sarah Frances Smith, " 'She moves the hands that move the world': Antebellum child-rearing. Images of mother and child in nineteenth-century periodicals for mothers," 2006 PhD dissertation, The University of Minnesota (Publication Number: ATT 3225774).

Elysa Ream Engelman, " 'The face that haunts me ever': Consumers, retailers, critics, and the branded personality of Lydia E. Pinkham," 2003 PhD dissertation, Boston University (Publication Number: AAT 3083834).

Suzanne Smythe, "The good mother: A critical discourse analysis of literacy advice to mothers in the 20th century," 2006 PhD dissertation, The University of British Columbia (Canada) (Publication Number: AAT NR19910).

Meghan McInnis-Dominguez, "Diagnosing empire: Refiguring disease in the early modern Hispanic world," 2006 PhD dissertation, The University of Pennsylvania (Publication Number: AAT 3246201).

Justin H. Pettegrew, "Onward Christian soldiers: The transformation of religion, masculinity, and class in the Chicago YMCA, 1857–1933," 2006 PhD dissertation, Loyola University (Publication Number: AAT 3243422).

David Patrick Nally, "The administration of hunger: Colonialism, biopolitics and the Great Irish Famine, 1845–1852," 2006 PhD dissertation, The University of British Columbia (Canada) (Publication Number: AAT NR19898).

Hoi-eun Kim, "Physicians on the move: German physicians in Meiji Japan and Japanese medical students in Imperial Germany, 1868–1914," 2006 PhD dissertation, Harvard University (Publication Number: AAT 3245153).

Patricia Nardi, "Mothers at home: Their role in childrearing and instruction in early modern England," 2007 PhD dissertation, The City University of New York (Publication Number: AAT 3245075).

Solsiree del Moral, "Race, science, and nation: The cultural politics of schools in colonial Puerto Rico, 1917–1938," 2006 PhD dissertation, The University of Wisconsin–Madison (Publication Number: AAT 3245688).

Richard James Bell, "Do not despair: The cultural significance of suicide in America, 1780–1840," 2006 PhD dissertation, Harvard University (Publication Number: AAT 3245108).

Kristin Burnett, "The healing work and nursing care of Aboriginal women, female medical missionaries, nursing sisters, public health nurses, and female attendants in southern Alberta First Nations communities, 1880–1930," 2006 PhD dissertation, York University (Canada) (Publication Number: AAT NR19781).

Robert J. Heynen, "Degeneration and revolution: Radical cultural politics and the politics of the body in Weimar Germany, 1914–1933," 2006 PhD dissertation, York University (Canada) (Publication Number: AAT NR19808).

Dane Christian Barca, "The human is flesh: Science and medicine in literature, 1780–1870," 2006 PhD dissertation, University of California, Riverside (Publication Number: AAT 3249733).

Jolie Alexandra Sheffer, "Imagining America: The psychology of race and gender in representations of the national family, 1880–1920," 2007 PhD dissertation, University of Virginia (Publication Number: AAT 3248107).

Sasha Mullally, "Unpacking the black bag: Rural medicine in the Maritime Provinces and northern New England states, 1900–1950," 2005 PhD dissertation, University of Toronto (Canada) (Publication Number: AAT NR22067).

Andrew McIlwaine Bell, "Mosquito soldiers: The impact of malaria and yellow fever during the American Civil War," 2007 PhD dissertation, The George Washington University (Publication Number: AAT 3248468).

James T. Downs, "Diagnosing Reconstruction: Sickness, dependency, and the Medical Division of the Freedmen's Bureau, 1861–1870," 2005 PhD dissertation, Columbia University (Publication Number: AAT 3249177).

Dennis Arthur Doyle, IV, "The universal mind assumption: Harlem and the development of a new racial formation in American psychiatry, 1938–1968," 2006 PhD dissertation, State University of New York at Stony Brook (Publication Number: AAT 3246819).

Sharon Lowe, "Behind the soothing mist: Women and opiate use in the mining West, 1860–1900," 2006 PhD dissertation, Union Institute and University (Publication Number: AAT 3248198).

Bobby A. Wintermute, "Waging health: The United States Army Medical Department and public health in the Progressive Era, 1890–1920," 2006 PhD dissertation, Temple University (Publication Number: AAT 3247320).

Olena Mykolayivna Prokopovych, "The institutional dynamics of health care reform: Organizational and class dimensions of policy-making at the Columbia-Presbyterian Medical Center, 1911–1998," 2007 PhD dissertation, Cornell University (Publication Number: AAT 3246730).

Nancy Anne Harris, "Alice Magaw: The mother of anesthesia," 2006 PhD dissertation, The University of Iowa (Publication Number: AAT 3248015).

Gayle Poinsette, "The Social Security Act of 1935: Religious and economic belief systems underlying the congressional debates," 2006 PhD dissertation, Union Institute and University (Publication Number: AAT 3251487).

Robert J. Brown, "Fateful alliance: The 1918 influenza pandemic and the First World War in the British context," 2006 PhD dissertation, Syracuse University (Publication Number: AAT 3251814).

Deborah McRaven, "Birth control women: Controlling reproduction in the South, 1933–1973," 2006 PhD dissertation, University of Kentucky (Publication Number: AAT 3250585).

Sally Kerry Hayward, "Managing death: Diagnosing the 'new' eugenics in Canadian legal discourses and narratives of disability," 2006 PhD dissertation, University of Alberta (Canada) (Publication Number: AAT NR23042).

Andrew Jonathan Noymer, "Studies in the historical demography and epidemiology of influenza and tuberculosis selective mortality," 2006 PhD dissertation, University of California, Berkeley (Publication Number: AAT 3254008).

Mike Esbester, "'Dead on the point of safety': Occupational safety on the Great Western Railroad, c. 1913–39," 2007 PhD dissertation, University of York (Great Britain).

Maryellen Riley, "The education of children with disabilities in Germany: From 1945–1970," 2007 PhD dissertation, Boston University (Publication Number: AAT 3254473).

Sarah Elizabeth Hinman, "Spatial and temporal structure of typhoid fever in Washington, D.C., 1895–1909: A geographic information systems exploration of urban health concerns," 2007 PhD dissertation, Louisiana State University and Agricultural & Mechanical College (Publication Number: AAT 3256331).

Tina Phillips, "Building the nation through women's health: Modern midwifery in early twentieth-century China," 2006 PhD dissertation, University of Pittsburgh (Publication Number: AAT 3255739).

So Young Suh, "Korean medicine between the local and the universal: 1600–1945," 2006 PhD dissertation, University of California, Los Angeles (Publication Number: AAT 3254794).

Nancy Stark Lee, "Curing consumers: How the patient became a consumer in modern American medicine," 2007 PhD dissertation, University of California, San Diego (Publication Number: AAT 3258828).

Samuel D. Jensen, "Epidemics, public health policies and their impact on biodefense and preparedness," 2007 PhD dissertation, George Mason University (Publication Number: AAT 3255685).